Orthopaedic Surgery Review

Questions and Answers

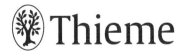

Thieme

Orthopaedic Surgery Review

Questions and Answers

Mark J. Sokolowski, MD
Trinity Orthopaedics SC
Oak Park, Illinois

Thieme
New York • Stuttgart

Thieme Medical Publishers, Inc.
333 Seventh Ave.
New York, NY 10001

Executve Editor: Kay D. Conerly
Managing Editor: J. Owen Zurhellen IV
Vice President, Production and Electronic Publishing: Anne T. Vinnicombe
Production Editor: Print Matters Inc.
Vice President, International Marketing and Sales: Cornelia Schulze
Chief Financial Officer: Peter van Woerden
President: Brian D. Scanlan
Compositor: The Manila Typesetting Company
Printer: King Printing Co., Inc.

Library of Congress Cataloging-in-Publication Data

Sokolowski, Mark J.
    Orthopaedic surgery review : questions and answers / Mark J. Sokolowski.
      p. ; cm.
    ISBN 978-1-60406-042-3 (alk. paper)
    1. Orthopedic surgery--Examinations, questions, etc. I. Title.
    [DNLM: 1. Orthopedic Procedures--methods--Problems and Exercises. WE 18.2 S683o 2009]
    RD732.6.S65 2009
    617.4'7076--dc22
                           2008043148

Important note: Medical knowledge is ever-changing. As new research and clinical experience broaden our knowledge, changes in treatment and drug therapy may be required. The authors and editors of the material herein have consulted sources believed to be reliable in their efforts to provide information that is complete and in accord with the standards accepted at the time of publication. However, in view of the possibility of human error by the authors, editors, or publisher of the work herein or changes in medical knowledge, neither the authors, editors, or publisher, nor any other party who has been involved in the preparation of this work, warrants that the information contained herein is in every respect accurate or complete, and they are not responsible for any errors or omissions or for the results obtained from use of such information. Readers are encouraged to confirm the information contained herein with other sources. For example, readers are advised to check the product information sheet included in the package of each drug they plan to administer to be certain that the information contained in this publication is accurate and that changes have not been made in the recommended dose or in the contraindications for administration. This recommendation is of particular importance in connection with new or infrequently used drugs.

Some of the product names, patents, and registered designs referred to in this book are in fact registered trademarks or proprietary names even though specific reference to this fact is not always made in the text. Therefore, the appearance of a name without designation as proprietary is not to be construed as a representation by the publisher that it is in the public domain.

Printed in the United States

5 4 3 2

ISBN: 978-1-60406-042-3

FSC
www.fsc.org
100%
Paper from well-managed forests
FSC® C103101

I dedicate this book to my wife, Margaret, to my children, Anna and Katherine, and to my parents, Wesley and Irene, who continue to make my life and my career rewarding everyday.

Contents

Preface

In preparing for examinations and surgeries, the contributors to this book, *Orthopaedic Surgery Review,* have used many different strategies and sought out many different sources of key orthopaedic information. This text was conceived to supplement the many different excellent sources of orthopaedic review information already available. *Orthopaedic Surgery Review* has a question-and-answer format, that facilitates convenient and rapid review of key material before examinations and surgeries. We anticipate this text will be useful for medical students, residents, and practicing orthopaedists.

Because of its "high-yield" format, *Orthopaedic Surgery Review* is necessarily concise. It is our suggestion that the reader consult the many excellent resources of the American Academy of Orthopaedic Surgeons, or a text such as Miller's *Review of Orthopaedics,* when a more comprehensive discussion of a topic is necessary. As you use this first edition of *Orthopaedic Surgery Review,* we sincerely welcome your comments, corrections, and suggestions for future editions.

Acknowledgments

This book is the result of the efforts of many individuals. In particular, I would like to thank my coauthors for their contributions to the development of this text. I also wish to thank the orthopaedic surgery faculty of Northwestern University, Children's Memorial Hospital, and Evanston Hospital, and the spine surgeons of the Twin Cities Spine Center, all of whom established the foundation of my orthopaedic education.

I am grateful to my Twin Cities co-fellows and to my partners at Trinity Orthopaedics, Victor Romano and Joseph Sheehan, who enabled me to dedicate time to this book.

I appreciate the contributions of the staff at Thieme Publishers. In particular, I thank Esther Gumpert for accepting this project, and J. Owen Zurhellen for guiding me through to its completion.

Finally, I wish to thank my wife and children for lovingly and patiently allowing me to devote many evenings and weekends to this text.

Contributors

Matthew J. Boardman, DO
Department of Orthopaedic Surgery
Philadelphia College of Osteopathic Medicine
Philadelphia, Pennsylvania

Michael Caravelli, MD
Department of Orthopaedic Surgery
Feinberg School of Medicine
Northwestern University
Northwestern Memorial Hospital
Chicago, Illinois

Leonard L. D'Addesi, MD
Orthopaedic Associates of Reading
West Reading, Pennsylvania

Steven E. Flores, MD
Assistant Professor, Sports Medicine
Department of Orthopaedic Surgery
Baylor College of Medicine
Houston, Texas

Najeeb Khan, MD
Department of Orthopaedic Surgery
Feinberg School of Medicine
Northwestern University
Northwestern Memorial Hospital
Chicago, Illinois

Amir A. Mehbod, MD
Orthopaedic Spine Surgeon
Twin Cities Spine Center
Mineapolis, Minnesota

Jason A. Nydick, DO
Department of Orthopaedic Surgery
Philadelphia College of Osteopathic
Medicine
Philadelphia, Pennsylvania

Nirav A. Shah, MD
Department of Orthopaedic Surgery
Feinberg School of Medicine
Northwestern University
Northwestern Memorial Hospital
Chicago, Illinois

Mark J. Sokolowski, MD
Trinity Orthopaedics SC
Oak Park, Illinois

Vineeta T. Swaroop, MD
Department of Orthopaedic Surgery
Feinberg School of Medicine
Northwestern University
Division of Orthopaedic Surgery
Rehabilitation Institute of Chicago
Chicago, Illinois

1

Spine

■ General Knowledge

Intervertebral Disk

1. What two changes occur in the vascular supply to the disk with aging?

2. What is the source of nutrients to the disk?

3. What two external factors decrease endplate permeability?

4. What factors increase permeability?

5. How does aging affect the disk's collagen content?

6. How does aging affect the disk's fibril diameter?

7. How does aging affect the disk's noncollagenous protein?

8. How does aging affect the disk's pH?

9. Magnetic resonance imaging (MRI): what are the rates of false-positive (asymptomatic) findings for patients <40 years old, >40 years old, and >60 years old?

1. Vessels begin disappearing after the age of 10 years
Endplates ossify

2. Diffusion through endplates

3. Smoking
Vibration

4. Exercise

5. Decreased collagen content

6. Increased fibril diameter and variability

7. Increased noncollagenous protein

8. Decreased pH

9. <40 years old: 25%
>40 years old: 60%
>60 years old: 90%

Biomechanics

10. What is the function of the anterior column and the posterior column?

11. An anteriorly placed graft is loaded in which two directions and unloaded in which two directions?

12. What effect does an anterior plate have on the axis of rotation?

13. … on the graft in extension?

14. … on the graft in flexion?

10. Anterior column: support
Posterior column: tension band

11. Loaded in compression, flexion
Unloaded in extension, traction

12. Moves axis of rotation anteriorly

13. Loads graft in extension

14. Unloads graft in flexion

15. What is the definition of terminal bending?

15. Moments at ends of a long construct

16. How can terminal bending be prevented?

16. With intermediate fixation points

17. How much lumbar torsional resistance is provided by facets, disk, and ligaments?

17. Facets: 40%
    Disk: 40%
    Ligaments: 20%

18. After a flexion-distraction injury, what is the status of the anterior longitudinal ligament (ALL) and the posterior longitudinal ligament (PLL disrupted)?

18. ALL intact
    PLL out

19. Which approach is biomechanically superior in this situation?

19. Posteriorly based fusions are superior to anteriorly based fusions

Anatomy

20. How are the cervical spine facets oriented in the sagittal plane?

20. Cervical: 45 degrees in the sagittal plane

21. Compare with thoracic and lumbar facet orientation.

21. Thoracic: vertical in sagittal plane (essentially in the coronal plane)
    Lumbar: sagittally aligned

22. The sinuvertebral nerve originates from which structure?

22. Sympathetic chain

23. What structures and elements does it supply?

23. Supplies structures within the spinal canal
    Supplies posterior elements

24. What other neurologic structure also innervates the posterior elements?

24. Primary dorsal ramus also contributes to innervation

25. Pattern of innervation example: the L3 nerve root innervates which facets?

25. L3 innervates the L3-4 facets

26. At which level is the pedicle diameter the smallest?

26. T5

27. What is the furcal nerve? What is its clinical significance?

27. Peripheral nerve often originating from L4 nerve root
    Can result in variable L4 dermatomal distribution

Infections and Malignancies

28. Infection versus malignancy: which generally destroys the disk?

28. Infection destroys the disk early
    Malignancy usually skips the disk

29. Compare with the effect of tuberculosis on the disk.

29. Tb skips the disk early, but may involve the disk late

30. What are the earliest plain radiographic findings of infection?

30. Disk space narrowing at 7 to 10 days

31. What is the natural history of disk space infection?

31. Spontaneous arthrodesis

32. What are the two usual treatment for osteomyelitis?

32. Intravenous antibiotics
    Brace

33. What are the three operative indications?

33. Failure of conservative treatment
Progressive neurologic deficit
Instability (e.g., fracture)

34. What are the two negative prognostic factors for infection?

34. Increased age
More cephalad involvement

35. What is the MRI appearance of malignancy on T1 and T2 sequences?

35. T1: low
T2: high

36. What three tumors classically involve the posterior elements?

36. ABC (aneurysmal bone cyst)
Osteoid osteoma/osteoblastoma
Osteochondroma

■ Cervical Spine

General Knowledge

37. Cervical spondylosis is most common at which two levels?

37. C5-6
C6-7

38. Degenerative cervical spondylolisthesis is most common at which two levels?

38. C3-4
C4-5

39. What are the most common levels of cervical trauma in the young?

39. C4 to C7

40. What are the most common levels of cervical trauma in the elderly?

40. C1, C2

41. What is Spurling's test? What is its clinical significance?

41. Rotation, lateral bend, vertical
    compression of neck
To identify cervical radiculopathy

42. What arm position classically relieves the symptoms of cervical radiculopathy?

42. Symptoms improve with the arm
    overhead

43. What is the ideal therapy regimen for radiculopathy? What percentage of patients improve?

43. Isometric exercises
75% improve

44. What is the finger escape test? What is its clinical significance?

44. Spontaneous small finger abduction
    secondary to weak intrinsics
Indicative of myelopathy

45. In what two ways does cervical myelopathy generally progress?

45. Long quiescent periods
Stepwise deterioration

46. What is Lhermittes sign?

46. Lightning sensation in arms with neck
    flexion

47. What does the C4 nerve root innervate?

47. Scapular muscles

48. What three roots correspond to reflexes within the upper extremities?

48. C5: biceps
C6: brachioradialis
C7: triceps

49. What is the significance of a hypoactive brachioradialis (BR) reflex?

49. Hypoactive BR reflex = lower motor
    neuron involvement (radiculopathy)

50. What is the significance of an inverted radial reflex (IRR)?

50. IRR: hypoactive BR reflex + concurrent
    finger flexion
Upper motor neuron involvement
    (myelopathy)

51. What is Power's ratio used for? What is its critical value?

51. Anterior atlanto-occipital (AO) dissociation
BC/AO >1: abnormal

52. What is the definition of Torg's ratio? What is its clinical significance?

52. Canal width divided by vertebral body width
For the identification of congenital stenosis

53. Compare normal and critical values of Torg's ratio?

53. Normal is 1.0
Critical value is <0.8

54. What three arteries contribute to the spinal cord blood supply?

54. Anterior spinal artery (two thirds from vertebrate artery)
Two dorsal spinal arteries (one third from posterior inferior cerebellar artery [PICA])

55. The watershed area of the cervical spinal cord is at which levels?

55. C5 to C7

56. What are the two classic symptoms of calcified disk disease in a child?

56. Neck pain
Torticollis

57. What is the treatment of choice?

57. Observation

58. What is the prognosis?

58. Likely to go on to spontaneous resolution

Radiographic Evaluation

59. What is the most common reason for a missed cervical spine injury?

59. Inadequate visualization of involved levels

60. At which two levels are injuries most often missed?

60. Cervicothoracic junction
Atlantooccipital junction

61. In an awake, alert patient without neck symptoms, what is required for C-spine clearance?

61. Clinical exam only
No films required

62. Compare with a patient with neck pain or neurologic deficits.

62. Three views of cervical spine with or without computed tomography (CT)

63. What is the normal atlantodens interval (ADI) in adults and in children?

63. Adults: <3.5 mm
Children: <4.0 mm

64. What are the normal and unstable values of a lateral mass overhang on an open mouth view? What is its clinical significance?

64. Normal = 0 mm overhang
Unstable = >6.9 mm
Relevant for Jefferson fracture

65. What are the two White/Panjabi instability criteria for subaxial C-spine on flexion-extension films?

65. Sagittal translation >3.5 mm or 20%
Sagittal rotation >20 degrees

66. ... on resting films?

66. Sagittal translation >3.5 mm or 20%
Relative sagittal angulation >11 degrees

67. On a pediatric lateral C-spine film, what is the normal C2 retropharyngeal space? Retrotracheal space?

67. <6 mm retropharyngeal
<14 mm retrotracheal

68. What level is most commonly involved in pseudosubluxation? What is its significance?

68. C2 on C3
May be a normal finding in children

69. What is the key radiographic landmark when evaluating for pseudosubluxation?

69. Check spinolaminar line

Surgical Anatomy: Atlas/Axis

70. What percentage of space is occupied by the cord? What makes up the remainder?

70. 33% cord
33% dens
33% empty (cerebrospinal fluid [CSF], fat)
Steele's rule of thirds

71. What percentage of head rotation occurs at C1-2?

71. 50%

72. The arterial arcade around the odontoid process is supplied by which two vessels?

72. Vertebral artery
External carotid artery

Surgical Anatomy: Anterior Approach

73. What are the anterior landmarks for levels C3, C4, C5, and C6?

73. C3: hyoid
C4, C5: thyroid
C6: cricoid

74. The carotid tubercle is at which level?

74. C6

75. What is the C7-T1 landmark?

75. Sternal notch

76. With an anterior cervical discectomy and fusion (ACDF), what is the first muscle encountered? What is the innervation?

76. Platysma
Facial nerve (cranial nerve [CN] VII)

77. With an ACDF, the interval for dissection lies between what two anatomical areas?

77. Carotid sheath
Trachea

78. What are the four contents of the carotid sheath?

78. Internal carotid artery (ICA)
Common carotid artery (CCA)
Internal jugular vein (IJV)
CN X (vagus)

79. What artery lies at the proximal extent of exposure? What is to be done with it?

79. Superior thyroid artery
It may be sacrificed

80. Where is the omohyoid muscle encountered? How should it be retracted?

80. Encountered on the medial side of the carotid sheath within pretracheal tissue
Retract medially, may divide if necessary

81. What are the origin, insertion, innervation, and function of the omohyoid muscle?

81. Origin: scapula
Insertion: hyoid bone
Innervation: ansa cervicalis (C1 to C3)
Function: depress hyoid bone and larynx

82. More proximal approaches put which nerve at risk? What is its clinical significance?

82. Superior laryngeal nerve
Responsible for high note phonation

83. Classically, there is increased recurrent laryngeal nerve risk with which approach? Why?

83. Right-sided approach
More variable on right (left goes around the aortic arch)

84. In which interval does the recurrent laryngeal nerve ascend?

84. Tracheoesophageal interval

85. What do recent data indicate about the side of approach and recurrent laryngeal nerve injury rate?

85. Right- and left-sided approaches have equivalent injury rates

86. What approach places the thoracic duct at risk? What is the treatment if the duct is injured?

86. Left-sided approach
If injured, ligate proximally and distally

87. Horner's syndrome is a risk at which level? Why?

87. C7-T1
Because of the inferior cervical ganglion

88. Vocal cord paralysis may also occur by which other mechanism? How can this be prevented?

88. Compression of larynx between retractor and endotracheal (ET) tube
Prevention: deflate ET tube after retractors are placed, allow tube to re-centralize

89. What does "SLAC Line" refer to?

89. The five capital letters in the acronym refer to the following structures (anterior to posterior):
Sympathetic chain
Longus coli
Artery (vertebral)
Cervical nerve root
Lateral mass

90. What is the preferred proximal cervical approach for a singer?

90. Anterior retropharyngeal approach

Surgical Anatomy: Posterior Approach

91. What is the key posterior triangle for the posterior approach?

91. Suboccipital triangle

92. What two structures does this triangle contain?

92. Vertebral artery
C1 nerve

93. What is the most superficial structure?

93. Greater occipital nerve (C2)

94. What is the size of the safe zone relative to the C1 spinous process?

94. 1.5 to 2 cm lateral from C1 spinous process to vertebral artery

95. With a posterior approach, which way should the nerve root be retracted?

95. Elevate root superiorly

96. What nerve root is at the highest risk for traction injury? Why?

96. C5 at highest risk
Straightest take-off

97. What is the best way to approach ossification of the posterior longitudinal ligament (OPLL)? What is the preferred surgical technique for decompression?

97. Posterior
Laminoplasty

98. What preoperative sagittal plane requirement is necessary for laminoplasty success?

98. Cervical lordosis

99. What is the principal complication of laminoplasty?

99. Decreased cervical range of motion (ROM) by 50 to 62%

100. The lateral mass includes which two structures?

100. Pedicle
Ipsilateral lamina

Outcomes and Surgical Decision Making

101. For a one-level ACDF, compare outcomes associated with allograft versus autograft use.

101. Equivalent outcomes

102. What two clinical conditions are the exceptions?

102. Multiple levels
Smokers

103. In performing a multiple-level ACDF, what should one consider preoperatively?

103. Strut graft
Plate
Adjunct posterior fusion

104. For smokers, is allograft or autograft preferred for one level? What about for two levels?

104. One level: always autograft
Two levels: autograft strut

105. A posterior approach should generally be included with anterior surgeries in excess of _____.

105. Two corpectomies

106. What are reported ACDF pseudarthrosis rates for one level?

106. 12%

107. What are reported ACDF pseudarthrosis rates for multiple levels?

107. 30%

108. What is the significance of the Hillibrand study?

108. 25% of ACDF patients required an additional procedure within 10 years for adjacent-level disease

109. What is the principal factor in determining adjacent-level degeneration?

109. Preoperative adjacent-level status

110. What is the treatment if the lateral femoral cutaneous nerve (LFCN) is cut with graft harvest?

110. Allow it to retract into the pelvis

111. What percentage of patients develop long-term pain at the graft site?

111. 25%

112. For the elderly patient, is an ACDF or a posterior approach generally better tolerated?

112. Posterior approach

113. Increased risk of dysphagia and respiratory compromise occur with which four factors?

113. Increased number of levels
Increased operative time
Increased blood loss
More proximal level of surgery

114. What complication is unique to an posterior approach?

114. Air embolism

115. When performing a multilevel posterior laminectomy, what else should one do? Why?

115. Instrumented fusion
To prevent postoperative kyphosis

Rheumatoid Arthritis

116. What is the order of relative frequency of the three rheumatoid-related disorders within the cervical spine?

116. 1: C1-2 instability
2: basilar invagination
3: subaxial subluxation

Atlantoaxial Instability

117. What are the criteria for atlantoaxial instability in the adult and in the child?

117. Adult: >3 mm motion
Child: >4 mm motion

118. What is the significance if >7 mm motion is seen at C1-2?

118. Alar ligaments also disrupted
Contraindication to elective orthopaedic surgery

119. A posterior atlanto-dens interval (PADI) smaller than ____ is an indication for surgery.

119. 14 mm

120. What are the expected surgical outcomes if PADI is 10 to 14 mm or <10 mm?

120. 10 to 14 mm: can expect neurologic improvement postoperatively
<10 mm: stabilize; improvement unlikely

121. What is the critical PADI value in flexed position?

121. Surgery indicated if <6 mm in flexion

122. What are the two additional operative indications at C1-2?

122. >10 mm motion
Myelopathy

123. What four surgical options are appropriate if C1-2 subluxation is reducible?

123. Gallie technique
Brooks technique
Transarticular screws
Harms technique

124. What three surgical options are appropriate if subluxation is irreducible? What is the key step to all three?

124. Posterior decompression with occiput–C2 fusion
Posterior decompression with C1-2 transarticular screws
Harms technique
Key step with all interventions: decompression!

125. What is the expected long-term consequence without surgery for instability?

125. On average, patients die within 8 years

126. What are the three criteria that indicate that surgery is less likely to be successful? What is the Ranawat category?

126. Objective weakness
Upper motor neuron (UMN) signs
Nonambulatory
Ranawat IIIB

127. Upon which two factors is the Nurick classification of myelopathy based?

127. Gait
Ambulatory function

Basilar Invagination

128. What anatomic line lies at the base of the foramen magnum? What is its clinical significance?

128. McRae's line across the base of the foramen magnum
Odontoid should always be below this line (if not, then invagination is present)

129. What is the most important operative indication for invagination?

Other indications include ...

130. ... Migration in excess of?

131. ... Cervicomedullary angle (CMA)?

132. ... Ranawat measurement?

133. ... McRae's line?

134. What two surgical options are appropriate for basilar invagination?

135. What are the only two current indications for a transoral approach?

136. What are the two classic symptoms of atlantoaxial arthritis? What is the treatment?

Subaxial Subluxation

137. What are the criteria for instability: (__ mm, __ degrees)?

138. Which gender is most commonly affected? What are the other three primary risk factors?

139. An increased risk of neurologic compromise exists with what two radiographic criteria?

140. What is the treatment of choice?

Surgical Techniques

Fusion to Occiput

141. Where is the skull thickest?

142. What structures are at risk with screws?

Comparison of Posterior Fusion Techniques

143. What is the Gallie technique?

144. How much relative resistance does the Gallie provide versus flexion, extension, and rotation?

145. Gallie should not be used in what situation?

146. What is the Brooks technique?

147. How much relative resistance does the Brooks provide versus flexion, extension, and rotation?

129. Neurologic compromise

130. >5 mm

131. <135 degrees

132. <13 mm

133. Odontoid proximal to McRae's line

134. Occiput to C2 fusion
Transoral odontoid resection

135. Cranial nerve deficits (brainstem compromise)
Solid posterior C1-2 fusion with persistent anterior cord compromise

136. Headache
Rotational pain
Treatment: posterior C1-2 fusion

137. >3.5 mm or 20% translation
>11 degrees (static film)
>20 degrees (flexion-extension films)

138. Male
History steroid use
RF+
Nodules

139. Subluxation >4 mm
Cervical height index >2

140. Posterior fusion and wiring

141. External occipital protuberance

142. Venous sinuses

143. Spinous process wiring with midline graft

144. Good versus flexion
Not good versus extension and rotation

145. Posteriorly displaced odontoid fracture

146. Posterior wiring with bilateral grafts

147. Good versus flexion
Better versus extension and rotation

148. With either the Gallie or Brooks, what must be applied postoperatively?

148. Halo vest

149. How effective are C1-2 transarticular screws against flexion, extension, and rotation?

149. Best versus flex, extension, and rotation

150. How can the vertebral artery be injured with a transarticular screw?

150. Screw too caudally directed

151. How can the occiput–C1 joint be injured?

151. Screw too cephalad

152. How can the hypoglossal nerve (CN XII) be injured?

152. Screw too long: too anterior to lateral mass

153. What are the two functions of the hypoglossal nerve?

153. Innervates muscles of tongue
Contributes to strap muscle innervation via ansa cervicalis

154. If considering transarticular screws, which study must be obtained preoperatively?

154. Preoperative thin-cut CT scan

155. What percentage of patients have anatomy that precludes C1-2 screws?

155. 15%

156. If an iatrogenic injury to one vertebral artery occurs, what is the next step?

156. Sublaminar wires and graft (Gallie/ Brooks type)

Vertebral Artery Injury

157. Vertebral artery injury may be seen in association with trauma at what location?

157. Facet joint injury

158. How can it be injured intraoperatively?

158. Lateral bone removal with burr

159. If a vertebral artery stroke occurs, what is the name of the resultant syndrome? What are its four features?

159. Wallenberg syndrome
Nystagmus
Diplopia
Dysphagia
Pain, temperature loss

160. What is the path of the vertebral artery? Above C1?

160. C6 foramen transversarium to C1
Up and medially through arcuate foramen above C1

161. What goes through the C7 foramen transversarium?

161. Accessory vein

■ Thoracic Spine

General Knowledge

162. Thoracic disk disease is most common at which levels?

162. T8 to T12 (especially T11-T12)

163. What is the classic mechanism of injury resulting in thoracic disk herniation (herniated nucleus pulposus [HNP])?

163. Torsion + bend

164. An HNP is most likely to be symptomatic in what two situations?

164. Scheuermann's disease
Calcified disk

165. What are the two indications for surgery?

165. Myelopathy
Pain with magnetic resonance (MR) correlation

166. What are the two surgical options?

166. Open/thoracoscopic (anterior)
Costotransversectomy (posterior)

167. What is the disadvantage of a posterior approach?

167. Decreased midline access from the posterior

168. If the HNP is calcified, there is an increased risk of what surgical complication?

168. Dural tear

169. For the approach, should the surgeon go over or under the rib? From right or left? Why?

169. Over rib
From right
Avoid artery of Adamkiewicz

170. What supplies the artery of Adamkiewicz?

170. Left posterior intercostals T9 to T11

171. Where is the watershed area for the thoracic spinal cord?

171. Middle T-spine

172. Where does the spinal cord end?

172. L1-2

173. What are the radiographic criteria for a diagnosis of disseminated idiopathic skeletal hyperostosis (DISH, diffuse idiopathic skeletal hyperostosis)?

173. Nonmarginal syndesmophytes >3 levels

174. What region of the spine is most commonly involved?

174. Right thoracic spine

175. Is the disk generally involved?

175. DISH generally spares the disk

176. What type of syndesmophytes are seen with ankylosing spondylitis?

176. Marginal syndesmophytes

Vertebral Compression Fractures

177. Are compression fractures more common in the thoracic or lumbar spines? Why?

177. Thoracic spine more common because it is kyphotic

178. A vacuum sign on x-ray implies what two characteristics of the fracture?

178. Osteonecrosis
Nonhealing

179. How can compression fracture acuity be best evaluated?

179. Short tau inversion recovery (STIR) MRI

180. What are the five risk factors (in descending significance) for a vertebral compression fracture?

180. Prior compression fractures
Decreased bone mineral density (BMD)
Family history
Premature menopause
Smoking

181. After taking bisphosphonates for 1 year, how much does a patient's risk of compression fracture decrease?

181. 60%

Hyperkyphosis and Related Osteotomies

182. On standing lateral films, where should the C7 plumb line fall?

182. Through the sacrum or within 2 cm anterior to the sacrum

183. What are the five common causes of kyphotic sagittal imbalance?

183. Scheuermann's disease
Ankylosing spondylitis
Neurofibromatosis
Traumatic (e.g., compression, burst fractures)
Iatrogenic (e.g., postlaminectomy, Harrington distraction instrumentation)

Smith-Petersen Osteotomy (SPO)

184. What is an SPO? What is the effect on the posterior, middle, and anterior columns?

184. Resection of posterior column between the facet joints
Posterior column shortened
Middle column = hinge
Anterior column lengthened

185. How much correction can be obtained, on average, per level?

185. 10 degrees

186. What additional procedure may potentially be necessary?

186. Anterior grafting if a gap opens in anterior disk space

Pedicle Subtraction Osteotomy (PSO)

187. What is a PSO? What is the effect on the posterior, middle, and anterior columns?

187. Wedge-shaped resection with apex anterior of vertebral body, pedicle, and posterior elements
Posterior column shortened
Middle column shortened
Anterior column = hinge

188. How much correction can be obtained, on average, per level? Which levels are preferred?

188. 30 degrees
L2, L3 probably safest

■ Thoracolumbar Spine

189. In thoracolumbar compression fractures, what is the indication for surgery? Why?

189. Fractures at >3 consecutive levels
Increased risk of kyphosis

Thoracolumbar Burst Fractures

190. What are the five surgical indications?

190. Unstable injury (posterior ligamentous complex disrupted)
>50% height loss
>50% canal compromise
>30 degrees kyphosis
Incomplete or progressive neurologic deficit

191. If a neurologic deficit is present, what is the preferred surgical approach?

191. Anteriorly to decompress, fuse

192. If posterior column involvement is present, what is the preferred surgical approach? What is the significance of a lamina fracture?

192. Posteriorly to fuse
Lamina fracture may entrap and compress nerve roots (go posterior)

193. What is the most common long-term complication of a thoracolumbar burst fracture?

193. Pain

194. Compare the reported outcomes of operative versus nonoperative treatment of stable burst fractures.

194. Equivalent outcomes

■ Lumbar Spine

General Knowledge

195. What four factors are prognostic for future back pain?

195. History of back pain
Smoker
>30 years old
Workmen's compensation case

196. In acute low back pain, when do 50% of patients recover? When do 90% of patients recover?

196. 50% recover at 1 week
90% recover at 3 months

197. In acute sciatica, when do 50% of patients recover?

197. At 1 month

198. A program consisting of what two factors has been demonstrated to result in the best return to work?

198. Education
Aerobic conditioning

199. What three Minnesota Multiphasic Personality Inventory (MMPI) findings are predictors of poor recovery?

199. Hysteria
Hypochondriasis
Depression

200. What are the aggravating positions for degenerative disk disease (DDD) and instability?

200. DDD: worse with flexion
Instability: worse with extension

201. What are the general surgical treatment principles for DDD and instability?

201. DDD: treat with interbody techniques (remove painful disk)
Instability: treat with instrumented posterolateral fusion

202. What are the two classic symptoms of lumbar instability?

202. "Catch" with extension
Back pain

203. What are the radiographic instability criteria at L1–L4?

203. >4 mm motion
10 degrees angulation

204. ... at L5-S1?

204. >6 mm motion
20 degrees angulation

205. What are the five Waddell signs? What is their clinical significance?

205. Tenderness
Simulation
Distraction
Regional disturbance (stocking-glove)
Overreaction
Significance: be wary if >3 positive

206. How are impairment and disability defined? Which determines compensation?

206. Impairment: deviation from normal function
Disability: inability to perform a specific function
Disability more important for compensation

207. What is the proven benefit of a corset? What is its effect on motion?

207. Decreased intradiskal pressure
No effect on motion

208. Compare Jewett versus thoracolumbar spinal orthosis (TLSO) for rotational control.

208. TLSO better

209. How can L5-S1 best be immobilized?

209. TLSO with thigh extension

Surgical Anatomy: Anterior Approach

210. Which levels are accessible in transperitoneal and retroperitoneal approaches?

210. Transperitoneal: L5-S1
Retroperitoneal: L1–sacrum

211. Where does the aorta bifurcate? Above this level, where does it lie?

211. Bifurcation at L4
In the midline above bifurcation

212. The inferior vena cava is on which side?

212. Right

213. Where do the segmental vessels come off?

213. Mid-body level (not at level of disk)

L4-L5, L5-S1 Approaches

214. Are the parasympathetic or sympathetic fibers at risk at these levels? Which plexus?

214. Sympathetic fibers at risk
Superior hypogastric plexus

215. What are the potential complications of injury to the sympathetics?

215. Retrograde ejaculation
Lower extremity temperature difference (chain injury)

216. Where are the parasympathetic fibers? What is their reproductive effect?

216. S2-3, S3-4, usually not disturbed
Control erection

217. What is the preferred direction of anterior dissection? Why?

217. Dissect from left to right
Plexus is more adherent on right

218. What is the most common level of vascular injury? How is it injured? What is the consequence?

218. L4-5 most common level
Injury with pituitary rongeur
Most commonly leads to arteriovenous (AV) fistula, but may lead to death

219. What vessel lies in the L4-5 interspace?

219. Iliolumbar vein

What Is the Relationship to the Psoas of …

220. …Ilioinguinal and iliohypogastric nerves?

221. … Genitofemoral nerve?

222. … Obturator and femoral nerves?

223. … Sympathetic chain?

224. At what level is the genitofemoral nerve? How can it be tested?

225. What is the most common complication of total disk arthroplasty?

220. Lateral border of psoas

221. On psoas

222. Deep to psoas

223. Medial to psoas

224. Near L2-3
Cremasteric reflex

225. Transient radiculopathy

Surgical Anatomy: Posterior Approach

226. The optimal lumbar pedicle screw starting point lies at the junction of what three anatomical entities?

227. Should one aim more medially or laterally as one moves caudally in the lumbar spine?

228. What is the No. 1 factor associated with lumbar screw pullout?

229. What is the No. 1 risk factor for postoperative interbody cage migration?

230. What two levels have the most lumbar lordosis?

226. Transverse process
Pars
Superior articular facet

227. More medially as one heads down

228. Osteoporosis

229. Posterior approach

230. L4-L5
L5-S1

Disk Herniation

231. Straight leg raise (SLR) versus femoral stretch tests identify HNPs at which levels?

232. What is the most specific clinical exam for HNP? Especially true in what situation?

233. What body position results in the lowest intradiskal pressure? Highest?

234. Lumbar disk herniations occur most commonly at which location (on axial imaging)?

235. How can referred pain be differentiated from lumbar radicular pain?

236. How does the orientation of the upper lumbar nerve roots differ from that of the lower roots?

231. Femoral stretch: L2-3 (hip flexors), L3-4 (quads, TA [tibialis anterior])
SLR: L4-5, L5-S1

232. Contralateral SLR
Especially for axillary herniation

233. Lowest: supine
Highest: sitting, flexed with weights in hands

234. Paracentral

235. Referred pain usually above knee

236. Upper roots have more direct takeoff (less room to manipulate)

237. What is the natural history motor recovery, pain resolution, and sensory deficits in HNP?

237. Motor generally recovers
Pain generally resolves
30% of sensory deficits persist

238. Pediatric herniations are *not* generally disk material; they consist of what?

238. Avulsion of ring apophysis of vertebral body

239. Is there a proven benefit to epidural steroids for HNP?

239. No

240. What patients are especially likely to have recurrent postoperative pain? What percentage of patients?

240. Large annular defect
Up to 15 to 20% have long-term backache

241. What is the reported re-herniation rate? What is the imaging study of choice to identify re-herniation?

241. 10%
MRI with gadolinium

242. What are the three components of the treatment algorithm for postoperative infection after lumbar diskectomy? When should surgery be performed?

242. MRI with gadolinium
Percutaneous biopsy and culture
IV antibiotics
Surgery for failure of antibiotic treatment

Cauda Equina Syndrome

243. Better outcomes can be expected if decompression is performed within what time frame?

243. 48 hours

244. Does early decompression benefit bladder function, motor recovery, or pain?

244. Improves bladder and motor recovery
No effect on pain resolution

Stenosis

245. What is the principal cause of lateral recess stenosis?

245. Superior articular facet hypertrophy

246. What are three causes of foraminal stenosis?

246. Foraminal HNP
Decreased disk height
Pars defect

247. In foraminal stenosis, what are the critical foraminal height and the critical posterior disk height?

247. Foraminal height <15 mm
Posterior disk height <4 mm

248. Are tension signs present with central or lateral stenosis?

248. Not generally

249. Why is hyperreflexia not seen with lumbar stenosis? What is the most common neurologic deficit on exam?

249. Lower motor neuron (LMN) problem, so no hyperreflexia
L5 most common root for weakness

250. Is there a proven benefit to epidural steroids?

250. No consistent benefit in controlled studies

251. What type of injection has most consistently demonstrated symptomatic benefit?

251. Transforaminal nerve block

252. What are the three indications for fusion after decompression of stenosis?

252. Degenerative spondylolisthesis
Instability/iatrogenic injury
Degenerative scoliosis

253. Is there a proven benefit to instrumentation for stenosis? How about symptomatic relief?

253. No proven benefit to instrumentation
Improved symptom relief *without* instrumentation

254. What age group has poorer decompression outcomes? Are there other prognostic factors?

254. Young patients do worse
Patients with multiple comorbidities do worse

255. What is the typical mechanism of extraforaminal L5 root compression? What is the ideal radiographic view to identify it?

255. L5 impingement between sacral ala and L5 transverse process
Ferguson's view

Spondylolisthesis

256. What are the six types of spondylolisthesis, and (where applicable) which level is most commonly affected by each?

256. Dysplastic (L5-S1)
Isthmic (L5-S1)
Degenerative (L4-L5)
Traumatic
Pathologic
Postsurgical

257. What nerve root is most commonly affected by spondylolisthesis?

257. L5

Dysplastic Spondylolisthesis

258. What are the two classic radiographic features?

258. Trapezoidal L5
Rounded S1

259. What is the normal value of sacral inclination? What is the significance of greater inclination?

259. Normal inclination >30 degrees
More vertical sacrum: increased risk of slip

260. How is the slip angle measured? What values are considered normal?

260. Lordosis at L5-S1
Normal <0 (kyphotic)

261. What nerve root is most commonly affected? Why are nerve root signs especially common with dysplastic spondylolisthesis?

261. L5 at risk
Especially common because posterior arch is intact

262. Is there a proven clinical benefit to spondylolisthesis reduction?

262. No

263. If a reduction is performed, when is the nerve root most likely to be injured?

263. During the last 50% of reduction

264. Is there a proven benefit to decompression?

264. No
Fusion with or without decompression leads to good outcomes

Isthmic Spondylolisthesis

265. What is the most sensitive imaging study for identification of a pars defect?

265. Single photon emission computed tomography (SPECT) scan

266. When is the listhesis thought to occur? To what grade?

266. At ages 4 to 6 years
Usually not to more than grade II

267. Which gender is most commonly affected?

267. Female

268. What effect does a unilateral pars defect have on risk of listhesis?

268. Unilateral defects generally do not result in a slip

269. Ideal brace?

269. Antilordotic brace

270. What are the treatment and activity restrictions for the various grades of adolescent slips?

270. Grade I: contact sports OK if patient asymptomatic
Grade II: no contact sports
Grade III/IV: fuse L4-S1 in situ

271. Is a laminectomy without fusion an option for children?

271. No!

272. Pars defect repair indications: age, grade, and level?

272. Young
Grade I or less
Above L5

273. For an adult patient, which levels should be fused if the L5-S1 slip is low grade or high grade?

273. Low grade: L5-S1
High grade: L4-S1

274. Is there a proven clinical benefit to using instrumentation with fusion? Is there another point to consider?

274. No proven benefit; uninstrumented outcomes are equivalent to instrumented outcomes
But instrumentation does increase fusion rates

275. If instrumentation is used, which approach has the best reported outcomes?

275. Best outcomes with circumferential instrumentation

Degenerative Spondylolisthesis

276. What race and which gender are at highest risk? What age group?

276. African-American female
>40 years

277. What radiographic feature is especially common among affected patients?

277. Transitional L5 vertebrae

278. What two factors may predispose to degenerative spondylolisthesis?

278. Pregnancy
Diabetes mellitus

279. Is there a proven benefit to fusion at the time of surgery?

279. Fusion outcomes significantly better than decompression alone

280. Is there a proven benefit to instrumentation?

280. None proven

Degenerative Scoliosis

281. What is the long-term effect of untreated degenerative scoliosis?

281. Increased back pain

282. What are the two factors that curve flexibility depend on?

282. Curve magnitude
Age

283. Compare general curve progression rates >50 degrees: thoracic versus thoracolumbar versus lumbar?

283. Thoracic: progresses 1 degree/year
Thoracolumbar: progresses 0.5 degrees/year
Lumbar: progresses 0.25 degrees/year

284. Are combined or staged surgical procedures generally preferred in adults?

284. Combined preferred, because staging leads to malnutrition between stages

285. If severe osteoporosis is present, what is the most secure point of fixation?

285. Lamina

286. What are surgical outcomes most dependent on?

286. Final coronal and sagittal balance

287. What are the three benefits to interbody device use at the caudal end of long lumbosacral fusion?

287. Increased construct stiffness
Decreased strain on posterior instrumentation
Increased fusion rate

Complications

288. What is the No. 1 complication of adult scoliosis surgery?

288. Pseudarthrosis

289. What is the No. 1 medical complication?

289. Urinary tract infection

290. What is the pulmonary consequence of thoracotomy in the adult?

290. Never returns to preoperative pulmonary function test (PFT) values

291. What is delayed postoperative paraplegia most often due to?

291. Cord ischemia (stretch)

292. What was the main problem with Harrington instrumentation?

292. Positive sagittal balance = flatback

293. Pedicle subtraction osteotomy (PSO) for flatback is generally performed at which levels?

293. L2 or below

294. What is a contraindication to PSO?

294. Anterior pseudarthrosis

Superior Mesenteric Artery (SMA) Syndrome

295. What are the three characteristic SMA syndrome symptoms?

295. Abdominal pain
Distention
Persistent vomiting

296. When does SMA syndrome occur? Why?

296. Within 1 week postop
Compression of third part of duodenum between aorta and SMA

297. How can SMA be differentiated clinically and radiographically from postoperative ileus?

297. Clinically: bowel sounds present
X-ray: upper gastrointestinal (GI) study

298. What are the two aspects to treatment for SMA syndrome?

298. Nasogastric (NG) tube
Intravenous (IV) fluids/alimentation

■ Spinal Cord Injury

General Knowledge

299. What grade of muscle strength indicates active muscle function against gravity?

299. 3 out of 5

300. What are the two ways in which the functional level of an SCI patient is determined?

300. Most distal intact sensory level
Most distal intact (3/5 or greater) motor level if next level is 5/5

301. What is the Frankel classification used for?

301. Grades motor function below injury level (A = none to E = full)

302. For what two capabilities has the ASIA (American Spine Injury Association) motor score been shown to be prognostic?

302. Functional improvement potential Performance in rehabilitation

303. What is the significance of the jaw jerk reflex?

303. Indicates injury proximal to the cervical spine

304. What result or time frame characterizes the end of spinal shock?

304. Return of bulbocavernosus reflex Or 48 hours passed since injury

305. Are reflexes present in spinal shock?

305. No reflexes (UMN or LMN) are present

306. Neurogenic shock is associated with injuries above which level? What is it due to?

306. Injury above T5 Disruption of descending sympathetics

307. What are the two components of the treatment algorithm for neurogenic shock?

307. 1st: fluids 2nd: pressors

308. What three MRI findings are poorly prognostic for recovery after SCI?

308. Hemorrhage Contusion Edema

309. What two factors are positively prognostic for recovery after SCI?

309. <30 years old <30% displacement on radiographs

310. What type of injury is most often associated with further deterioration after admission?

310. Rotational fracture dislocation

Current Steroid Protocol

311. If steroids are started within 3 hours, they should be continued for how long? What if they are started within 8 hours of injury? What if they are started more than 8 hours after injury?

311. Start within 3 hours, continue for 24 hours Start within 8 hours, continue for 48 hours After 8 hours, no steroids

312. Should steroids be administered with a penetrating wound?

312. No

313. What roots are involved with a conus medullaris injury? What functions are lost?

313. Roots S2, S3, S4 Lost: bowel, bladder function only

314. What anatomic levels of injury are most likely to result in conus injury? What is the differential diagnosis?

314. Anatomic level of injury: T12-L1 or T11-T12 Important differential: cauda equina syndrome

Intraoperative Neural Monitoring

315. Motor evoked potentials (MEPs) monitor which area of the spinal cord?

315. Anterior column only

316. Somatosensory evoked potentials (SSEPs) monitor which area of the spinal cord? What is the downside?

316. Dorsal column only May miss anterior column injury

317. What degree of SSEP amplitude change is concerning?

317. 50% drop

318. What degree of SSEP latency change is concerning?

318. 10% increase

319. What does electromyography (EMG) monitor?

319. Nerve root irritation

320. What two modalities are best during scoliosis correction? What modality is best during spondylolisthesis reduction?

320. Scoliosis: SSEP, motor evoked potential (MEP)
Spondylolisthesis reduction: EMG

321. If intraoperative SSEP changes occur during scoliosis surgery, what two steps should be taken?

321. Increase blood pressure
Stagnara wake-up test

322. If the changes persist, then what?

322. Remove instrumentation

Operative Complications

323. What are the treatment and activity restrictions for an intraoperative dural tear? Is a drain necessary?

323. Primary watertight repair
48 hours of bedrest postoperatively
No drain necessary

324. What are the treatment and activity restrictions for a dural tear discovered postoperatively? Should it be re-explored?

324. Subarachnoid drain
Bedrest
Re-explore if symptoms persist 3 to 4 days

325. What three symptoms are associated with dural tear?

325. Nausea
Headache
Photophobia

326. What test is used to determine if drain output is CSF?

326. CSF is β2-transferrin positive

Gunshot Wounds to the Spine

327. Should antibiotics be administered after gunshot to the spine?

327. If associated with perforated viscus, broad spectrum antibiotics for 1 week

328. What are the two indications for intervention by general surgery?

328. Esophageal perforation
Bowel perforation

329. What two conditions justify surgery to remove bullet fragments?

329. Incomplete SCI
Bullet fragments causing compression

330. Bullet removal results in improved motor recovery below which level?

330. Motor recovery improves below T10

331. When should a laminectomy be performed?

331. Only if lamina fracture present

Incomplete SCI

332. What two factors have been shown to predict motor recovery?

332. Age
Injury type

333. Is there a proven benefit to early surgical intervention?

333. No

334. Is there a proven benefit to decompressing stenosis not associated with fracture?

334. No

335. Which incomplete SCI syndrome has the best prognosis? Which has the worst prognosis?

335. Best: Brown-Séquard (ipsilateral motor/sensory loss, contralateral pain/temperature loss)
Worst: anterior column

336. With posterior cord syndrome, what is required for successful postinjury ambulation? Why?

336. Requires intact vision for ambulation
Because proprioception is absent

337. The presence of which sensory quality is a good prognostic factor after SCI?

337. Pinprick sensation

Complete SCI

338. With complete SCI, is erection possible? Is ejaculation possible?

338. Reflex erection possible, not psychogenic
Normal ejaculation not possible

339. After 1 year, how much additional recovery is expected with cervical SCI versus thoracolumbar SCI?

339. Cervical: 1 additional level
Thoracolumbar: 0 additional levels

340. What adaptive equipment is required for a patient with an SCI level of C4?

340. C4: high back, head support

341. ... of C5?

341. C5: mouth-driven electric wheelchair

342. ... of C6?

342. C6: manual wheelchair with wrist/hand orthoses

343. ... of C7?

343. C7: can live independently

344. For C5 SCI patients, which tendon transfers will provide C6- or C7-type function?

344. C6: BR to extensor carpi radialis brevis (ECRB) transfer; BR = brachioradialis
C7: deltoid to triceps transfer

Brain Injuries

345. What is the treatment of an open skull fracture? Why? If closed?

345. Elevate depressed fragment if open
Decrease risk of infection
If closed, leave alone

346. What is the anticipated recovery period after traumatic brain injury?

346. 12 weeks

347. What extremities are most affected by an anterior cerebellar artery (ACA) stroke? What extremities are most affected by a middle cerebellar artery (MCA) stroke?

347. ACA stroke: lower extremities most affected
MCA stroke: upper extremities most affected

Mild Concussion

348. What is the definition of a mild concussion?

348. No loss of consciousness (LOC)

349. What are the three grades of mild concussion?

349. I: confusion, no amnesia
II: retrograde amnesia
III: amnesia after impact

350. What is the recommended time period before return to play (RTP) for each grade?

350. I: when patient is asymptomatic
II: 1 week
III: 1 month

Classic Concussion

351. What is the definition of classic concussion?

351. Associated with loss of consciousness

352. What circumstance justifies a postconcussion head CT?

352. LOC lasts longer than 5 minutes

353. What is the recommended time period before return to play (RTP) after first classic concussion?

353. 1 week to 1 month

354. What is the recommended time period before RTP after second classic concussion?

354. No RTP that season

355. What is the definition of diffuse axonal injury? What is the RTP recommendation?

355. LOC >6 hours
No RTP

356. Compare the symptoms of a burner to those of transient quadriplegia?

356. Burner: unilateral, upper plexus
Transient quadriplegia: axial load, bilateral, lasts up to 36 hours

Other Athletic Injuries

Transient Quadriplegia

357. What four factors may predispose to the development of transient quadriplegia?

357. Stenosis
Instability
Herniated nucleus pulposus (HNP)
Congenital fusions

358. If a patient sustains a traumatic HNP, what is the timing for RTP?

358. May return when asymptomatic

359. What are the two contraindications to return to play?

359. Instability
Neurologic symptoms >36 hours

360. Does prior transient quadriplegia predict future injury?

360. No

361. What are the two key features of spear tackler's spine?

361. Stenosis
Loss of lordosis

362. Once spear tackler's spine has been diagnosed, are contact sports allowed?

362. No

363. What is the most common SCI mechanism in an athlete?

363. Flexion-compression (burst)

364. What is an absolute contraindication to contact sports? Example?

364. Congenital anomalies of the upper cervical spine
Example: os odontoideum

Common Fracture Questions

365. What is a safe alternative to endotracheal (ET) intubation in C-spine trauma patients? Is there an exception?

365. Nasotracheal intubation
Exception: patients in respiratory arrest

366. What is a safe alternative to ET intubation in a patient with spine trauma and facial fractures?

366. Cricothyroidotomy

367. What is the recommended treatment for Jefferson fracture? What must be checked at the conclusion of treatment?

367. Halo with or without traction
Once treatment is completed, check C1-2 stability with flexion-extension films

Hangman's Fracture (Traumatic Spondylolisthesis)

368. How is traumatic spondylolisthesis classified?

368. I: minimally displaced
II: anterior translation >3 mm, angulated
IIa: increased angulaion with minimal translation
III: also C2-3 facet dislocation

369. Type I: What are the two criteria for acceptable reduction? What is the recommended treatment?

369. <4 mm displacement
<10 degrees angulation
Collar for treatment

370. Type II/IIa: What is the recommended treatment? What is a critical consideration in a type IIa patient?

370. Treat with halo
IIa: Do *not* apply traction!

371. Type III: What are the three acceptable treatment options?

371. Anterior C2-3 fusion
Posterior C1 to C3 fusion
Bilateral pars screws

372. In odontoid fractures, what two factors increase the risk of nonunion?

372. Displacement >5 mm
Angulation >10 degrees

373. What is a salvage option for odontoid nonunion?

373. Posterior fusion, no screws

374. How should a cervical facet fracture be treated? Compare nondisplaced versus floating facet injuries.

374. Nondisplaced facet fracture: collar
Floating facet: open reduction with internal fixation (ORIF) with lateral mass plate

Facet Dislocations

375. What mechanism of injury most commonly results in facet dislocation?

375. Flexion-distraction

376. How can unilateral and bilateral dislocations be distinguished radiographically?

376. Unilateral <50% translation
Bilateral ≥50% translation

377. If a pre-reduction MRI shows herniated disk, what is the necessary treatment?

377. Must approach anteriorly to decompress and fuse if herniated disk

378. What is the recommended treatment for bilateral dislocation with an HNP?

378. Approach posteriorly

379. What is the treatment of a stable lateral mass fracture? What is the treatment of a unstable lateral mass fracture?

379. Stable: collar
Unstable: surgery

380. What is the usual treatment for a subaxial compression fracture?

380. Collar

381. Is halo treatment generally effective for the subaxial spine?

381. No, a halo poorly immobilizes subaxial spine

382. What is the treatment for a subaxial burst fracture with nerve injury and an *intact* posterior element?

382. ACDF

383. What is the treatment for a subaxial burst fracture with nerve injury and *unstable* posterior elements?

383. Anterior and posterior fusions

Halo Treatment

384. Where should the anterior pin be placed?

384. Lateral one-third of brow

385. What structure is at risk if an anterior pin is placed too medially?

385. Supraorbital nerve

386. When applying a halo to a child, what is the key preoperative imaging study?

386. CT scan to assess skull thickness

387. When applying a halo to a child, how many pins should be placed?

387. Eight

388. At what torque?

388. 4 pounds

389. When applying a halo to an adult, how many pins should be placed and at what torque?

389. 4 pins at 8 pounds

Chance Fractures

390. What is the most common injury mechanism?

390. Flexion distraction

391. What is the associated visceral injury? What is the treatment to avoid in patients with abdominal injuries?

391. Associated with abdominal injury and ileus
Avoid extension bracing

Pelvic and Sacral Fractures

392. What is the bone scan appearance of sacral insufficiency fracture?

392. H-shaped uptake

393. A vertical shear pelvic fracture causes tension on which ligaments? What fracture may result?

393. Tension on iliolumbar ligaments
Classic x-ray finding: L5 transverse process fractures (check the pelvis!)

■ Pediatric Spine

Commonly Tested Clinical Conditions

Rotatory Atlantoaxial Subluxation

394. What is Grisel's syndrome?

394. Retropharyngeal bursitis preceding rotatory subluxation

395. Early treatment for Grisel's consists of?

395. Traction/bracing

396. What is the general classification of rotatory subluxation?

396. I: rotation, no anterior displacement
II: rotation with anterior displacement 3 to 5 mm
III: rotation with anterior displacement >5 mm
IV: rotation with posterior displacement

397. What is the imaging study of choice?

397. Dynamic CT

398. What is the treatment of traumatic subluxation <1 week in duration?

398. Soft collar

399. ... 1 week to 1 month in duration?

399. Cervical traction

400. ... >1 month in duration?

400. Fusion

401. What is the treatment for a late presentation?

401. C1-2 fusion

Os Odontoideum

402. Os odontoideum may appear radiographically similar to what condition?

402. Type II odontoid fracture

403. What are the three surgical indications?

403. Instability >10 mm
SAC <13 mm (SAC = space available for the cord)
Neurologic deficit

404. What is the procedure of choice for symptomatic os odontoideum?

404. Posterior C1-2 fusion

405. Are contact sports permitted with an os odontoideum?

405. No

Spinal Cord Injury Without Radiologic Abnormality (SCIWORA)

406. What injury mechanism is generally responsible?

406. Hyperextension leading to posterior cord compression

407. What imaging study is necessary for diagnosis of SCIWORA? What percentage of studies will appear normal?

407. MRI
25%

408. What is the treatment of cervical SCIWORA?

408. Cervical collar

409. What is a common long-term complication of paraplegia/quadriplegia?

409. Paralytic scoliosis

Adolescent Idiopathic Scoliosis (AIS)

410. Where is the apex of normal thoracic kyphosis?

410. T5 to T8

411. What is the average annual spinal growth rate per segment? What is the approximate total?

411. 0.07 cm per year per segment
1 cm per year total

412. What is the recommended scoliometry threshold for referral for spine surgery evaluation?

412. 7 degrees on Adams forward bend

413. Curve progression best corresponds with which measure?

413. Peak growth velocity

414. Peak growth velocity generally occurs at which Risser stage? How about menarche?

414. Peak growth velocity at Risser 0
Menarche occurs before Risser 1

415. What are five indications for obtaining an MRI in the adolescent scoliosis patient?

415. Left thoracic curve
Abnormal neurologic exam, especially asymmetric abdominal reflexes
Excess kyphosis (conider neurofibromatosis)
Onset <11 years old (think infantile, juvenile)
Pain

416. How are stable vertebrae and neutral vertebrae defined?

416. Midsacral line bisects the stable vertebrae
Neutral vertebrae have no rotation and symmetric-appearing pedicles

417. What is the usual sagittal alignment at the apical vertebrae with AIS?

417. Apical vertebrae usually hypokyphotic

418. What are the six components of the Lenke classification for AIS?

418. Main thoracic
Double thoracic
Double major
Triple major
Thoracolumbar/lumbar
Thoracolumbar/lumbar—main thoracic

419. What is the definition of a structural curve? Why are structural curves clinically significant?

419. Structural curves do not bend out to less than 25 degrees
All structural curves should be incorporated in fusion

420. What three aspects make the progression of neuromuscular scoliosis unique?

420. More rapid
Continues after maturity
Pelvic obliquity

421. In general, at what age should fusion surgery be undertaken for neuromuscular scoliosis?

421. 10 to 12 years

General Scoliosis Treatment Principles

422. If the apex is proximal to T7, what brace is needed?

422. Milwaukee brace

423. Bracing has been prospectively shown to be effective for which population?

423. Females with 25- to 35-degree curves

424. An anterior spinal fusion alone may suffice for which curve type?

424. Thoracolumbar curves

425. What are the two classic advantages of an anterior fusion in this population? Is there an important caveat?

425. Save levels
Improve correction
Caveat: pedicle screws may negate these advantages

426. What are the three general indications for a combined anterior and posterior fusion?

426. Curves >75 degrees
Crankshaft prevention (females <10 years old, males <13 years old)
Neuromuscular scoliosis

427. Why are some neuromuscular conditions treated with posterior fusion alone?

427. To avoid compromising already fragile pulmonary function

428. What are three examples of neuromuscular disorders treated with posterior fusion only?

428. Muscular dystrophy
Spinal muscular atrophy
Werdnig-Hoffmann

429. What should the distal extent of fusion ideally be in the adolescent idiopathic population?

429. L3 or above

430. What are the two risk factors for neurologic injury?

430. Excessive correction
Sublaminar wires

431. What is the ideal pedicle screw depth?

431. 80% of vertebral body depth

Pseudarthrosis in AIS

432. In what percentage of patients do pseudarthroses develop?

432. 2%

433. How is an asymptomatic pseudarthrosis treated?

433. Observation

434. If symptomatic?

434. Revision with compression instrumentation

435. What graft type increases pseudarthrosis risk in adult scoliosis patients?

435. Freeze-dried allograft

436. In general, what are the two surgical options for flatback correction?

436. Posterior closing wedge osteotomy (at L2 or below)
Anterior release and fusion

Scoliosis Literature: Key Points

437. Untreated AIS patients are more likely to suffer from which two conditions as adults?

437. Dyspnea
Back pain

438. What are treated AIS patients more likely than the general population to suffer from?

438. Back pain

439. Has the magnitude of Cobb angle correction ever been associated with patient satisfaction?

439. No

440. What is the preferred tool for evaluation of patient postoperative satisfaction?

440. SRS-22 has been validated as an outcome measure

Infantile and Juvenile Idiopathic Scoliosis

Infantile Idiopathic Scoliosis

441. What age group is affected by infantile idiopathic scoliosis?

441. <3 years of age

442. What gender is most commonly affected?

442. Male

443. With which two musculoskeletal conditions is infantile scoliosis associated?

443. Plagiocephaly (flat skull)
Congenital defects

444. What percentage of patients have associated spinal cord disease?

444. 20%

445. What is the most common curve pattern?

445. Left thoracic curve

446. What is the difference between phase I and phase II? What is the clinical significance?

446. Phase I: no rib/vertebral overlap
Phase II: rib/vertebral overlap is present
All phase II curves progress

447. For phase I curves, what two conditions indicate that spontaneous resolution is likely?

447. Curve <25 degrees
Rib–vertebral angle difference (RVAD) <20 degrees

448. Where should the RVAD be measured?

448. Curve convexity

449. What does surgical treatment entail?

449. Combined anterior and posterior fusion

450. Under which two conditions may a preoperative brace be of benefit?

450. To delay surgery until greater maturity
If RVAD is increasing

451. What is the treatment if RVAD >20 degrees and if it progresses?

451. If RVAD >20 degrees, then brace
If progresses, then operate

Juvenile Idiopathic Scoliosis

452. What age group is affected by juvenile idiopathic scoliosis?

452. 3 to 10 years old

453. What is the most common curve type?

453. Right thoracic

454. How does the risk of progression compare with the risk of AIS?

454. Increased

455. What are the two general treatment options?

455. Growing rods (unfused)
Combined anterior/posterior spinal fusion

Congenital and Other Developmental Conditions of the Spine

Congenital Scoliosis

456. With congenital scoliosis, the defect occurs at how many weeks of gestation?

456. 4 to 6 weeks

457. Patients must also be evaluated for which two conditions? Why?

457. Renal anomalies (abdominal ultrasound)
Heart disease
Because these systems develop at same point in gestation

458. What are the two components of the general classification of congenital scoliosis?

458. I: failure of segmentation (bar)
II: failure of formation (hemivertebra)

459. Which type has the best prognosis? Which has the worst?

459. Best: block vertebrae (bilateral failure of segmentation)
Worst: unilateral unsegmented bar with contralateral fully segmented hemivertebra

460. What is the treatment for unilateral unsegmented bar with contralateral fully segmented hemivertebra?

460. Fuse at presentation with combined anterior/posterior procedure

461. What is the treatment for other types of congenital scoliosis?

461. Await progression

462. What is the classic form of treatment? What is the notable exception?

462. Classically, posterior spinal fusion in situ
Exception: combined anterior/posterior fusion if significant crankshaft risk

463. What are the two other surgical options and their associated criteria?

463. Hemivertebra excision (curve >40 degrees; especially L4, L5)
Anterior/posterior hemiepiphysiodesis (curve >40 degrees)

Congenital Kyphosis

464. Which type has the worst prognosis? Why?

464. Failure of formation (type I)
Because it is most likely to result in paraplegia

465. What is the surgical procedure of choice?

465. Posterior spinal fusion (because crankshaft is desirable)

466. An anterior approach should also be considered with curves of which magnitude?

466. >55 degrees

Diastematomyelia

467. What is the definition of diastematomyelia?

467. Longitudinal cleft in cord

468. With what condition is diastematomyelia associated?

468. Cord tethering

469. What is a key radiographic feature suggestive of diastematomyelia?

469. Intrapedicular widening

470. What is the treatment if asymptomatic?

470. Observation

Sacral Agenesis

471. How can sacral agenesis be differentiated from myelomeningocele?

471. Protective sensation present, but motor function still absent

472. What is the classic physical exam finding?

472. Dimpling of buttocks

473. What is the characteristic gait pattern of these patients?

473. Trendelenburg

474. What are the two treatment options?

474. Amputation
Spinal-pelvic fusion

Scheuermann's Disease

475. What are the two diagnostic criteria?

475. >45 degrees thoracic kyphosis
>5 degrees anterior wedging of three sequential vertebrae

476. Scheuermann's may be associated with what three spinal conditions?

476. Spondylolysis
Scoliosis
Schmorl's nodes

477. Which gender is most commonly affected?

477. Male

478. What are the two indications for bracing?

478. Kyphosis <75 degrees
Skeletally immature patient

479. What are the three criteria for surgical intervention?

479. Skeletally mature patient
Kyphosis >75 degrees
Does not correct to <55 degrees (relatively inflexible curve)

480. What is the surgical procedure of choice?

480. Posterior spinal fusion with or without anterior release and fusion

481. What levels should be included in the fusion? What are the proximal and distal extents?

481. T2 proximally
One level beyond lordosis distally

482. What are the two common complications of operative treatment?

482. SMA syndrome
Junctional kyphosis

2

Trauma Principles and Pelvic Trauma

■ Principles of Trauma

Evaluation Principles

Primary Survey

1. What are the two purposes of the primary survey?

   1. Find causes of hemodynamic instability and respiratory impairment
   Restore cardiorespiratory function

2. What are the five components of the primary survey?

   2. A—airway
   B—breathing
   C—circulation
   D—disability
   E—environmental exposure

Secondary Survey

3. What is the secondary survey?

   3. Traditional history and physical examination after initial resuscitation

Routine Imaging

4. What is the most common reason for missed fractures in polytrauma patients?

   4. Inadequately imaged extremities

5. With polytrauma, what two radiographs are obtained during the primary survey?

   5. Anteroposterior (AP) chest
   AP pelvis

6. What radiographs are usually obtained during the secondary survey?

   6. Cervical spine films: lateral view including the superior endplate of T1, AP cervical spine, and AP odontoid view

Calculations and Prognostic Indicators

7. How is the Injury Severity Scale (ISS) score calculated? In what situation is it not prognostic?

7. $(AIS)^2 + (AIS)^2 + (AIS)^2$ for the three most severely injured systems
Not prognostic for severely affected single system

8. What are the mortality rates for an ISS score >16? >40?

8. ISS >16: 10% mortality
ISS >40: 50% mortality

9. Increased ISS is associated with what three outcomes?

9. Greater disability
Higher rate of unemployment
Lower quality of life

10. Increased short-term mortality rates are associated with what two factors?

10. Advanced age
Increased severity of injury

11. What are the components of the Glasgow Coma Scale (GCS)?

11. Eye opening
Verbal response
Motor response

12. How is eye opening scored?

12. 1, no eye opening
2, eye opening to pain
3, eye opening to verbal command
4, eyes open spontaneously

13. How is verbal response scored?

13. 1, no verbal response
2, incomprehensible sounds
3, inappropriate words
4, confused
5, orientated

14. How is motor response scored?

14. 1, no motor response
2, extension to pain
3, flexion to pain
4, withdrawal from pain
5, localizing pain
6, obeys commands

15. How is the GCS score arrived at? What is the definition of coma?

15. Score is the sum of all three sections
A GCS score <8 indicates coma

16. The GCS score is prognostic of what outcome?

16. Future neurologic function

Shock, Resuscitation, and Systemic Inflammatory Response Syndrome

17. With hypovolemic shock, what happens to cardiac output (CO) and peripheral venous resistance (PVR)? Do veins constrict or dilate? What is the preferred treatment?

17. CO decreases
PVR increases
Veins constrict
Treatment: resuscitation with crystalloid and colloid, control of ongoing losses

18. What is the effect of cardiogenic shock on CO, PVR, and the venous system?

18. CO decreases
PVR increases
Venous dilation

19. What is the effect of vasogenic shock on arteries and veins?

19. Arteries constrict
Veins dilate

20. What is the effect of neurogenic shock on arteries and veins? What is the treatment?

20. Arteries dilate
Veins dilate
Treatment: restore intravascular volume and vasopressors after hypovolemia excluded

21. What is the effect of septic shock on CO, PVR, and heart rate (HR)?

21. CO increases
PVR decreases
HR increases
Also fever and leukocytosis

Stages of Hemorrhagic Shock

22. Class I: What percentage of blood volume is lost? How are HR and blood pressure (BP) affected?

22. <15% lost
HR <100
Normal BP

23. Class II: What percentage of blood volume is lost? How are HR and BP affected?

23. 15 to 30% lost
HR >100
Normal BP

24. Class III: What percentage of blood volume is lost? How are HR and BP affected? Are there other changes?

24. 30 to 40% lost
HR >100
Low BP
Decreased urine output, slight mental status changes

25. Class IV: What percentage of blood volume is lost? How are HR and BP affected? Are there other changes?

25. >40% lost
HR >100
Low BP
No urine output, lethargy, confusion

Resuscitation Pearls

26. What are the seven criteria for adequate resuscitation of the polytrauma patient?

26. Hemodynamically stable
Stable oxygen saturation
Lactate level <2 mmol/L
International normalized ratio (INR) <1.25
Normal body temperature
Adequate urine output
Not requiring inotropic support

27. What are the adult and pediatric goals for urine output after resuscitation?

27. Adult: 0.5 mL/kg/hour
Pediatric: 1 mL/kg/hour

28. At what level should thrombocytopenia be treated in the setting of polytrauma?

28. <50,000/mL

Common Calculations

29. How is pO_2 expected (exp) calculated?

29. $7 * FiO_2 - pCO_2$

30. If expected (exp) pO_2 is less than observed (obs), then calculate what? How?

30. Calculate Aa gradient = pO_2 (exp) – pO_2 (obs)

31. Aa gradient/20 = ?

31. Percent physiologic shunt

Systemic Inflammatory Response Syndrome (SIRS)

32. What is the key interleukin (IL) in SIRS?

32. IL-6

33. In what four clinical situations is IL-6 released?

33. Systemic inflammatory response
Femoral nailing (releases IL-6 and IL-8)
Myeloma (secreted by plasma cells along with MIP-1α); MIP = macrophage inflammatory protein
Periprosthetic loosening (secreted by fibroblasts)

34. Orthopaedic dissection also releases what clotting factor?

34. Thromboplastin (factor 3), which activates the clotting cascade

35. IL-6 concentrations above what level may be diagnostic of SIRS?

35. >200 pg/ml

36. What is the key characteristic of the ebb phase of systemic inflammation?

36. Cardiovascular instability

37. What are the four characteristics of the flow phase?

37. Muscle wasting
Fever
Glucose intolerance
Gluconeogenesis

Key Points for Specific Injury Conditions

Skeletal Injury

38. How much blood can an unsplinted closed femur fracture lose?

38. Up to 4 units

39. What is the incidence of femoral neck fracture associated with femoral shaft fracture?

39. 1 to 9%
20 to 50% are missed on initial radiographs

Open Fractures

40. Coverage within what time period has been shown to result in improved outcomes?

40. 72 hours

41. What is the recommended antibiotic for Gustillo stage I and II open fractures?

41. Cephalosporin

42. What are the two recommended antibiotics for Gustillo stage III open fractures?

42. Cephalosporin
Aminoglycoside

43. Which antibiotic should be added with heavy contamination, farm injury, or anaerobic risk?

43. Penicillin or ampicillin

44. For how long should antibiotic therapy be continued?

44. 72 hours after each debridement, and 72 hours after definitive wound closure

45. In addition, what should all open fractures be treated with?

45. Tetanus booster on immunoglobulin based on immunization history

Soft Tissue Injury

46. When should soft tissue injuries in the setting of open fractures be closed?

46. Either local flap or free vascularized flap should be performed within 72 hours of injury

47. In what six clinical situations should a "damage control" approach be considered?

47. Polytrauma with ISS score >20 and a thoracic trauma AIS of >2
Polytrauma with abdominal/pelvic injury and hemorrhagic shock
ISS >40
Chest radiograph or computed tomography (CT) evidence of bilateral pulmonary contusion
Initial mean pulmonary arterial pressure of >24 mm Hg
Pulmonary artery pressure increase during intramedullary (IM) nailing >6 mm Hg

Spine and Spinal Cord Injury (SCI)

48. What is the rate of noncontiguous injury in a spine-injured patient?

48. 5 to 20%

49. Diagnosis of complete SCI can only be made after what condition resolves? What is the key reflex?

49. Spinal shock
Bulbocavernosus reflex

Chest Trauma

50. What chest x-ray finding is characteristic of lung injury?

50. Pulmonary edema

51. What are the three physical exam findings of tension pneumothorax?

51. Mediastinal shift
Ipsilateral absent breath sounds
Hyperresonant percussion in the setting of hypoxia

52. What are the two components of treatment for tension pneumothorax?

52. Insert large-bore needle in second intercostal space at the midclavicular line
Follow by placement of a chest tube

53. What are the two components of treatment for an open pneumothorax?

53. Occlusive dressing over the wound sealed on three sides
Place a chest tube as far from the wound as possible

54. In the setting of massive hemothorax, what are two indications for thoracotomy?

54. More than 1500 mL of blood is obtained with chest tube placement
Drainage of more than 200 mL/hour for 2 hours

55. What are the series of events leading to acute respiratory distress syndrome (ARDS) after initial lung injury? Then what happens?

55. Pulmonary effusion and respiratory failure
Complement activation and progression

56. Which test is best for diagnosing ARDS?

56. Arterial blood gas (ABG)

57. How is ARDS treated?

57. High peak end-expiratory pressure (PEEP) ventilation

Abdominal Trauma

58. What two organs are most commonly affected with blunt trauma?

59. What is the advantage of abdominal ultrasound over CT scan? What is the disadvantage?

60. What are the three contraindications to an abdominal ultrasound?

Vascular Injury

61. What is the role of the ankle-brachial index (ABI) in diagnosis of vascular injury? What is the gold standard?

Rhabdomyolysis

62. In what two ways can rhabdomyolysis be diagnosed on urinalysis?

63. How is rhabdomyolysis treated?

Fat Embolism

64. What are the three clinical signs of fat embolism?

65. In what three places are the petechiae found?

66. How is fat embolism treated?

Gunshot Injuries

67. What is the threshold velocity for determining low- versus high-velocity gunshot wound?

68. What are the general indications for removal of a retained projectile?

---

58. Kidney
Spleen

59. Fast
Operator dependent

60. Obesity
Subcutaneous air
Prior abdominal surgery

61. An ABI of 0.9 or higher generally excludes arterial injury
Arteriography is still the gold standard

62. Presence of heme
Absence of red blood cells

63. Administration of bicarbonate

64. Hypoxemia
Central nervous system (CNS) depression
Petechiae

65. Axilla
Conjunctivae
Palate

66. High PEEP ventilation

67. Low: <2000 ft/sec
High: ≥2000 ft/sec

68. Subcutaneous position in a pressure area where painful when sitting or lying
Visible bulge beneath the skin
In a joint space
In the globe of the eye
In a vessel lumen causing ischemia or embolic risk to heart, lungs, or periphery
Impinging on a nerve or nerve root and causing pain
Localized abscess formation
Required for forensic investigation if no expected increase in pain or suffering
Documented elevated lead levels

Burn and Frostbite Injuries

69. How are burn injuries classified, and what is the status of the vascular supply for each?

69. I (coagulation): most damaged, no blood flow
II (stasis): sluggish blood flow
III (hyperemia): capillary leakage

70. Copper sulfate is a treatment for what type of burn?

70. White phosphorus

71. Calcium gluconate is a treatment for what type of burn?

71. Hydrofluoric acid

72. At what temperature range should extremity frostbite injuries be rewarmed?

72. 104° to 107°F

Miscellaneous

73. What factor is most important in heterotopic ossification development after polytrauma?

73. Duration of ventilation

74. What is the principal risk factor for secondary posttraumatic brain injury? If it occurs, with what outcome measure is it associated?

74. Hypotension
Correlates with increased mortality

■ Pelvic Trauma

Unstable Pelvic Fracture

75. What is the first step in treatment of an unstable pelvic fracture?

75. Trauma ABC (airway, breathing, circulation)

76. What is the next step?

76. Pelvic binder

77. If the fracture is a vertical shear type, what else should be applied?

77. Skeletal traction pin

78. What are the three complications of military antishock trousers (MAST) treatment?

78. Respiratory compromise
Compartment syndrome
Lactic acidosis

79. What is the indication for an angiogram in the setting of pelvic fracture?

79. Persistent hemodynamic instability despite 4 units of packed red blood cells (PRBCs)

80. Arterial hemorrhage comprises what fraction of pelvic bleeding? What two vessels are most commonly affected?

80. 5% of pelvic bleeding is arterial
Internal pudendal artery
Superior gluteal artery

81. With concurrent pelvic and abdominal bleeding, what is the order of intervention?

81. First: angiogram
Second: laparotomy

82. What is the best measure of resuscitation in the first 6 hours? What does it correlate with? What is elevation due to?

82. Base deficit
Correlates with mortality
Elevated due to lactic acid

83. What pelvic fracture type is associated with the highest volume of blood lost?

83. APC III; APC = anteroposterior compression

84. What two vessels are susceptible to injury with a lateral compression (LC) pelvic injury?

84. Obturator artery
Internal pudendal artery

85. The corona mortise is the junction of which two vessels? Where is it located relative to the symphysis?

85. External iliac artery
Obturator artery
7 to 9 cm from symphysis

86. What are the five operative indications for pelvic fracture?

86. >2.5 cm symphyseal diastasis
Sacroiliac (SI) joint displacement >1 cm
Sacral fracture displacement >1 cm
Vertical hemipelvis displacement
Open fracture

87. What neurologic injury is associated with a vertical shear fracture?

87. Lumbosacral plexus traction injury

88. An open pelvic fracture generally requires what general surgical intervention?

88. Diverting colostomy

89. If anterior and posterior ring fractures are present, which is generally treated first?

89. Generally fix posterior ring first
Then evaluate anterior ring

90. If only the anterior rami are fractured, what is the surgical indication?

90. Fix if residual displacement >2 cm

91. What two ligaments are injured with an APC II type of pelvic injury?

91. Sacrospinous
Sacrotuberous

92. What is the long-term complication of residual displacement >1 cm?

92. 75% of patients report chronic pain

93. What factor best correlates with pelvic fracture outcomes?

93. Initial instability

94. What are the two most frequent complications of displaced pelvic fractures in females?

94. Urinary difficulties
Sexual dysfunction

Urologic Injuries

95. In a retroperitoneal bladder injury, what is the treatment if approaching the pelvis anteriorly? If not?

95. If approaching anteriorly, repair bladder
If not, leave bladder alone

96. What is the preferred treatment of urethral injury?

96. Early endoscopic realignment

97. What is the treatment for postpartum pelvic diastasis? What is the indication for surgery?

97. Binder for treatment
Diastasis >4 cm: operative treatment recommended

Management of Specific Injury Patterns

Sacroiliac (SI) Joint Dislocation

98. What are the two components of the preferred technique for open reduction with internal fixation (ORIF) of SI joint dislocation?

98. Anterior plate
Percutaneous SI screws

99. An anterior approach should be avoided in which four clinical situations?

99. Ipsilateral marginal sacral lip fracture
Obese patient
Anterior external fixator
Colostomy

100. What construct type is preferred for posterior ring fixation? Explain.

100. Triangular osteosynthesis
Plate with pedicle sacral screw and two ilium screws at 90 degrees

Sacroiliac Screws

101. What nerve root is most commonly injured by SI screws? What nerve root is closest anatomically?

101. L5 most often injured
L4 closest anatomically

102. What are the two contraindications to the use of SI screws?

102. Transitional vertebrae
Hypoplastic sacral segments

103. What is the definition of an SI fracture-dislocation? What are the two components of the ORIF technique as it is generally performed?

103. Definition: ilium fracture and SI dislocation
Posterior plate
Transiliac bars

Sacral Fracture

104. What are the indications for surgical treatment of sacral fracture? An injury to what zone results in this clinical picture?

104. Bowel or bladder dysfunction
Zone III (because bilateral involvement of sacral roots is generally necessary for dysfunction)

105. What is the preferred approach for ORIF of a sacral fracture? Why?

105. Approach posteriorly
Better visualization and ability to decompress

106. A U-shaped sacral fracture may result in what deformity?

106. Kyphosis

107. During posterior iliac crest graft harvest, where can the cluneal nerves be found?

107. 8 cm lateral to posterior superior iliac spine (PSIS)

3

Hip and Femur

■ Hip: General Knowledge

Anatomy

Femoral Head Blood Supply

1. What three vessels comprise the main femoral head blood supply from birth to 4 years?

2. What two vessels comprise the main femoral head blood supply from 4 years to adulthood? What surgical technique may potentially compromise this supply?

3. What vessel comprises the main femoral head blood supply in the adult?

4. The medial and lateral femoral circumflex vessels are branches of what vessel?

5. What four vessels contribute to the cruciate anastomosis? Where is the anastomosis found?

Lumbosacral Plexus

6. The lumbosacral plexus is composed of the ventral rami of which roots?

7. The lumbosacral plexus lies posterior to what structure?

8. The lumbosacral plexus lies on the surface of what structure?

1. Medial femoral circumflex
   Lateral femoral circumflex
   Posterior branch of obturator artery (ligamentum teres)

2. Medial femoral circumflex to lateral epiphyseal artery
   Piriformis nail may injure blood supply

3. Medial femoral circumflex to posterosuperior/posteroinferior retinacular arteries

4. Profunda femoris

5. First perforating artery
   Inferior gluteal artery
   Medial femoral circumflex
   Lateral femoral circumflex
   At inferior edge of quadratus femoris

6. T12 to S3

7. Psoas

8. Quadratus lumborum

9. What nerve roots contribute to the femoral nerve?

9. L2 to L4

10. What nerve roots contribute to the superior gluteal nerve?

10. L4 to S1

11. What nerve roots contribute to the inferior gluteal nerve?

11. L5 to S2

12. What nerve roots contribute to the sciatic nerve?

12. L4 to S3

13. What division of the sciatic nerve is lateral? Why is this important?

13. The peroneal division is lateral
Most commonly injured

14. What is the only peroneal division innervated muscle above the knee?

14. Short head of biceps

15. The peroneal nerve runs under what muscle in the thigh?

15. Long head of biceps

16. What two structures exit the greater sciatic foramen (GSF) above the piriformis?

16. Superior gluteal artery
Superior gluteal nerve

17. What is the mnemonic for the six structures that exit the GSF below the piriformis?

17. POPS IQ
*P*udendal nerve
Nerve to *o*bturator internus
*P*osterior femoral cutaneous nerve
*S*ciatic nerve
*I*nferior gluteal artery and nerve
Nerve to *q*uadratus femoris

18. What three muscles contribute to hip flexion? What is their innervation?

18. Iliopsoas
Rectus femoris
Sartorius
Innervation: femoral nerve

19. What two muscles extend the hip? What is their innervation?

19. Gluteus maximus (innervation: inferior gluteal nerve)
Hamstrings (innervation: sciatic)

20. What two muscles abduct the hip? What is their innervation?

20. Gluteus medius
Gluteus minimus
Innervation: superior gluteal nerve

21. What four muscles adduct the hip? What is their innervation?

21. Adductor magnus (innervation: sciatic, posterior branch obturator)
Adductor brevis (innervation: posterior branch obturator)
Adductor longus (innervation: anterior branch obturator)
Gracilis (innervation: anterior branch obturator)

22. What three nerves supply the external rotators of the hip?

22. Nerve to obturator internus
Nerve to quadratus femoris
Nerve to piriformis

23. What two structures does the nerve to the obturator internus innervate?

23. Obturator internus
Superior gemellus

24. What two structures does the nerve to the quadratus femoris innervate?

24. Quadratus femoris
Inferior gemellus

25. What structure does the nerve to the piriformis innervate?

25. Piriformis

26. What innervates the obturator externus?

26. Nerve to obturator externus

27. What muscle is the primary internal rotator of the hip?

27. Gluteus medius

28. Where does the long head of the biceps originate?

28. Ischial tuberosity

29. What is the origin of the short head of the biceps?

29. Linea aspera

30. Between what two structures does the sciatic nerve exit the GSF?

30. Piriformis
    Superior gemellus

31. What three muscles attach to the anterior superior iliac spine (ASIS)?

31. Sartorius
    Transverse abdominal muscle
    Internal abdominal muscle

32. What two structures are attached to the anterior inferior iliac spine (AIIS)?

32. Rectus femoris
    Y ligament of Bigelow

33. What is the origin of the obturator internus muscle? Through what foramen does it pass? Where does it insert? What vessels lie underneath?

33. Origin: internal pelvic wall
    Passes through lesser sciatic foramen
    Insertion: medial greater trochanter
    Obturator artery and nerve
       underneath

34. How does the nerve to the obturator internus exit the pelvis? How does it reenter? What else travels this way?

34. Exits through greater sciatic foramen
    Reenters lesser sciatic foramen
    Pudendal nerve and internal pudendal
       artery also travel out GSF and in
       lesser sciatic foramen (LSF)

35. What separates the greater and lesser sciatic foramina?

35. Sacrospinous ligament

36. How does the obturator nerve exit the pelvis?

36. Through the obturator foramen

37. Between what two structures does the femoral nerve lie?

37. Iliacus
    Psoas

38. How might a psoas abscess present? What position generally provides relief?

38. Psoas abscess may cause femoral or
       sciatic symptoms
    Hip flexion may provide temporary
       relief

39. What nerve is associated with hip pain referred to the knee?

39. Anterior branch of obturator nerve

Surgical Approaches

Smith-Petersen (Anterior)

40. What is the interval for dissection?

40. Sartorius/tensor fascia lata (TFL)

41. What two structures are at risk?

41. Lateral femoral cutaneous nerve
    Lateral femoral circumflex artery
       (ascending branch, ligate)

42. What are two common uses for the Smith-Petersen approach?

42. Congenital hip dislocation
    Hemiarthroplasty

Watson-Jones (Anterolateral)

43. What is the interval for dissection?

43. TFL/gluteus medius

44. What three structures are at risk?

44. Femoral nerve with excessive traction
    Superior gluteal nerve if >5 cm above acetabulum
    Lateral femoral circumflex artery (descending branch)

45. What is the most common use for the Watson-Jones approach?

45. Total hip arthroplasty

Hardinge (Lateral)

46. What is the interval for dissection?

46. Split vastus lateralis and gluteus medius (no true plane)

47. What two structures are at risk?

47. Femoral nerve
    Superior gluteal nerve if >5 cm above acetabulum

48. What is the most common use for the Hardinge approach?

48. Total hip arthroplasty

49. What are the postoperative total hip precautions for a lateral approach? What approach has the same precautions?

49. Avoid excess extension and external rotation
    Same as for anterior approach

Medial Approach

50. What is the interval for dissection?

50. Adductor longus/gracilis

51. What three structures are at risk?

51. Obturator nerve
    Medial femoral circumflex artery
    Deep external pudendal artery

52. What is the most common use for the medial approach?

52. Congenital hip dislocation

Heterotopic Ossification (HO)

53. What hip approach is most often associated with heterotopic ossification?

53. Direct lateral approach

54. What is the prophylactic radiation dose for HO prevention? Within how many hours must it be administered?

54. 700 cGy (centigray)
    Within 48 hours

55. What is the recommended indomethacin dose for HO prevention? For how long?

55. 75 mg daily
    For 6 weeks

56. Have bisphosphonates been shown to be effective in preventing HO?

56. No

■ Hip: Pathologic States

Avascular Necrosis (AVN)

57. What is the first step in the development of AVN?

57. Osteocyte death

58. What are the next three steps? What stage is weakest and thus most likely to result in collapse?

58. Inflammation
New woven bone laid onto dead trabeculae
Dead trabeculae resorbed and remodeled (weakest stage)

59. What percentage of AVNs are bilateral?

59. 50 to 80%

60. What Ficat/Steinberg stage corresponds to subchondral collapse?

60. III

61. The Association Research Circulation Osseous (ARCO) classification also classifies AVN progression based on what parameter?

61. Percentage of head involvement

62. What is the radiographic sign of subchondral collapse? What does it actually represent?

62. Crescent sign
Space between articular surface and subchondral bone

63. What imaging study has the highest sensitivity and specificity for detecting early AVN?

63. Magnetic resonance imaging (MRI)

64. What is the recommended treatment for pre-collapse AVN? Which patients respond poorly?

64. Core decompression
Poor response in patients with history of taking steroids

65. Does a history of steroids adversely affect the outcome of vascularized fibular grafting?

65. Steroid history does not worsen outcomes

66. What are the two principal complications of free fibula graft harvest?

66. Sensory deficit
Valgus instability

67. What is the 5-year failure rate after vascularized fibular grafting?

67. 33% convert to total hip arthroplasty (THA) in 5 years

68. What is the maximum percentage of head involvement for consideration of osteotomy?

68. 50%

69. What is the preferred treatment for advanced AVN? What two complications are more likely in AVN patients?

69. Total hip arthroplasty
Loosening
Dislocation

Transient Osteoporosis of Hip

70. What patients have been classically associated with transient hip osteoporosis?

70. Pregnant women

71. What patient population is actually most commonly affected?

71. Young males

72. What diagnostic imaging modality is safe even in pregnancy?

72. MRI

73. How can transient osteoporosis be differentiated from AVN on MRI?

73. Not sharply demarcated like AVN

74. What does the medical treatment of transient osteoporosis consist of?

74. Nonsteroidal antiinflammatory drugs (NSAIDs)

75. What is the weight-bearing status on the affected extremity?

75. Non–weight bearing (NWB)

76. What is the usual natural history?

76. Spontaneous resolution

Acetabular and Femoral Osteotomies: Adults

77. What are the three general causes of excess femoral anteversion in adults?

77. Residual developmental dysplasia of the hip (DDH)
Total hip replacement with subsequent HO development (pelvis flexed)
Miserable malalignment syndrome

78. What acetabular osteotomy is preferred for adults? What is the effect on the medial/lateral acetabular position?

78. Ganz
Medializes the acetabulum

79. What is an indication for femoral varus derotational osteotomy (VRDO) in an adult?

79. Dysplasia with coxa valga

80. With what percentage of head involvement with AVN should one consider intertrochanteric osteotomy?

80. <50% head involvement for osteotomy
Varus osteotomy if lateral head intact
Valgus osteotomy if medial head intact

81. After Perthes disease, where does the femoral head generally impinge? What is the treatment?

81. Impinges laterally (at osteophyte)
Treatment: valgus intertrochanteric osteotomy

82. What osteotomy is preferred after slipped capital femoral epiphysis (SCFE)? Is there a caveat?

82. Valgus flexion osteotomy
Caveat: no anterior closing wedge for flexion osteotomy

Hip Arthroscopy and Femoro-Acetabular Impingement

Hip Arthroscopy

83. The anterior portal for hip arthroscopy lies at the intersection of what two landmarks?

83. Vertical line from ASIS
Horizontal line from the greater trochanter

84. What two structures are at risk with the anterior portal?

84. Lateral femoral cutaneous nerve
Femoral vessels

85. What other two portals are commonly used and where do they lie?

85. Anterolateral portal
Posterolateral portal
On either side of greater trochanter

86. What two structures are at risk with the anterolateral portal?

86. Superior gluteal nerve
Lateral femoral cutaneous nerve

87. What two structures are at risk with the posterolateral portal?

87. Sciatic nerve

88. What patients are at highest risk for developing labral tears?

88. Those with acetabular dysplasia

Femoro-Acetabular Impingement

89. What is the fundamental problem? How does this relate to acetabular version?

89. Anterior over-coverage
Excess acetabular retroversion

90. What is the usual location of the corresponding labral injury?

90. Anterosuperior labral tear

91. What is the rate of osteonecrosis after anterior dislocation for open resection of osteophytes?

91. <2%

92. If osteophyte resection is unsuccessful, what is the surgical alternative? Especially in what situations?

92. Reverse acetabular osteotomy
Especially if deficient posterior
  coverage

Syndromes Common Among Athletes

Athletic Pubalgia: "Sports Hernia"

93. What injury mechanism is postulated to result in athletic pubalgia?

93. Repetitive extension-abduction

94. Where does the injury actually occur?

94. Adductor origin

95. What are the classic symptoms?

95. Abdominal and groin pain after exertion

96. Athletic pubalgia must be differentiated from what other common condition?

96. True hernia

97. What is the recommended treatment?

97. Pelvic floor reconstruction

Snapping Hip Syndromes

98. What is the etiology of iliotibial band syndrome? What examination maneuver is diagnostic?

98. Running on banked surfaces
Test with hip in adduction; flex and
  extend hip

99. What examination maneuver tests for iliopsoas syndrome?

99. Move hip from flexion/external
  rotation to extension/internal
  rotation

100. What is the most common etiology of ilioinguinal nerve entrapment?

100. Abdominal muscle hypertrophy

101. What is the definition of piriformis syndrome?

101. Sciatic nerve entrapment by piriformis
  muscle

■ Trauma

Hip: Femoral Side

Hip Dislocation

102. What is the most common direction of traumatic dislocation?

102. Posterior

103. What direction of dislocation is associated with impaction fracture of femoral head?

103. Anterior

104. ... with transchondral fracture?

104. Posterior

105. ... with the highest rate of osteonecrosis?

105. Anterior

106. ... with acetabular fracture?

106. Posterior

107. After reducing a traumatically dislocated hip, what are the next two steps?

107. Assess stability clinically
Obtain computed tomography (CT) scan

108. After reduction, if the hip is stable without fracture, what is the treatment? What is the principal complication?

108. Protected weight bearing for 2 to 4 weeks
AVN is most common complication

109. What is the most common complication of traumatic fracture-dislocation of the hip?

109. Posttraumatic osteoarthritis

Femoral Head Fractures

110. What are the four components of the Pipkin classification of femoral head fracture?

110. I: infrafoveal
II: suprafoveal
III: with femoral neck fracture
IV: with acetabular fracture

111. What is the treatment for nondisplaced types I and II?

111. Touchdown weight bearing for 6 weeks

112. What are the three operative indications for femoral head fracture?

112. >1 mm displacement
Loose bodies in joint
Pipkin III, IV

113. What Pipkin class is associated with the highest rate of osteonecrosis?

113. III

114. When indicated, how are Pipkin I and II fractures generally approached?

114. Anterior approach

Femoral Neck Fractures

115. What are the two components of the treatment for compression side femoral neck stress fractures in runners?

115. Cross-training
Stop running

116. What is Pauwel's classification? What is the clinical significance of a Pauwel type III?

116. I: fracture line <30 degrees from horizontal
II: <50 degrees
III: <70 degrees (highest rate of osteonecrosis [ON], nonunion)

117. In a femoral shaft fracture with associated neck fracture, what is the typical neck fracture pattern? What is the preferred treatment?

117. Neck fracture often vertical
Treated with DHS (dynamic hip screw)

118. What is the only proven indication for the use of the fourth screw for femoral neck internal fixation?

118. Posterior comminution

119. What two factors increase the risk of osteonecrosis after femoral neck fracture?

119. Increased displacement
Delayed reduction

120. What is the 1-year mortality rate for elderly patients with femoral neck fractures?

120. 30%

121. Do cemented or uncemented hemiarthoplasties have better published outcomes for femoral neck fracture treatment?

121. Cemented

122. What patients should undergo a THA for fracture? What is the significance of acetabular wear? What complication is particularly common when a THA is performed for fracture?

122. Active elderly
Regardless of acetabular wear
Complication: increased dislocation rates

Intertrochanteric Fractures

123. What two factors principally determine how much sliding occurs with a dynamic hip screw?

123. Screw angle
Length of the screw in the barrel

124. What complication is more common with cephalomedullary nailing than with a dynamic hip screw for a standard intertrochanteric fracture?

124. Lag screw cutout

Fractures of the Acetabulum

125. Acetabulum fracture outcome has been demonstrated to correlate with what four factors?

125. Accuracy of reduction
Age
Complexity
Femoral head damage

126. What is the significance of vertical versus horizontal fracture lines on axial CT?

126. *Vertical* fracture line = *transverse* fracture
Horizontal fracture line = *column* injury (anterior or posterior)

Posterior Wall Fractures

127. Posterior wall fractures are generally stable if <__% of the wall is involved, and generally unstable if >__% of the wall is involved?

127. <33% generally stable
>50% generally unstable

128. Posterior wall fracture outcomes depend most heavily on what factor?

128. Accuracy of reduction

129. If the reduction is anatomic, then the outcome has been shown to be dependent on what three factors?

129. Delay/osteonecrosis
Patient age
Comminution

Both-Column Fractures

130. What radiographic sign is suggestive of a both-column fracture of the acetabulum?

130. Spur sign on obturator oblique

131. An extensile approach is recommended instead of an ilioinguinal approach in what three circumstances?

131. Posterior comminution
Older than 2 weeks
Displaced sacroiliac (SI) fracture

Other Fracture Patterns

132. How can T-type acetabular fractures be differentiated from transverse?

132. Obturator ring also fractured in T-type

133. What are the two possible approaches for open reduction with internal fixation (ORIF) of a T-type fracture?

133. Anterior/posterior
Extensile

134. What is the recommended treatment for a nondisplaced transtectal acetabular fracture?

134. 6 weeks touchdown weight bearing

135. An extensile approach should be considered for a transverse fracture in what circumstance?

135. Associated roof impaction

Ilioinguinal Approach to Acetabulum

136. Where is the lateral window of the ilioinguinal approach? To what two areas does it provide access?

136. Posterior to iliopectineal fascia
Access to iliac fossa, anterior SI joint

137. Between what structures is the middle window? To what two areas does it provide access?

137. Between iliopectineal fascia/external iliac artery
Access to pelvic brim, superior pubic ramus

138. Where is the medial window? To what two areas does it provide access?

138. Medial to external iliac artery, spermatic cord
Access to quadrilateral plate, retropubic space

Femoral Trauma: Surgical Approaches and Management

139. What is the dissection interval for a posterolateral approach to the femur?

139. Vastus lateralis/hamstrings

140. What is the interval for a posterior approach to the thigh? What is the most common use for this approach? What structure is particularly at risk?

140. Biceps/vastus lateralis
To explore sciatic nerve
Posterior femoral cutaneous nerve at risk

141. What is the dissection interval for an anteromedial approach to the distal femur?

141. Vastus medialis/rectus

142. What two structures are at risk with this approach?

142. Medial superior geniculate artery
     Infrapatellar branch of the saphenous nerve

Femoral Nailing

143. In patients with an Injury Severity Scale (ISS) score >18, what are the three proven advantages of early stabilization?

143. Decreased rate of acute respiratory distress syndrome (ARDS)
     Fewer pulmonary complications
     Shorter intensive care unit (ICU) stay

144. Intramedullary (IM) nailing releases what two interleukins (ILs)?

144. IL-6
     IL-8

145. It is generally preferred to do IM nailing in most patients early, except those with ___.

145. Closed head injuries (consider external fixator first)

146. Convert from external fixator to nail by ___ days to minimize risk of infection.

146. 21

147. What is the main advantage of the IM nail over external fixator in adult femoral fracture?

147. Improved knee range of motion

148. What is the biomechanical advantage to plate/screw construct for femur fracture? What is the principal disadvantage?

148. Plate/screw fixation results in increased torsional stiffness
     Disadvantage: requires more extensive soft tissue stripping

149. In what patient population is reaming not recommended? Is there another consideration?

149. In those with bilateral chest injury
     But reaming has not been shown to cause ARDS even with chest trauma

150. What is the preferred proximal locking screw orientation for femoral IM nailing? Why?

150. Oblique preferred
     Transverse screws are prone to failure

151. How long after femoral shaft fracture treatment can an athlete return to competition?

151. Can return when circumferential bridging callus is seen on radiograph

152. What is the preferred treatment of femoral nonunion after nailing? What other alternative might be considered if the nonunion is atrophic?

152. Reamed exchange nailing
     If atrophic, ORIF with grafting is an alternative

153. What is the most frequent complication of IM nailing for femur fracture? Is there another consideration?

153. Heterotopic ossification (HO)
     But only very rarely is the HO clinically important

154. What position of malunion is classically seen with a trochanteric starting point for a femoral nail?

154. Varus malunion

■ Total Hip Arthroplasty

Bearing Surfaces and Clinical Applications

General Principles

155. What is the coefficient for friction for a native hip? What is the primary lubrication method?

155. 0.002 to 0.04
Elastohydrodynamic lubrication (surface deforms slightly)

156. Hard-on-soft bearings generate particles of what size? Hard-on-soft bearings are primarily lubricated by what method? What head sizes tend to generate the least volumetric wear?

156. 0.2 to 7 µm
Boundary lubrication (contact between high points on surfaces)
Smaller head minimizes volumetric wear

157. Hard-on-hard bearings generate particles of what size? Hard-on-hard bearings are primarily lubricated by what method? What head sizes tend to generate the least volumetric wear?

157. <0.12 µm
Mixed lubrication (boundary and hydrodynamic)
Larger head minimizes volumetric wear

158. Compare the annual wear rates of ultra high molecular weight polyethylene (UHMWPE), metal–metal, and ceramic–ceramic?

158. UHMWPE: 100 µm/year
Metal–metal: 5 µm/year
Ceramic–ceramic: 2.5 µm/year

159. What type of wear is particularly problematic for polyethylene-titanium articulations?

159. Volumetric wear

Polyethylene (PE)

160. What manufacturing process for polyethylene is generally most favored?

160. Direct compression molding

161. What manufacturing process is viewed least favorably?

161. Heat processing

162. What is the optimal crystallinity for PE?

162. 50%

163. Has the addition of calcium stearate to PE been helpful or detrimental in terms of wear?

163. Detrimental

164. At what doses is highly cross-linked PE irradiated?

164. 5 to 15 megarads

165. Polyethylene irradiation leads to the development of what structures?

165. Free radicals

166. If free radicals cross-link in an oxygen-free environment, what are the upside and downside?

166. Upside: decreased wear rates
Downside: decreased mechanical properties

167. If free radicals cause chain scission, what is the possible negative clinical consequence?

167. Delamination

168. How are residual free radicals removed?

168. Heat annealing

169. What is the most common cause of polyethylene wear?

169. Third-body wear

Metal-on-Metal

170. What is the problem with titanium bearing surfaces? This is also referred to as what?

170. Easily scratched
Notch sensitivity

171. The premature development of osteolysis in metal-on-metal THA may suggest what condition?

171. Patient with metal sensitivity

Ceramics

172. Are larger or smaller grain sizes associated with improved ceramic strengths?

172. Smaller

173. Is alumina or Zirconia the preferred ceramic? Why?

173. Alumina
Zirconia undergoes phase change to tetragonal configuration

174. When revising a ceramic THA, what procedure must also be performed?

174. Synovectomy

175. What three factors are predictive of worse outcomes in ceramic revisions?

175. Retained acetabular component
Young patient
Stainless steel head used

Stem Designs and Clinical Applications

Uncemented Stems

176. For an ingrowth component, what are the optimal pore size, porosity, and gaps? What is the rule?

176. Pore size: 50 to 150 μm
Porosity: 50%
Gaps: <50 μm
Rule of "50"

177. What is the upper limit of micromotion for successful bony ingrowth? Otherwise what happens?

177. Micromotion <150 μm
Otherwise fibrous ingrowth

178. For an ongrowth component, what is the most important factor? What is the biggest disadvantage?

178. Surface roughness (determines interface strength)
Fixation at surface only increases susceptibility to shear

179. What is the demonstrated benefit of a hydroxyapatite coating? What is required?

179. Decreased time to biologic fixation
Requires increased crystallinity

180. What two characteristics of the prosthesis determine degree of stress shielding?

180. Extent of porous coating
Stem stiffness

181. Upon what three factors is stem stiffness most dependent?

181. Modulus
Radius[4]
Stem geometry

182. What is the most common postoperative complication after use of an uncemented stem?

182. Thigh pain

183. Are sharp corners on the prosthesis associated with better or worse outcomes?

183. Worse

184. What manufacturing method is preferred: forging or casting?

184. Forging

Cemented Stems

185. What is the ideal size of the cement mantle?

185. 2 mm or one third of canal diameter

186. When cementing, is it better or worse to use a stiffer stem?

186. Better

187. What is the effect of osteopenia on cementing?

187. Osteopenia increases relative porosity of bone

188. What three changes are seen in polymethylmethacrylate (PMMA) volume as it hardens?

188. Volume contracts (polymerization)
Volume expands (increasing temperature)
Volume contracts (cooling)

189. How long after stem insertion do levels of monomer peak in the bloodstream?

189. 3 minutes

190. How is the monomer cleared?

190. Via the lungs

191. What pulmonary change is seen during cementing? What are two potential systemic effects?

191. Increased pulmonary shunting
Hypotension
Hypoxia

Acetabulum: Clinical Applications

Screw Placement

192. What two quadrants are safest for screw placement?

192. Posterosuperior
Posteroinferior

193. What two structures are at risk posterosuperiorly?

193. Sciatic nerve
Superior gluteal artery

194. What two structures are at risk posteroinferiorly?

194. Sciatic nerve
Inferior gluteal artery

195. What structure is at risk anterosuperiorly?

195. External iliac vessels

196. What structure is at risk anteroinferiorly?

196. Obturator nerve

197. What structure is at risk with retractors under traverse acetabular ligament?

197. Obturator nerve

Total Hip Stability and Mechanics

198. What two structures does the abductor complex consist of? What is more medial?

198. Gluteus medius
Gluteus minimus
Minimus is more medial

199. How is offset measured?

199. From the center of the femoral head to the greater trochanter

200. How is neck length measured?

200. Center of head to lesser trochanter

201. What are the two potential disadvantages of decreased neck length?

201. Lax abductor complex
Trochanteric impingement

202. What surgical option exists if THA components are well aligned but remain unstable?

202. Trochanteric advancement

203. What three surgical options are available in abductor deficient patients?

203. Large head
Constrained (polyethelene) PE liner
Hemiarthroplasty

204. What effect on hip joint reaction force (JRF) does each of the following factors have? Trendelenburg gait?

204. Decreased abductor moment and decreased JRF

205. A contralateral cane?

205. Decreased JRF

206. A varus positioned femoral implant? What is the downside of varus?

206. Decreased JRF
Downside: increased shear

207. What is the advantage of increased offset? What is the disadvantage?

207. Decreased JRF
Increased loosening

208. Quick review: What are four key ways to decrease hip joint reaction force?

208. Cane in contralateral hand
Trendelenburg gait
Varus component
High offset

209. With a valgus positioned femoral component, what is the effect on offset?

209. Decreased offset

210. … on joint reaction force?

210. Increased JRF

211. … on shear?

211. Decreased shear

212. Therefore, is a varus or valgus femoral implant position preferred and why?

212. Valgus
Varus placement results in loosening because PMMA poorly resists shear

Revision Surgery: General Points

Acetabular Revision

213. What implant type is preferred for acetabular revision?

213. Porous coated hemispherical cup

214. What are the two requirements for use of a porous hemispherical cup?

214. Good rim fit
Two thirds of rim are intact

215. What two surgical options are available for large segmental defects?

215. Allograft and cage reconstruction
Trabecular metal cup

216. In what clinical situation has increased failure with cage reconstruction been observed?

216. Constrained polyethylene liner cemented to cage

Femoral Revision

217. What is the preferred removal technique for well-fixed cemented stem? Why?

217. Extended trochanteric osteotomy
Keeps gluteus/vastus lateralis intact; maintains blood supply for healing

218. What type of implant is preferred for femoral revision?

218. Uncemented porous coated modular stem

219. How can large segmental defects be addressed?

219. Supplement with allograft struts

220. What are the two indications for impaction grafting?

220. Large ectatic canal
Thin cortices

221. What are the two principal complications of impaction grafting?

221. Subsidence
Periprosthetic fracture

Hip Arthrodesis

222. What is the principal site of adjacent degeneration after hip arthrodesis?

222. Lumbosacral spine most affected

223. What is the optimal position for hip fusion?

223. 30 degrees flexion, 0 abduction, 0 to 15 external rotation

224. After hip arthrodesis, how much does energy expenditure with ambulation increase?

224. 30%

225. In what patients can a fusion *not* be converted to a total hip arthroplasty?

225. Absent abductors

Common Complication Questions

226. Are THA dislocation rates higher in males or females?

226. Females

227. What two populations are at especially high risk of nerve palsy with THA?

227. Females with DDH
CMT (Charcot-Marie-Tooth)

228. What THA complication is especially common in patients with prior acetabular fracture?

228. Loosening

229. If planning a THA after acetabular fracture, what is the advantage of performing ORIF?

229. Decreased need for bone graft

230. What complication is particularly common in THA patients with contralateral hip fusion?

230. Loosening

231. Ankylosing spondylitis is associated with what THA two complications? Why is acetabular component positioning often difficult in this patient population?

231. Decreased functional outcomes
Increased heterotopic bone
Flexion contractures of hips may lead to excess anteversion

232. Why is femoral component positioning often difficult in patients with Paget's disease?

232. Femoral bow may lead to varus malalignment

233. What THA is particularly likely in patients with severe coxa vara? Why?

233. Dislocation
Inadequately restored offset

234. What effect does hip protrusion have on hip center of rotation? What is the implication for THA?

234. Moves hip center medially and posteriorly
Must restore normal center of rotation at time of THA

235. What is the likely cause of late failure and sudden pain with modular acetabular components?

236. What is the benefit of foot/ankle exercises in the prevention of deep venous thrombosis (DVT)?

235. Liner dissociation secondary to failure of locking ring

236. 20% increase in venous outflow

Total Hip Arthroplasty After Fracture

237. What three factors are associated with increased mortality for THA after femoral neck fracture?

238. What is the principal THA complication in elderly patients with failed femoral neck ORIF?

239. What is the principal THA complication in patients with pathologic fracture?

237. Female
Elderly
Cemented stem

238. Highest dislocation rates

239. Deep infection

Intraoperative Complications

240. What is the principal cause of intraoperative acetabular fracture? What is the treatment if stable? If unstable?

241. What are the three treatment options for intraoperative femoral fracture?

242. At what intraoperative stage do DVTs start to form?

243. What three intraoperative events are associated with fat embolization?

244. Most orthopaedic surgical cases present what level of cardiac risk? What does this mean?

245. Increased cardiac risk is present if patient can't perform ___ metabolic equivalent tasks (METs)? Cite three example activities.

246. What are the two demonstrated benefits of perioperative beta-blockers?

240. Underreaming
Stable: ignore
Unstable: ORIF

241. Longer stem
Cerclage
Locking plate

242. At time of femoral canal preparation

243. Insertion of cemented stem
Relocation of the hip
Use of intramedullary guides

244. Intermediate cardiac risk
<5% chance of cardiac event

245. 4 METs
Do light housework
Climb one flight of stairs
Walk on level ground at 4 mph

246. Increased survival
Decreased perioperative events

Postoperative Nutritional Complications

247. What is the best clinical indicator of preoperative nutritional status?

248. What is the preferred treatment for a malnourished patient at risk of multiorgan failure?

247. Arm circumference

248. Enteral protein

249. What is Ogilvie's syndrome? What is its relevance? What is its associated electrolyte abnormality? What is its treatment?

249. Cecal distention >10 cm
Can occur after arthroplasty
Associated with hypokalemia
Treat with colonoscopic
    decompression

Infections

250. Acute infections occur within what time frame? What are the two components of treatment?

250. 3 weeks
Washout and polyethylene exchange
IV antibiotics for 6 weeks

251. What is the most common etiologic organism overall?

251. *Staphylococcus epidermidis*

252. What is the most common organism after infection from dental source?

252. *Peptostreptococcus*

253. What laboratory tests are highly specific for postoperative infection?

253. C-reactive protein (CRP)
Erythrocyte sedimentation rate (ESR)

254. What laboratory test is highly sensitive?

254. ESR

255. What is the problem with the use of aspiration as a diagnostic test?

255. High rate of false-positives (15%)

256. What is the most accurate diagnostic test?

256. Tissue culture

257. What is the bone scan appearance of infection?

257. Diffusely positive

Chronic Infections

258. If components are removed to treat a chronic infection, what is the duration of intravenous (IV) antibiotics?

258. 6 weeks

259. What are the three criteria that must be met before replacement of arthroplasty components?

259. Normal clinical exam
ESR, CRP normal
Aspiration negative

260. What must be considered if significant soft tissue compromise exists at the time of replacement?

260. Arthrodesis

261. What is the long-term success rate of chronic antibiotic suppression?

261. 20 to 40%

262. In an uninfected total joint, high postoperative CRPs may also be predictive of what?

262. Increased HO risk

4

Knee and Tibia/Fibula

■ Knee: General Knowledge

Surgical Anatomy

Medial Layers of Knee

1. What are the two components of layer I?

2. What two structures lie between layers I and II?

3. What are the four components of layer II?

4. What are the two components of layer III?

1. Sartorius and associated fascia
   Medial patellar retinaculum

2. Gracilis
   Semitendinosus

3. Superficial medial collateral ligament (MCL)
   Posterior oblique ligament (POL)
   Medial patellofemoral ligament (MPFL)
   Semimembranosus

4. Deep MCL
   Capsule

Lateral Layers of Knee

5. What are the three components of layer I?

6. What are the two components of layer II?

7. What are the four components of layer III?

5. Iliotibial (IT) band
   Biceps
   Fascia

6. Patellar retinaculum
   Patellofemoral ligament

7. Arcuate ligament
   Fabellofibular ligament
   Capsule
   Lateral collateral ligament (LCL)

Posteromedial Corner

8. What three structures make up the posteromedial corner?

8. Semimembranosus insertions
   POL (adductor tubercle origin)
   OPL (oblique popliteal ligament)

9. What is the function of the posteromedial corner?

9. Rotatory stability

Posterolateral Corner (PLC)

10. What five structures make up the posterolateral corner?

10. Popliteus
Popliteofibular ligament
Lateral capsule
Arcuate ligament
Fabellofibular ligament

11. What exam finding is suggestive of disrupted PLC? What if the posterior cruciate ligament (PCL) is also disrupted?

11. Asymmetric external rotation (ER) at 30 degrees knee flexion: isolated PLC injury
Asymmetric ER at 30 and 90 degrees: PLC and PCL injuries

Menisci

12. What is the orientation of the superficial fibers?

12. Radial

13. What is the orientation of the deep fibers?

13. Predominantly circumferential
Interspersed radial "tie fibers"

14. What type of cartilage makes up the meniscus?

14. Fibroelastic cartilage

15. What is the predominant collagen type present within the meniscus?

15. Predominantly type I collagen

16. What cell type makes up the meniscus?

16. Fibrochondrocytes

17. How is the meniscus innervated? Where is the meniscus especially well innervated?

17. Peripheral two thirds innervated with type I and II nerve endings
Especially well innervated in the posterior horn (mechanoreceptors)

18. What vessels provide the meniscal blood supply?

18. Geniculates supply blood to peripheral one third

19. What percentage of force does the meniscus transmit in extension? What percentage is transmitted in flexion?

19. 50% in extension
90% in flexion

20. Is the medial or lateral meniscus more mobile? Why? Why is this clinically important?

20. Lateral meniscus is more mobile
Because popliteus interrupts lateral meniscal attachment
May contribute to more common medial tears

21. What is the classic magnetic resonance imaging (MRI) appearance of a displaced bucket-handle tear of the posterior horn of the medial meniscus?

21. Double PCL

Meniscofemoral Ligaments

22. Between what structures do the meniscofemoral ligaments run?

22. Posterior horn of lateral meniscus to medial femoral condyle with PCL

23. Which of the meniscofemoral ligaments is anterior? Which is posterior?

23. Humphrey's (anterior)
Wrisberg (posterior)

Anterior Cruciate Ligament (ACL)

24. What are the two main collagen types within the ACL and what is the relative proportions of each?

24. 90% type I
0% type II

25. What vessel supplies the ACL? What supplies the fat pad?

25. Middle geniculate supplies ACL
Inferior geniculates supplies fat pad

26. What is the strength of the native ACL?

26. 2100 N

27. What are the two bundles of the ACL?

27. Anteromedial
Posterolateral

28. At what flexion angle is the anteromedial bundle at maximum tension?

28. 60 degrees

29. At what flexion angle is the posterolateral bundle at maximum tension?

29. 15 degrees

Posterior Cruciate Ligament (PCL)

30. What are the two bundles of the PCL?

30. Anterolateral
Posteromedial

31. At what flexion angle should the anterolateral bundle be tensioned intraoperatively?

31. 90 degrees

32. At what flexion angle should the posteromedial bundle be tensioned?

32. 30 degrees

Collateral Ligaments

33. How can the MCL or LCL be tested in isolation? What happens in extension?

33. Valgus or varus stress at 30 degrees flexion isolates the respective collateral ligament
In extension, the PCL also contributes to stability

34. What is the better restraint against valgus stress: superficial or deep MCL?

34. Superficial

Arterial Supply

35. What two structures does the superior geniculate (lateral, medial branches) supply?

35. Patella
PCL

36. What three structures does the middle geniculate supply?

36. ACL
PCL
Collaterals

37. What two structures does the inferior geniculate (lateral, medial branches) supply?

37. Menisci
Fat pad

38. In what interval does the lateral branch of the superior geniculate lie? With what procedure is this branch most commonly at risk?

38. Femur/vastus lateralis
At risk with lateral release

39. The inferior geniculate branch lies posterior to what anatomic landmark?

39. Posterior to LCL

40. Where does the tibial nutrient artery enter?

40. Below PCL insertion

Patellar Anatomy

41. What three facets make up the articular surface of the patella?

41. Lateral facet
Medial facet
Odd facet

42. What is the Wiberg classification?

42. Type I: medial and lateral facets are equal
Types II and III: medial facet smaller than lateral
Type IV (Jagerhut patella): no medial facet present

43. What are the two most likely sites of bony injury following lateral patellar dislocation?

43. Medial facet of patella
Superior lateral condyle of femur

Surgical Approach Pearls

44. Over what structure is the medial knee approach centered?

44. Adductor tubercle

45. Over what structure is the lateral knee approach centered? What is the interval for dissection?

45. Centered over Gerdy's tubercle
Interval: iliotibial (IT) band/biceps femoris

Other Key Facts

46. How far distal does the knee capsule extend? Where is the most distal extent?

46. 15 mm distal extent
Most distal extent is posterior to fibula

47. Within what tendon does the fabella lie?

47. Lateral gastrocnemius

48. The peroneal nerve lies at the posterior border of what structure?

48. Biceps femoris

Biomechanics

49. What is the screw home mechanism?

49. Femur internal rotation during the last 15 degrees of knee extension

50. Where does the lower extremity mechanical axis pass through the knee?

50. Medial to the medial tibial spine

51. Starting at vertical, what is the relationship of the mechanical and anatomic axes?

51. Mechanical axis lies in 3 degrees of valgus
Anatomic axis is 9 degrees of valgus
So, anatomic axis is 6 degrees of valgus relative to mechanical axis

52. How is the Q angle measured?

52. Anterior superior iliac spine (ASIS) to patella to tibial tubercle

53. What is the approximate normal value of the Q angle in extension? In flexion?

53. 15 degrees in extension
8 degrees in flexion

54. The highest joint reaction forces in the knee are experienced where? At what phase of gait?

54. Medially
Stance phase

55. Where is the highest joint reaction force experienced in the patella?

55. Laterally

■ Knee: Pathologic States

Meniscal Injuries and Repair

56. What injury is associated with meniscal cyst development?

56. Horizontal cleavage tear of the lateral meniscus

Baker's Cyst

57. In which interval can Baker's cysts generally be found?

57. Between semimembranosus and medial gastrocnemius

58. What are the two conservative treatment options for Baker's cyst?

58. Nonsteroidal antiinflammatory drugs (NSAIDs)
Compression sleeve

59. If conservative treatment fails, what are the next steps?

59. MRI to evaluate for associated intraarticular pathology (e.g., meniscal tear)
Operative treatment

Discoid Meniscus

60. How are discoid menisci classified? What are the three types?

60. Watanabe classification
I: Incomplete coverage of lateral tibial plateau
II: Complete coverage of lateral tibial plateau
III: Wrisberg type

61. How does the posterior attachment differ between the types of discoid menisci?

61. Incomplete and complete discoid menisci have intact posterior meniscotibial ligaments
Wrisberg variant has no meniscotibial ligament attachment to posterior horn

62. What is the clinical significance of this difference?

62. Incomplete and complete discoid menisci generally do *not* have abnormal motion and are asymptomatic unless torn
Wrisberg discoid moves abnormally and is often symptomatic even without tear

63. What two radiographic features are suggestive of discoid meniscus?

63. Square lateral condyle
Widened lateral joint space

64. What is the MRI appearance of a discoid meniscus?

64. Bow-tie appearance on more than two consecutive sagittal images

65. What are the two indications for surgery for discoid meniscus?

65. Symptomatic tears of the incomplete and complete discoid types
Restoration of meniscal stability to a symptomatic Wrisberg type, even if not torn

Meniscectomy

66. Does medial or lateral partial meniscectomy lead to earlier degenerative changes?

66. Lateral

67. Three years after total meniscectomy, what percentage of patients has clinical osteoarthritis?

67. 20%

68. … radiographic osteoarthritis?

68. 70%

69. Total meniscectomy decreases the contact area by what amount?

69. 75%

Meniscal Repair

70. What is the "gold standard" approach? What is the suture technique? Why?

70. Inside-out
Vertical mattress
Highest number of circumferential fibers captured

71. What structure is at risk medially? How can injury be prevented?

71. Saphenous nerve
Identify and retract nerve and infrapatellar branch before tying sutures

72. What structure is at risk laterally? How can injury be prevented?

72. Peroneal nerve
Prevent by placing sutures anterior to biceps

73. What are the three general criteria for meniscal tears that do *not* need repair?

73. Longitudinal tear <8 mm in length that cannot be displaced >3 mm
Stable partial tear
Shallow radial tear <3 mm in depth

74. What are the six general indications for meniscal repair?

74. Complete longitudinal tear >10 mm length

Tear within peripheral one third of the meniscus or within 3 to 4 mm of meniscocapsular junction

Unstable tear that can be displaced by probing

Tear without secondary degeneration or deformity

Tear in an active patient

Tear identified during ligament stabilization procedure

75. What four factors have been proven to enhance meniscal repair?

75. Trephination
Synovial rasping
Fibrin clot
Hyaluronic acid

76. Does immobilization improve meniscal repair outcomes?

76. No

77. What is a possible complication of operative intervention in a patient with calcium pyrophosphate deposition disease?

77. May precipitate acute pseudogout attack

Meniscal Transplantation

78. What two factors must be present for meniscal transplantation to succeed?

78. Well-aligned knee
Intact cruciate ligaments

79. What are the five contraindications to meniscal allograft transplantation?

79. Varus or valgus malalignment 2 to 4 degrees greater than contralateral knee

Mechanical axis passes through the meniscus-deficient compartment

Knee instability

Age >50

Osteophyte formation

Untreated Outerbridge class IV lesions

Anterior Cruciate Ligament Injuries and Reconstruction

80. What is the most common mechanism of ACL injury?

80. Noncontact pivot

81. What gender is most at risk for sustaining an ACL injury?

81. Female

82. How often does an acute bloody knee effusion correlate with a ruptured ACL?

82. 75%

83. What test is most sensitive on physical examination for ACL rupture?

83. Lachman test

84. What is a clinically significant KT-1000 (arthometry) difference side-to-side?

84. 3 mm

85. Once the ACL is disrupted, what is the primary restraint to anterior translation?

85. Meniscus

86. What plain radiographic finding is classically associated with an ACL injury?

86. Segond fracture

87. What is the MRI appearance of a bloody effusion? Nonbloody effusion?

87. Bloody: high T1, low T2
Non-bloody: low T1, high T2

Preoperative and Intraoperative Considerations

88. What are the three preoperative requirements to minimize the risk of arthrofibrosis?

88. Full range of motion (ROM)
No effusion
Good quadriceps function

89. With a preoperative varus thrust, what procedure should be considered before ACL reconstruction?

89. High tibial osteotomy (HTO)

90. Of the graft options, which has the highest ultimate tensile load?

90. Quadrupled hamstring

91. What two hamstring tendons are used as graft for reconstruction?

91. Gracilis
Semitendinosus

92. What nerve is at risk with hamstring harvest?

92. Sartorial branch of the saphenous nerve

93. What graft option has strength characteristics most similar to those of the native ACL?

93. Bone–patellar tendon–bone

94. What nerve is at risk with patellar tendon harvest?

94. Infrapatellar branch of saphenous nerve

95. In which direction is an intraoperative patellar fracture generally oriented?

95. Vertical

96. In which direction is a postoperative patella fracture generally oriented?

96. Horizontal

97. How can the strength of the graft be increased by about 30%?

97. Rotate 90 degrees

98. What is the benefit of preconditioning the graft?

98. Reduces stress relaxation by 50%

99. What are the two most reliable tibial tunnel landmarks?

99. Just anterior to PCL
Native ACL footprint

Postoperative Considerations

100. At 6 weeks after surgery, what percentage of original graft strength has returned? At 1 year?

100. <20% of original at 6 weeks
<50% of original at 1 year

101. After ACL, what rehabilitation exercises are preferred? What is the goal of rehabilitation? What type of training is emphasized? Are prone hangs permissible?

101. Closed chain, weight bearing as tolerated (WBAT) exercises
Safe quadriceps strengthening
Emphasizes proprioceptive training
Prone hangs are OK

102. What is the worst ACL postoperative exercise? What is the ideal PCL postoperative exercise?

102. Worst ACL: active extension 15 to 30 degrees
Ideal PCL: active extension 90 to 0 degrees

103. What four factors have been associated with good 2-year outcomes after ACL reconstruction?

103. Accurate tunnel placement
Strong grafts
Solid graft fixation
Rational rehabilitation program

Potential Complications

104. What is the most common cause of immediate postoperative ACL failure?

104. Failure of fixation

105. What is the most common operative complication overall?

105. Aberrant tunnel placement

106. What is the upper limit of acceptable screw divergence?

106. 20 degrees

107. What is the consequence of a too anterior femoral tunnel? … tibial tunnel?

107. Femoral tunnel too anterior: decreased flexion
Tibial tunnel: impingement in extension

108. If the femoral tunnel is too far back (over top), what is the consequence in flexion? … extension?

108. Lax in flexion
Tight in extension

Posterior Cruciate Ligament Injuries and Reconstruction

109. What two injury mechanisms are associated with PCL injury?

109. Knee hyperflexion with plantarflexed foot
Posteriorly directed force to proximal tibia with flexed knee

110. What are the definitions of grade I, II, and III injuries?

110. I: <5 mm motion (plateau remains anterior to medial femoral condyle)
II: 5 to 10 mm motion (plateau flush with condyle)
III: >10 mm motion (plateau can be displaced posterior to the condyle)

111. In general, what is the treatment of an isolated PCL injury? How about in high-performance athletes?

111. Nonoperative in general
Even in high-performance athletes, 5 to 10 mm laxity may be well tolerated

112. For grade I and II injuries, what is the weight-bearing status? When should rehabilitation start?

112. Protected weight bearing
May start quads rehab immediately

113. What are the two components of the treatment for grade III PCL injury?

113. Immobilize in extension 2 to 4 weeks
Then begin quads rehab

114. What is the ideal exercise to rehabilitate quadriceps after PCL injury?

114. Active extension 90 to 0 degrees

115. What is the long-term consequence of chronic PCL deficiency?

115. Medial femoral condyle wear
Patellofemoral wear

Preoperative and Intraoperative Considerations

116. What are the two indications for surgery after PCL injury?

116. Functional instability
Multi-ligament injury

117. For the inlay technique, how is PCL insertion exposed? What other condition uses the same interval?

117. Between semimembranosus and medial gastrocnemius
Same interval as for Baker's cyst

118. What structure lies directly posterior to the PCL insertion (potential injury with tunnel)?

118. Popliteal artery

Other Ligamentous Injuries and Combined Injuries

119. What is the most common location of knee MCL injury?

119. Femoral insertion

120. What radiographic finding is indicative of chronic MCL injury?

120. Pellegrini-Stieda lesion (calcified MCL insertion)

121. When should a posterolateral corner injury be repaired?

121. Acutely

122. What is the general technique for posterolateral corner repair?

122. Primary repair with or without augmentation with allograft or autograft

Combined Injury (Suggestive of Dislocation)

123. By definition, how many ligaments are involved in a combined injury?

123. Three or more

124. What two structures are most commonly injured with knee dislocation?

124. ACL
PCL

125. What is the incidence of vascular injury after anterior dislocation?

125. 30 to 50%

126. What is the first-line test to exclude arterial injury with knee dislocation? What is the safe value?

126. Ankle-brachial index (ABI)
Safe if ABI >0.9 and good pulses are present

127. If a knee dislocation is irreducible, what is the most likely direction of dislocation? Why?

127. Posterolateral rotatory
Because condyle has button-holed through the capsule

128. What is the preferred timing of surgery after knee dislocation? What is it imperative to check?

128. Operate 5 to 12 days after injury
Check vascular integrity

129. What two posterior structures should be repaired?

129. PCL
PLC

130. What are the two principal risk factors for heterotopic ossification (HO) development after knee dislocation?

130. Mechanical ventilation
Elevated Injury Severity Scale (ISS) score

131. What possible intraoperative complication must one be alert for? Why?

131. Fluid extravasation
May lead to compartment syndrome

Patellofemoral Syndromes

132. The highest patellofemoral contact pressures occur in what knee position?

132. 0 to 30 degrees of extension

133. What is the primary restraint to lateral patellar translation?

133. Medial patellofemoral ligament (MPFL)

134. How can lateral patellar compression syndrome be differentiated from patellar tilt?

134. Compression syndrome has no patellar tilt on sunrise view

135. What is the indication for lateral release?

135. Compression or tilt unresponsive to rehab

136. What is the recommended treatment for a young athlete with single patellar dislocation?

136. Acute MPFL repair with or without lateral release (if tilt)

137. What is the recommended treatment for skeletally mature, recurrent dislocators? Contraindication?

137. Realignment procedure if necessary with or without MPFL repair
Contraindication: presence of proximal medial arthrosis

138. What are the three components of miserable malalignment syndrome?

138. Excess femoral anteversion
Genu valgum
Pronated feet

139. What is the first line surgical treatment for symptomatic bipartite patellar nonunion?

139. Lateral release

140. What is the surgical treatment for patellar tendinosis in athletes?

140. Excise necrotic area of tendon

Other Syndromes Involving the Knee and Leg

Osteochondritis Dissecans (OCD)

141. What is the most common site of OCD injury?

141. Lateral aspect of medial femoral condyle

142. In what two locations are prognoses particularly poor?

142. Lateral femoral condyle
Patella

143. What is the initial treatment if the physes are still open?

143. Observation, non–weight-bearing for minimum of 6 weeks

144. If the physes are closed, how is an in-situ lesion treated? What are the options if detached?

144. In situ: retrograde drilling
Detached: repair, microfracture, osteochondral allograft, etc.

Pigmented Villonodular Synovitis (PVNS)

145. What is the typical clinical presentation?

145. Hemarthrosis, possible mass

146. PVNS is associated with deposits of what substance?

146. Hemosiderin

147. What is the recommended treatment? How often does PVNS recur?

147. Synovectomy
High recurrence rate after synovectomy

148. Compare the efficacy of arthroscopic versus open treatment for PVNS?

148. Equivalent

149. What adjunctive measure can be used to lower recurrence rate?

149. Radiation

150. What is the treatment for PVNS with a single nodular mass?

150. Excision of the mass alone is often effective

151. How does PVNS compare to the clinical presentation of synovial chondromatosis?

151. Synovial chondromatosis generally has loose bodies within the knee.

152. What is the MRI appearance of PVNS of the hips?

152. "Bulging" hemarthrotic hip joints

Atraumatic Avascular Necrosis (AVN) of Condyle

153. What population is particularly at risk for condylar AVN?

153. Elderly women

154. What is the likely outcome if <50% of condyle involved?

154. Spontaneous healing

155. If >50% of the condyle is involved, there is an increased risk of what complication?

155. Collapse

Other Conditions Associated with Participation in Athletics

156. What physical exam test best identifies IT band friction syndrome? How is it performed?

156. Ober test for tight IT band
Examine hip in abduction and hyperextension

157. What are the four components of the differential diagnosis of a runner with leg pain?

157. Tibial stress fracture
Medial tibial stress syndrome
Popliteal artery entrapment syndrome
Exercise-induced compartment syndrome

158. What is the cause of medial tibial stress syndrome?

158. Periostitis

159. Where is the pain generally located?

159. Posteromedial tibial border, middle to distal

160. Does rest generally relieve medial tibial stress syndrome symptoms?

160. Yes

161. What is the recommended treatment?

161. Nonoperative rehabilitation

162. What are the criteria for the diagnosis of exercise induced compartment syndrome?

162. >30 mm Hg at 1 minute post exercise
>20 at 5 minutes
>15 at 15 minutes

Quick Review of Key Material from Other Chapters

163. What pediatric physeal injury of the knee must be carefully excluded? How?

163. Salter Harris II of distal femur
Obtain stress radiographs

164. These injuries have a tendency to fall into which direction?

164. Varus

165. The resultant amount of deformity is related to what factor?

165. Degree of displacement

Osteotomies

166. What is the best osteotomy level at which to correct tibial deformity?

166. At or below level of tibial tubercle

167. What is the first structure at risk posteriorly at the level of the tibial tubercle?

167. Popliteus

168. What is the maximum correction attainable with a high tibial osteotomy (HTO)? What is the goal of correction?

168. Maximum correction of 20 degrees
Goal: overcorrect to 8 to 10 degrees valgus

169. Is an open or closing wedge osteotomy preferred for HTO?

169. Opening

170. What is the expected longevity of symptomatic relief from HTO?

170. 6 years

171. There are better outcomes if the preoperative alignment is ____ and if the postoperative alignment is ____.

171. Preoperative: <9 degrees varus
Postoperative: >7 degrees valgus

172. What patients are at increased risk of long-term failure after HTO?

172. Overweight patients

173. Is HTO an option for patients with inflammatory arthritis?

173. No osteotomies for inflammatory arthritis

174. What are the three most common complications of HTO?

174. Return of deformity
Change in tibial slope
Patella baja

175. What is the correction goal of a distal femoral varus producing osteotomy?

175. Correct to neutral alignment

176. Is there an effective nonoperative option for unicompartmental arthritis?

176. Lateral wedge insoles have been shown to be effective

■ Trauma

Fractures About the Knee

Supracondylar Femur Fracture

177. Compare union rates with intramedullary (IM) nail versus plate use for supracondylar fracture?

177. Plate union rates are greater than for the IM nail

178. Into what direction of malalignment does a supracondylar malunion generally fall?

178. Varus malunion

Tibial Plateau Fracture

179. What is the treatment for a nondisplaced Schatzker I fracture? What is the recommended adjunct?

179. Immobilization
Consider arthroscopy to examine uniformity of articular surface

180. What two Schatzker types are associated with the greatest degrees of soft tissue injury?

180. II
IV

181. What Schatzker type is most commonly associated with MCL injury?

181. II

182. What Schatzker type is most commonly associated with meniscal injury?

182. IV

183. What direction of knee instability results in worse clinical outcomes?

183. Varus

184. Therefore, on which side should a unilateral external fixator be placed?

184. Place the external fixator medially to prevent varus.

Comminuted Patellar Fracture

185. When performing partial patellectomy for fracture, where should the patellar tendon be reattached?

185. Anteriorly

Tibial Trauma

Metaphyseal Proximal Tibia Fracture

186. Into what two directions of deformity does a metaphyseal proximal tibia fracture fall?

186. Apex anterior
Apex medial

187. In what two ways should the intramedullary nail starting point be adjusted to minimize deformity risk?

187. Slightly more posterior
More lateral

188. What knee position should be maintained while nailing?

188. Semi-extended

189. If blocking screws are used, where should they be placed?

189. Posterior and lateral

190. What are two options for maintaining the reduction while nailing?

190. Unicortical plate
Temporary external fixator

191. A percutaneous plating technique places what nerve at risk? How?

191. Superficial peroneal nerve
Percutaneous insertion of distal screws may result in nerve injury

192. Quick review: What is the most commonly injured vessel with displaced physeal injury of the proximal tibia and resultant compartment syndrome?

192. Anterior tibial artery

Tibial Shaft Fracture

193. Compare the outcomes of external fixator versus nail treatment for open tibia fracture.

193. Similar clinical outcomes

194. How do overall complication rates compare for both techniques with open fracture?

194. IM nail has lower overall complication rate

195. What is the reported advantage to reaming an open fracture? Open fractures up to what grade can generally be reamed safely?

195. Decreased rate of hardware failure
Can ream up to grade IIIB open tibial shaft fracture

196. What is the reported advantage of reaming a closed fracture?

196. Better clinical outcomes

197. How is "reaming to fit" performed?

197. Ream to 1 mm over isthmic diameter
Insert nail 1 to 1.5 mm smaller than biggest reamer used

198. Which complication of open tibia fracture is more common: nonunion or infection?

198. Nonunion

199. What are the three reported risk factors for nonunion development with a tibial shaft fracture?

199. Open fracture
Persistent gap
Transverse fracture pattern

200. If a tibial nonunion develops, what should be the first attempt at treatment? Compare with femoral shaft.

200. Dynamization of tibial nail
Dynamization not advocated for femur

201. What is the most common mechanism of hardware failure in nonunion? What fails first?

201. Fatigue fracture
Locking screws fail first

202. What is the No. 1 complication of IM nailing of the tibia? It is especially common in what patients?

202. Knee pain
The young

203. What is the No. 1 closed treatment complication?

203. Ankle stiffness

Tibial Stress Fracture

204. Why are anterior stress fractures particularly difficult to treat?

204. Because the anterior tibia is the tension side

205. What is the radiographic indication for IM nailing of a tibial stress fracture?

205. Plain radiographic "black line" appearance

206. Should the nail be reamed or unreamed?

206. Reamed

207. When should bone grafting be considered?

207. If unhealed at 6 months

208. What is the preferred approach for bone grafting of a tibial shaft nonunion? What is the interval?

208. Posterolateral (Harmon) approach
Interval between flexor hallucis longus (FHL)/soleus and peroneals

209. What does deep dissection involve?

209. Elevate posterior tibialis

210. The posterior tibialis protects what two neurovascular structures?

210. Posterior tibial artery
Tibial nerve

Pilon Fractures

211. What is the most common complication after open reduction with internal fixation (ORIF) of pilon fracture?

211. Posttraumatic arthrosis

212. What is the postoperative deep infection rate?

212. 4 to 35%

213. What clinical finding best correlates with deep infection development? What clinical finding does not correlate with deep infection development?

213. Postoperative skin slough
Whether the fracture was initially open

214. In a prospective randomized comparison of ORIF versus external fixator with limited ORIF for pilon fracture, which treatment modality had the better short-term outcome score?

214. Equivalent

215. Which had the greater number of complications?

215. ORIF

216. Which had the better long-term outcome?

216. Both groups did poorly long-term, but ORIF outcomes were better long-term

217. When placing an external fixator for pilon fracture, how far proximally does the joint capsule extend?

217. 12.2 mm

■ Total Knee Arthroplasty

Preoperative Planning and Decision Making

General Points on Total Knee Arthroplasty (TKA) Design

218. Why is a metal-backed tibial component used? What is the clinical significance?

218. Decreases compressive force on tibial plateau
Minimizes osteolysis

219. What are the reported outcomes for tibial component with cement only under the metaphysis and a press fit stem?

219. Increased risk of loosening relative to cementing entire component

220. Is a metal-backed patellar component routinely used?

220. No, as it has increased wear
All polyethylene patellar components are routinely used

Cruciate Retaining Total Knee Arthroplasty

221. What is the theoretical advantage of cruciate retaining total knee arthroplasty?

221. Allows for physiologic rollback of femur on tibia

222. Has this been borne out in radiographic studies?

222. Fluoroscopic studies have found cruciate retaining knees do not exhibit physiologic rollback

223. The most normal knee kinematics are actually seen with what knee design?

223. Unicompartmental total knee arthroplasty

224. What are the three symptoms of late cruciate failure after cruciate-retaining TKA?

224. Effusion
Flexion instability
Pain

Cruciate Substituting Posterior Stabilized (PS) Knees

225. In what four situations is a posterior stabilized knee indicated instead of cruciate retaining?

225. Patellectomy
Inflammatory arthritis
PCL absent or over-released
Prior HTO

226. What are the two theoretical advantages of a PS knee?

226. Improved flexion
Mechanical rollback achieved

227. Use of a PS knee requires careful attention to what to prevent what complication?

227. Well-balanced knee required to prevent dislocation

228. Hyperflexion of a PS knee may lead to what complication?

228. Dislocation

229. What are the two causes of cam impingement?

229. Hyperextension
Femoral component flexion

230. Moving the joint line in what direction increases the chance of impingement?

230. Joint line elevation may lead to patella baja and increased chance of impingement

231. A patellar clunk is classically associated with PS knee in what position? What generally causes it?

231. Extension
A superior nodule

Mobile Bearing Knee

232. How does mobile bearing articular conformity compare with standard TKA?

232. Improved

233. How do mobile bearing interface stresses compare with those in a standard knee?

233. Decreased

234. Have improved clinical outcomes been demonstrated with mobile bearing knees?

234. No

235. What two factors increase the risk of mobile bearing knee dislocation?

235. Valgus alignment
Older patient

Unicompartmental Total Knee Arthroplasty

236. What are the four preoperative criteria for unicompartmental knee arthroplasty?

236. Correctable valgus/varus deformity (not fixed deformity)
Flexion >90 degrees
<10-degree flexion contracture
No inflammatory arthritis

237. With medial unicompartmental replacement, what is the desired postoperative alignment?

237. 0 to 3 degrees valgus

238. What is the reported advantage of a minimally invasive unicompartmental knee replacement?

238. Faster rehabilitation

239. How do failures from fixed bearing unicompartmental knees typically present?

239. Component failure

240. What is the presentation of failure after mobile bearing unicompartmental knee?

240. Disease progression

Other Preoperative Considerations

241. In general, in what situation should bilateral total knees be staged?

241. If patient has many medical comorbidities

242. What is the most common complication of simultaneous bilateral total knee arthroplasty?

242. Deep venous thrombosis (DVT)

243. What is the short-term benefit to a subvastus approach? Is there a long-term benefit?

243. Improved early range of motion (ROM)
No long-term benefit

244. What is the observed clinical effect of patella baja in total knee arthroplasty?

244. Decreased flexion

245. In general, what are the four treatment options for patella baja?

245. Lower the joint line
Use small superior patellar dome
Cut patellar polyethylene at impingement points
Do not resurface the patella

246. In general, what are the outcomes of TKA in the setting of arthrofibrosis?

246. Unpredictable

Key Techniques and Intraoperative Decision Making

Standard Cuts and Technique

247. The goal is to make the distal femoral cut perpendicular to what?

247. Mechanical axis of femur

248. How much should the distal femoral cut angle measure?

248. 6 degrees valgus

249. How much should the external rotation angle for the femoral component measure?

249. 3 degrees external rotation

250. What three landmarks can be used to assess femoral component rotation?

250. Whiteside's line
Epicondylar axis
Posterior condylar axis (3 to 5 degrees shy of neutral)

251. The femoral component should be placed in line with what landmark (medial-lateral)?

251. Lined up with the lateral cortex to prevent component medialization

252. Has notching been shown to affect TKA outcomes?

252. Notching has not been demonstrated to have a significant effect on outcomes
May have some association with periprosthetic fracture risk

253. The goal is to make the tibial cut perpendicular to what?

253. Tibial mechanical axis

254. When should an IM rod not be used for a tibial cut?

254. If the tibial mechanical axis is not the same as the anatomic axis

255 Defects up to 1 cm can be filled with what? What about larger defects?

255. ≤1 cm: cement
>1 cm: metal augments

256. What is the minimum acceptable tibial ultra high molecular weight polyethylene thickness?

256. 8 mm

257. How can the patellar cut compromise patellar tracking?

257. Excessive lateral facet cut can lead to subluxation

258. Is a deeper trochlea better for tracking?

258. Yes

259. What is the minimum acceptable patellar thickness after cut?

259. 12 mm

Balancing: Varus Deformity

260. With a varus deformity, what two structures should be released first?

260. Osteophytes
Deep MCL

261. If the knee is still not balanced, what two structures should be released next?

261. Posteromedial corner
Semimembranosus

262. If all else fails, what structure can finally be released?

262. Superficial MCL

263. What happens if the MCL is inadvertently over-released?

263. Constrained total knee required

Balancing: Valgus Deformity

264. With a valgus deformity, what two structures should be released first?

264. Osteophytes
Lateral capsule

265. What are the next steps if the knee remains tight in extension? What if it remains tight in flexion?

265. Extension tight: release IT band
Flexion tight: release popliteal tendon

266. If the valgus deformity is severe, release of which structure may provide additional improvement? Then what is needed?

266. Release LCL
Then need constrained prosthesis

267. What is the potential complication of overcorrecting valgus knees?

267. Peroneal nerve stretch

268. Peroneal palsy most often occurs with what two preoperative features?

268. Valgus knee
Flexion contracture

Other Key Operative Points

269. What is the ideal position in which to close the knee?

269. Closing in flexion achieves equivalent ROM as with postoperative continuous passive motion (CPM) device use

Key Points on Postoperative Course and Common Complications

270. What is the best outcome measure after a total knee arthroplasty?

270. Pain relief

Acute Complications

271. What is the most likely cause of a cold, pulseless foot immediately after surgery?

271. Embolized atherosclerotic plaque

272. What is the treatment for postoperative slough of soft tissue over patellar tendon?

272. Medial gastrocnemius flap

273. What is the treatment for slough of soft tissue over patella itself?

273. Debridement and skin graft

Infection

274. What are the four reported risk factors for infection after total knee arthroplasty?

274. Rheumatoid arthritis
Male
Compromised skin
Elevated international normalized ratio (INR)

275. What effect do drains have on risk of infection?

275. Drains increase risk of infection

276. What is the problem with using polymerase chain reaction (PCR) to detect infection?

276. High rate of false-positives

Limited Postoperative Range of Motion

277. What is the principal determinant of postoperative stiffness?

277. Preoperative stiffness

278. Postoperative knee flexion due to hamstring overpull can last how long?

278. Up to 6 months

279. At what time should one manipulate the postoperative total knee?

279. 4 to 6 weeks

280. Where are adhesions most commonly found?

280. Within the gutters

281. Increased risk of heterotopic ossification after TKA has been associated with what patient characteristic?

281. Increased weight

282. What laboratory marker is associated with increased risk of HO after TKA?

282. Postoperative C-reactive protein (CRP) values

Complications Associated with Disease States

283. What two TKA complications have been associated with rheumatoid arthritis?

283. Infection
Stiffness

284. What two complications have been associated with hemophilia?

284. Infection
Stiffness

Periprosthetic Fracture

285. What are the five reported risk factors for periprosthetic fracture after TKA?

285. Osteoporosis
Stress shielding
Femoral notching
Osteonecrosis
Wear-related osteolysis

286. How are distal femoral periprosthetic fractures classified?

286. Lewis and Rorabeck system
I: nondisplaced, intact prosthesis
II: displaced, intact prosthesis
III: displaced, loose prosthesis

287. How are proximal tibial periprosthetic fractures classified and subclassified?

287. Felix, Stuart, and Hanssen system
I: tibial plateau
II: adjacent to stem
III: distal to prosthesis
IV: tibial tubercle
Subclassification A to C describes relative stability of prosthesis

288. When planning revision surgery for periprosthetic fracture, what are the three key considerations?

288. Fracture displacement
Stability of the prosthesis
Bone quality

Revision Surgery: General Points

289. In general, if a patient has a painful TKA with good ROM and normal x-rays, what is the expected outcome of revision? Why?

289. Generally quite poor
Outcomes of revisions are better if patient has preoperative pain and limited ROM

Revision Surgery Pearls

290. If there are multiple prior incisions about the knee, which should be used for surgery? Why?

290. Choose the most lateral
Blood supply goes from medial to lateral

291. When performing polyethylene exchange alone, which possible complication may occur?

291. Potential locking mechanism failure

292. What component is generally loose in a revision situation?

292. Tibial component

293. What is a general landmark for establishing the location of the joint line?

293. 1.5 cm above fibular head

294. What is the maximum acceptable joint line change?

294. 8 mm

295. What should be done for massive bone loss encountered during reconstruction?

295. Use structural allograft

296. In what three ways can the extensor mechanism be best protected during surgery?

296. Quadriceps (rectus) snip
Tubercle osteotomy
V-Y quadricepsplasty

297. What two salvage procedures are available for a disrupted extensor mechanism?

297. Semitendinosus autograft
Augment with allograft

298. What common clinical problem may persist despite extensor reconstruction?

298. Extensor lag

299. What three salvage procedures are available for an incompetent MCL?

299. Posterior tibial tendon allograft
Advance MCL
CCK (constrained condylar knee)

Constrained Nonhinged Total Knee Arthroplasty

300. How do constrained nonhinged TKAs work?

300. Large central post substitutes for MCL/LCL

301. What are the three indications for their use?

301. MCL attenuation
LCL deficiency
Flexion gap laxity (because it has a tall post)

302. Why is the use of a constrained nonhinged knee controversial if MCL totally absent?

302. Risk for post breakage

Constrained Hinged and Rotating Platform Total Knee Arthroplasty

303. What are the three surgical indications for use of constrained hinged rotating TKA?

303. All ligaments gone
Knee resection
Hyperextension instability (e.g., polio)

304. If using a constrained total knee, what else should always be used?

304. Intramedullary device

5

Foot and Ankle

■ Anatomy of the Ankle and Foot

Anatomy of the Ankle: Key Points

Bony Anatomy

1. What is more proximal: the medial or lateral malleolus?

2. Is the center of ankle rotation externally or internally rotated?
3. With which direction of fibular motion is ankle dorsiflexion associated?

Muscular Anatomy

4. What peroneal tendon hugs the fibula?
5. What peroneal tendon has a more distal muscle belly?
6. The os peroneum lies within what peroneal tendon?
7. What peroneal tendon attaches to the base of the fifth metatarsal?
8. The groove within the talar body houses what tendon?
9. What structure is found lateral to the flexor hallucis longus tendon?
10. The groove within the calcaneus houses what tendon?
11. What ligament is found in close proximity?
12. The groove within the cuboid houses what tendon?
13. What is the associated syndrome at this location?

1. Medial malleolus is more proximal
   A line drawn from medial to lateral malleolus is at an 8 degree angle to the horizontal
2. 23 degrees externally rotated

3. External rotation

4. Peroneus brevis
5. Peroneus brevis

6. Peroneus longus

7. Peroneus brevis

8. Flexor hallucis longus (FHL)

9. Os trigonum

10. The FHL coursing underneath the sustentaculum tali

11. Calcaneonavicular (spring) ligament

12. Peroneus longus

13. POPS (painful os peroneum syndrome)

14. What tendon inserts on the navicular?
15. This insertion must be repaired after what surgical procedure?

14. Posterior tibial tendon
15. Resection of an accessory navicular

Ligamentous Anatomy

16. What are the four components of the distal tibiofibular (tib-fib) joint?

16. Anterior inferior tib-fib ligament (AITFL)
    Posterior inferior tib-fib ligament (PITFL)
    Interosseous ligament (IO)
    Transverse ligament

17. The AITFL is most commonly involved in what two types of injuries?
18. What is the clinical significance of the PITFL?

17. Syndesmotic injuries
    Tillaux fractures
18. Attached to the posterior malleolar fracture fragment in a trimalleolar fracture

19. What are the two components of the superficial deltoid ligament?
20. What are the two components of the deep deltoid ligament?
21. What is the clinical significance of the deep deltoid ligament?
22. What deep deltoid component exhibits hypertrophy with recurrent ankle sprains?

19. Tibionavicular
    Tibiocalcaneal
20. Anterior tibiotalar
    Posterior tibiotalar
21. Primary restraint to anterolateral talar displacement
22. Anterior tibiotalar

Surgical Anatomy

23. What is the interval for the anterior approach to the ankle?

23. Between extensor hallucis longus (EHL) and extensor digitorum longus (EDL)

24. What structure must be identified and protected with this approach?
25. Where does the sural nerve generally cross the Achilles tendon?

24. Superficial peroneal nerve (SPN)
25. 10 cm proximal to the insertion

Physical Examination

26. In what position should the foot be placed when testing the posterior tibial tendon (PTT)?

26. Eversion
    Plantar flexion

27. In what position should the foot be placed when testing the calcaneofibular ligament?
28. In what position should the foot be placed when testing the anterior talofibular ligament (ATFL)?
29. In what position should the foot be placed when testing for subluxing peroneal tendons?

27. Inversion
    Dorsiflexion
28. Plantar flexion
    Perform anterior drawer test
29. Dorsiflexion
    Eversion

Anatomy of the Foot: Muscular and Nervous Anatomy

Layers of the Plantar Foot

30. What muscle layers are considered intrinsic?

30. 1
3

31. What muscle layers are considered extrinsic?

31. 2
4

32. Layer 1: what are the three components of the musculature and what is their innervation?

32. Abductor hallucis (medial plantar nerve [MPN])
Flexor digitorum brevis (MPN)
Abductor digiti minimi (lateral plantar nerve [LPN])

33. Layer 2: what are the four components of the musculature and what is their innervation?

33. Quadratus plantae (LPN)
Lumbricals (MPN, LPN)
Flexor digitorum longus (tibial nerve)
Flexor hallucis longus (tibial nerve)

34. Layer 3: what are the three components of the musculature and what is their innervation?

34. Flexor hallucis brevis (MPN)
Adductor hallucis (LPN)
Flexor digit minimi brevis (LPN)

35. Layer 4: what are the four components of the musculature and what is their innervation?

35. Dorsal interosseous muscles (LPN)
Plantar interosseous muscles (LPN)
Peroneus longus (superficial peroneal nerve)
Posterior tibialis (tibial nerve)

36. In what layer and at what locations do the medial and lateral plantar nerves lie?

36. Layer 2
MPN lies deep to the abductor hallucis muscle
LPN lies deep to the quadratus plantae muscle

37. What is the significance of the extensor digitorum brevis (EDB)? What is its innervation?

37. Dorsal intrinsic muscle
Innervated by the deep peroneal nerve

38. What is the origin of the flexor digitorum brevis (FDB)?

38. Medial calcaneal tubercle

39. What is the insertion of the FDB?

39. Middle phalanges

40. What is the origin of the plantar aponeurosis?

40. Plantar medial calcaneus

41. Where does the plantar aponeurosis insert?

41. Toe flexors

42. What are the three main functions of the aponeurosis?

42. Increase arch height as toes dorsiflex
Major support of medial longitudinal arch
Aid hindfoot inversion

43. What is the effect of hindfoot inversion on the transverse tarsal joints?

43. Hindfoot inversion locks the transverse tarsal joints

44. What nerve provides sensation to the dorsomedial great toe?

44. Dorsomedial cutaneous branch of superficial peroneal nerve (SPN)

45. This nerve runs across what structure?

45. Extensor hallucis longus (EHL)

Surgical Approaches to the Foot

46. What is the interval for the lateral approach to the hindfoot?

46. Between peroneus tertius (deep peroneal nerve) and peroneus brevis (SPN)

47. What structure must be reflected with this approach?

47. Extensor digitorum brevis (EDB)

48. What deeper structure must be identified and protected?

48. Flexor hallucis longus (FHL)

49. What structure must be released for the anterolateral approach to the midfoot?

49. EDB

50. What deeper structure must be identified and protected with this approach?

50. Spring ligament

Anatomy of the Foot: Vascular Anatomy

51. What two arteries comprise the major vascular supply to the foot?

51. Dorsalis pedis (especially the dorsum of the foot)
Posterior tibial artery

52. What is the main branch of the dorsalis pedis and where is it found?

52. Deep plantar artery
Between the first and second metatarsals

53. What are the two major branches of the posterior tibial artery?

53. Medial plantar artery
Lateral plantar artery

54. Together, the deep plantar artery and the lateral plantar artery form what structure?

54. Plantar arch

55. In what layer of the foot is the plantar arch found?

55. 4th

56. Dorsal ulceration and weak pulses are suggestive of what clinical problem?

56. Arterial insufficiency

Vascular Supply to the Talus

57. The artery of the tarsal canal is principally supplied by what?

57. Posterior tibial artery

58. What region of the talus does it supply?

58. Body

59. Then it contributes to what artery?

59. Deltoid artery

60. What does the deltoid artery supply?

60. Medial one third of the talus

61. Disruption of the deltoid artery is associated with what delayed complication?

61. Varus collapse of the talus

62. The artery of the tarsal sinus is principally supplied by what two entities?

62. Dorsalis pedis
Peroneal artery

63. What two regions of the talus does it supply?

63. Head and neck (antegrade)
Body (retrograde)

■ The Gait Cycle

Normal Gait

64. What percentage of the gait cycle does the stance phase comprise?

64. 60%

65. What are the three divisions of the stance phase?

65. Heel strike
Foot flat
Toe off

66. What is the position of the hindfoot at heel strike?

66. Inverted

67. What is the position of the hindfoot at foot flat?

67. Everted (subtalar joint unlocked)

68. What is the position of the hindfoot at toe off?

68. Inverted

69. What is the principal invertor of the subtalar joint?

69. Posterior tibial tendon

70. What effect does subtalar inversion have on the talus?

70. Talus externally rotates

71. What effect does subtalar inversion have on the tibia?

71. Tibia externally rotates

72. Most gait cycle muscle activity is of what type?

72. Eccentric

73. What is the principal muscle activity during heel strike?

73. Tibialis anterior (TA) eccentric contraction (controlled plantar flexion)

74. What is the principal muscle activity during foot flat?

74. Gastrocnemius eccentric contraction (controlled dorsiflexion)

75. What is the principal muscle activity during toe off?

75. Gastrocnemius concentric contraction (active plantar flexion)

76. Where is the normal center of pressure at heel strike?

76. Heel pressure

77. Where is the normal center of pressure at foot flat?

77. Second metatarsal head

78. Where is the normal center of pressure at toe off?

78. Toes

Deviations from Normal Gait

79. How does hallux valgus alter the pressure distribution in foot flat?

79. Hallux bears less weight than predicted
Center of pressure moves laterally

80. In what two ways does hallux valgus alter the pressure distribution in toe off?

80. Increases pressure centrally from medial to lateral
Unloads toes

81. What are the two characteristics of an antalgic (painful) gait pattern?

81. Shorter stance on the painful side
Contralateral swing phase more rapid

82. What is the gait pattern of a patient with an absent anterior cruciate ligament (ACL) called?

82. Quadriceps avoidance gait

■ Pathologic States

Cavus Foot and Associated Conditions

83. What fraction of cavus feet is idiopathic?

83. One third

84. What four disorders comprise the major differential diagnosis for the remaining two thirds?

84. Charcot-Marie-Tooth
Tethered cord/other spine condition
Friedreich's ataxia
Dejerine-Sottas
(and others)

Charcot-Marie-Tooth (CMT)

85. What are the two major types of CMT?

85. I: hands also involved
II: early onset, associated with axonal atrophy

86. What type is generally autosomal recessive?

86. II

87. If family CMT inheritance pattern is autosomal dominant (AD), what chromosome may be responsible?

87. Chromosome 17

88. What gene?

88. *PMP22*

89. What is the resulting defect?

89. Abnormal myelin production

90. *PMP22* abnormalities may also affect production of what substance?

90. Connexin

91. In which gender is CMT generally more common?

91. Male

92. In which gender is CMT generally more severe?

92. Female

93. Is CMT associated with sensory loss?

93. Sensory and proprioceptive losses may be present; it is variable

94. What are the four clinical findings of CMT foot?

94. Cavus foot
Plantarflexed first ray
Hindfoot varus
Claw toes

95. With CMT, what is the relative muscle strength of the tibialis anterior?

95. Weak

96. … of the peroneus brevis?

96. Weak

97. … of the peroneus longus?

97. Strong

98. … of the intrinsics?

98. Weak

99. What is the net result of this relative muscle imbalance?

99. Plantarflexed first ray

100. What clinical test can reliably differentiate fixed and flexible hindfoot deformity?

100. Coleman block test

101. In general, what is the first-line treatment for most CMT patients (especially adolescents)?

101. Trial of bracing

102. If bracing is unsuccessful, what are the two general surgical principles for the patient with supple hindfoot deformity?

102. Forefoot corrective procedures alone usually suffice
May consider adding calcaneal slide/osteotomy to protect soft tissue transfers

103. Specifically, surgery includes what five procedures?

103. Plantar fascia release
Dorsiflexion osteotomy of the first ray
Peroneus longus to peroneus brevis transfer
Achilles tendon lengthening
Possible calcaneal slide/osteotomy (to protect soft tissue transfer)

104. One might also consider performing the Jones procedure: what two components does it include?

104. Transfer of EHL to first metatarsal neck
Fusion of the first interphalangeal (IP) joint

105. How might a Jones procedure be beneficial?

105. Helps a weak tibialis anterior with dorsiflexion of the first ray

106. In general, what is the surgical principle if the hindfoot deformity is fixed?

106. Must include calcaneal osteotomy for correction

107. What surgical option exists for a patient with fixed hindfoot deformity and degenerative changes?

107. Triple arthrodesis

108. What is an important caveat in this population? Why?

108. Triple arthrodesis is a procedure of last resort
Poor outcomes have been reported in CMT patients

109. What two other musculoskeletal manifestations of CMT may be present?

109. Scoliosis
Developmental hip dysplasia

Calcaneocavus Foot

110. A calcaneocavus foot is associated with what disease process?

110. Polio

111. Calcaneocavus deformity is due to the imbalance of what three muscles?

111. Weak gastrocnemius
Strong tibialis anterior
Strong posterior tibialis

Hallux Valgus

112. What is the primary stabilizer of the first metatarsophalangeal (MTP) joint?

112. Plantar plate

113. What is the range of normal for DMAA (distal metatarsal articular angle)

113. <15 degrees

114. What are the five components of the hallux valgus progression of events?

114. Valgus >15 degrees
Abductor hallucis moves from medial to plantar
Shifts adductor hallucis, flexor hallucis brevis, FHL laterally
Sesamoids dislocate and fibular sesamoid falls into the first intermetatarsal space
Deformity progresses

115. What are the intermetatarsal (IM) angle and the hallus valgus (HV) angle indications for soft tissue procedures alone?

115. IM angle <13 degrees
HV angle <25 degrees

116. What are the IM angle and HV angle indications for a chevron osteotomy?

116. IM <13 degrees
HV <30 degrees

117. What are the indications for a biplanar chevron?

117. DMAA >15 degrees

118. How much angular correction can a chevron achieve for every 1 mm of translation?

118. 1 degree

119. If a chevron osteotomy results in avascular necrosis, what is the salvage option?

119. Fusion

120. What are the IM angle and HV angle indications for MT shaft and proximal procedures?

120. IM <20 degrees
HV <50 degrees

121. What are three examples of shaft and proximal osteotomies?

121. Scarf
Ludloff
Mau

122. In general, can greater correction be obtained with a shaft or with a proximal osteotomy?

122. Generally greater correction with proximal than with shaft

123. What are the IM angle and HV angle indications for a Lapidus procedure?

123. IM <20 degrees
HV <50 degrees

124. In particular, the Lapidus is indicated for patients with what two characteristics?

124. Hypermobile
Medially slanted surface at the metatarsocuneiform joint

125. What are the IM angle and HV angle indications for resection arthroplasty?

125. IM <13 degrees
HV <45 degrees

126. For what patient population would a resection arthroplasty be a consideration?

126. Low-demand elderly patients

127. What is the most common complication of a metatarsal osteotomy?

127. Malunion, which leads to transfer metatarsalgia

128. Of all the hallux valgus procedures, which has the highest nonunion rate?

128. Tarso-metatarsal fusion

Juvenile Hallux Valgus

129. What patient population is particularly at risk for juvenile hallux valgus?

129. Females with generalized ligamentous laxity

130. With juvenile hallux valgus, in which position is the first metatarsal generally found?

130. Primus varus

131. How does the DMAA differ from normal?

131. Increased

132. What is a common associated finding at the IP joint?

132. Hallux interphalangeus

133. Juvenile HV usually requires what surgical procedure?

133. Single or double (corrects DMAA) osteotomy of the first metatarsal

134. At what age can these procedures be performed?

134. Once physes are closed

135. What is the treatment for severe deformity in a child with open physes?

135. First cuneiform opening wedge osteotomy

Deformities of the Lesser Toes

Claw Toe

136. Why does a claw toe develop in patients with Charcot-Marie-Tooth?

136. Flexor spasticity

137. Why does a claw toe develop in patients with head injury?

137. Extensor spasticity

138. Why does a claw toe develop in patients with no obvious pathologic cause?

138. Volar plate laxity

139. What is the most common cause leading to the development of volar plate laxity?

139. Second MTP joint synovitis

140. What are two common clinical signs of second MTP synovitis?

140. Swelling
Positive drawer test

141. If caught at an early phase, what two treatment options are available?

141. Metatarsal bar
Stiff shoe

142. If these conservative measures fail, what two treatment options are available?

142. Synovectomy
Capsular reconstruction

143. Regardless of etiology, what is the sequence of five events that results in the clinical development of a claw toe?

143. Metatarsophalangeal joint extension
Dorsal interosseous muscle subluxation
Extensor digitorum longus hyperextends the MTP and cannot extend the proximal interphalangeal (PIP) joint or distal interphalangeal (DIP) joint
Intrinsics slide dorsally and cannot flex the MTP
Flexors flex the PIP and DIP

144. What are the three preferred treatments if the MTP joint is reducible?

144. Plantar plate release
Collateral release
Flexor to extensor tendon transfer

145. What is the preferred treatment if the MTP joint is irreducible? During this procedure, which structures must be preserved?

145. Weil osteotomy
Must take care to preserve collaterals

146. What are the two primary complications associated with Weil procedures?

146. Recurrent dorsal contracture
Floating toe (extended toe because intrinsics slip dorsally)

147. Are transfer lesions commonly associated with Weil procedures?

147. No, rarely

148. A claw toe associated with a mallet toe may result in which clinical deformity?

148. Crossover toe

149. What is the preferred treatment in that clinical situation?

149. Same as reducible/irreducible algorithm above

150. For isolated fifth toe clawing (cock-up deformity), what is the preferred treatment?

150. Proximal phalangectomy (Ruiz–Mora procedure)

Mallet Toe

151. If conservative treatment of mallet toe fails, then which procedure is preferred at the joint? At flexor digitorum longus (FDL)?

151. DIP joint arthrodesis or arthroplasty
FDL tenotomy

Hammer Toe

152. If conservative treatment of hammer toe fails, then which procedure is preferred at the joint? At FDL?

152. PIP arthrodesis or arthroplasty
FDL flexor to extensor tendon transfer

Curly (Underlapping) Toe

153. What is the surgical treatment of choice for curly toe?

153. Flexor tenotomy

Fifth Toe Bunionette

154. What 4,5 intermetatarsal (IM) angle is considered normal?

154. 5 to 6 degrees

155. If a normal IM angle is present, what is the preferred treatment for fifth toe bunionette?

155. Lateral eminence resection

156. If IM angle is abnormal, how does the treatment differ?

156. Metatarsal osteotomy is required

157. What is the preferred fifth metatarsal osteotomy?

157. Oblique diaphyseal osteotomy

158. What type of metatarsal osteotomy must be avoided?

158. Proximal osteotomies

159. Quick review: Proximal osteotomies of the first metatarsal must be avoided in what patients?

159. Hallux valgus patients with open physes

160. What is the treatment of choice for a crossover fifth toe?

160. Proximal phalanx excision

161. In idiopathic plantar keratosis, a discrete callus is usually due to pressure from what structure?

161. Lateral condyle of metatarsal head

Sesamoid Disorders and Related Conditions

162. Sesamoiditis is associated with what clinical condition?

162. FHB tendonitis

163. Which sesamoid is most commonly injured?

163. Tibial sesamoid

164. Which sesamoid is most commonly bipartite?

164. Tibial (bipartite in 10%)

165. Compare the treatment of sesamoid fracture in an elite athlete versus general population.

165. Elite athlete: sesamoidectomy
General population: immobilization

166. At the time of surgery, one must be careful to avoid injury to what structure?

166. Plantar nerve

167. What structure should be repaired at the time of the procedure?

167. FHB

Freiberg's Infarction

168. What patient population is particularly at risk for Freiberg's infarction?

168. Females

169. If identified early, what are the two treatment options?

169. Cast immobilization
Metatarsal bar

170. If nonoperative treatment fails, then what?

170. Operative debridement

171. What is the surgical treatment if Freiberg's is identified late (with dorsal flattening)?

171. Rotational osteotomy

172. What is the treatment for end-stage arthritis?

172. Metatarsal head arthroplasty

Compressive Neuropathies and Associated Syndromes

Tarsal Tunnel Syndrome

173. In what percentage of patients is there a specifically identifiable cause for tarsal tunnel syndrome?

173. 60% are associated with a specific cause

174. What are the two symptoms of tarsal tunnel syndrome?

174. Pain, which may radiate distally
Worst at night

175. What is the test of choice on physical exam?

175. Tinel's sign is indicative of posterior tibial nerve irritation

176. What is the positive predictive value of a consistent history and positive electromyography (EMG) study?

176. 90%

177. If tarsal tunnel is associated with limited subtalar motion, what must be considered? Why?

177. Must consider middle facet coalition
Because it results in fixed valgus deformity and nerve stretch

178. What potentially coexistent neurologic condition must one consider?

178. Neuroma

179. What patients are expected to have the best outcomes from surgical intervention?

179. Those with symptoms for less than 1 year

180. Operative treatment consists of releasing what three structures?

180. Flexor retinaculum
Fascia of lower leg
Abductor hallucis fascia (because medial plantar nerve runs underneath): must follow and release medial and lateral branches

181. What nerve branch passes through the retinaculum?

181. Medial calcaneal nerve

Anterior Tarsal Tunnel Syndrome

182. What nerve is involved with anterior tarsal tunnel syndrome?

182. Deep peroneal nerve below inferior extensor retinaculum (IER)

183. What are the common presenting symptoms?

183. Pain and paresthesias in the first dorsal web space

184. Atrophy of what muscle may be observed?

184. EDB

185. Distally, where does the deep peroneal nerve run?

185. Just lateral to the extensor hallucis brevis (EHB) tendon

186. What two nonoperative treatments of anterior tarsal tunnel syndrome might be tried?

186. Shoe-wear modification
Rocker sole steel shank shoe

187. How much inferior extensor retinaculum should one release surgically?

187. <50%

Other Compressive Neuropathies

188. What is the most common site of superficial peroneal nerve (SPN) entrapment?

188. Fascial defect about 12 cm proximal to the lateral malleolus

189. Is EMG/nerve conduction velocity (NCV) generally helpful for diagnosing SPN entrapment?

189. No

190. Quick review: For which neurologic condition of the *upper* extremity is an EMG/NCV not particularly helpful either?

190. Radial tunnel syndrome

191. What is the most common site of saphenous nerve entrapment?

191. Hunter's canal

192. What nerve is involved in the condition known as "jogger's foot"?

192. Medial plantar nerve

193. What is the most common site of entrapment?

193. Knot of Henry (site of FDL, FHL crossover)

Morton's Neuroma

194. What gender is particularly at risk for developing Morton's neuroma?

194. Female

195. What is the most commonly involved web space? Why?

195. Third web space is more commonly involved than the second
Because third web space is the site of LPN, MPN merger

196. Are any additional tests necessary beyond clinical exam?

196. No, clinical diagnosis is generally sufficient

197. What percentage of patients fail conservative treatment?

197. 20%

198. What is the reported success rate of surgery?

198. 85%

199. What are the two classic pathologic examination findings of Morton's neuroma specimen?

199. Perineural fibrosis
Renaut bodies

Disorders of the Plantar Fascia

Plantar Fasciitis

200. What nerve is associated with plantar fasciitis?

200. First branch of the lateral plantar nerve (also called Baxter's nerve)

201. What muscle does this nerve innervate?

201. Abductor digit minimi

202. Plantar fasciitis has been shown to have an association with what systemic condition?

202. Recent weight gain

203. Where is the patient generally tender?

203. Medially under the abductor hallucis longus

204. After giving off Baxter's nerve, under what structure does the LPN continue?

204. Under the quadratus plantae

205. How much of the plantar fascia should one release operatively?

205. No more than one third of the fascia

Plantar Fibroma

206. What is the preferred treatment of plantar fibroma in a nonweightbearing area?

206. Observation and use of an accommodative orthosis

207. What is the preferred treatment of plantar fibroma in a painful weightbearing area? Why?

207. Excise the entire plantar fascia
Decreased rate of recurrence if entire fascia excised

Other Conditions Affecting the Plantar Surface of the Foot

208. Overall, what is the most common malignancy of the foot?

208. Plantar melanoma

209. What is the most common malignancy of the hand?

209. Squamous cell carcinoma

210. When shaving a wart, how do you know when you have gone far enough?

210. Presence of punctate bleeding

Achilles Tendon Injuries and Repair

211. The tendon fibers spiral 90 degrees such that the gastrocnemius inserts where in relation to the soleus?

211. Gastrocnemius fibers insert lateral to the soleus

212. What is the preferred treatment technique for Achilles tendinosis?

212. Eccentric stretching

213. Quick review: What is the preferred treatment technique for myositis ossificans?

213. No passive stretching

214. For an acute Achilles rupture, what are the two advantages of surgical treatment?

214. Decreased rate of rerupture
Best plantar flexion strength restoration

215. What are the two disadvantages of surgical treatment?

215. Wound complications
Decreased range of motion (ROM)

216. For nonoperatively treated patients, what is the advantage of a functional brace over a cast?

216. Improved ROM

217. What are the two main disadvantages of percutaneous repair techniques?

217. Weaker repair
Increased risk of sural nerve injury

218. Where is the sural nerve particularly at risk with a surgical approach?

218. 10 cm proximal to the Achilles insertion

219. In general, what is the desired position of ankle immobilization after Achilles repair?

219. 20 degrees of plantar flexion

220. What is the preferred treatment for chronic Achilles rupture if separation <4 cm?

220. Tendon lengthening technique and primary repair

221. What is the preferred treatment for chronic Achilles rupture if separation ≤4 cm?

221. Turndown flap and augmented repair

Haglund Exostosis

222. What is a Haglund exostosis?

223. A Haglund exostosis is also commonly known as what?

224. In what plane does a retrocalcaneal bursa develop?

225. If an exostosis is refractory to shoe-wear modification, what is the operative treatment?

226. How much of the Achilles tendon can be released without need for repair?

222. Bony prominence at the posterosuperior calcaneus

223. Pump bump

224. Posterior to Haglund exostosis
Anterior to the Achilles tendon

225. Open exostectomy

226. Up to 50%

Peroneal Tendon Pathology

227. What peroneal tendon is associated with retrofibular pathology?

228. What two disorders are associated with the brevis in the retrofibular groove?

229. What is the magnetic resonance imaging (MRI) appearance of a torn peroneus brevis?

230. What is a nonoperative treatment option for an acute tear?

231. Will most patients be satisfied with nonoperative treatment?

232. What peroneal tendon is associated with subfibular pathology?

233. What peroneal tendon is associated with cuboid tunnel pathology?

234. What are the three components of the treatment for a torn peroneus longus within the cuboid tunnel?

227. Brevis

228. Tear
Subluxation

229. "Three" peroneal tendons: brevis splits around the longus (also called peroneal split syndrome)

230. Immobilization in plantar flexion

231. No, most will require surgery

232. Longus

233. Longus/os peroneum

234. Excise tear
Side-to-side PL (peroneus longus) to PB (peroneus brevis) repair above retinaculum
Consider performing calcaneal osteotomy or Brostrom procedure

---

■ Trauma and Associated Conditions

Ankle Sprains and Associated Injuries

Lateral Ankle Sprains

235. On computed tomography (CT) studies of the ankle, what two features have been associated with ankle instability?

236. Of the lateral ankle ligaments, which is the weakest?

235. Hindfoot varus
Fibula further posterior than average

236. ATFL

237. What two ligaments demonstrate inflammatory changes with repeated sprains?

237. AITFL
Deltoid

238. What two changes are seen in the deltoid ligament?

238. Hypertrophy
Impingement

239. What band of the deltoid is particularly affected by recurrent sprains?

239. Tibiotalar band

240. What are the two components of operative treatment for hindfoot varus and associated lateral instability?

240. Valgus calcaneal osteotomy
Brostrom procedure

241. What is the principal cause of recurrent ankle sprains in dancers?

241. Peroneal weakness

Syndesmotic Ankle Sprains

242. With a syndesmotic injury, is the AITFL or PITFL injured first?

242. AITFL

243. What clinical exam finding is particularly useful in the diagnosis of a subtle syndesmotic injury?

243. Inability to perform a single leg hop

244. What radiographic view is best for identifying a syndesmotic injury?

244. External rotation stress view

245. In general, what should the weight-bearing status during treatment be?

245. Non–weight-bearing

246. What is the anticipated time to resolution of an isolated syndesmotic injury?

246. Generally twice that of a lateral ankle sprain

247. How does the treatment differ in an elite athlete with radiographic syndesmotic diastasis?

247. Syndesmotic screw placement preferred

248. What is the biomechanical effect of a syndesmotic screw?

248. Decreased ankle external rotation

249. What is the ideal position for syndesmotic screw placement?

249. 1.5 to 3 cm proximal to the ankle joint

250. With respect to bioabsorbable screws, what is the disadvantage of PGA relative to PLA (polyactide)?

250. Increased effusion with PGA (polyglycolide)

Ankle Fractures: Key Points

Fractures of the Medial and Lateral Malleoli

251. What is the preferred treatment for unimalleolar Weber A (Lauge-Hansen supination-adduction) and Weber B (supination-external rotation; pronation-abduction) fractures?

251. Weight bearing as tolerated

252. A malreduction with 1 mm of talar shift leads to what change in tibiotalar contact area?

252. 42% decrease in contact area

253. What ligament tends to pull the posterior malleolus fracture fragment into reduction with traction?

253. PITFL

254. According to the Boden study, if the fibular fracture is within ___ cm of the ankle joint, there is a very low likelihood of associated syndesmotic injury.

254. 4.5

255. What fibular approach is least likely to result in superficial peroneal nerve injury?

255. Posterolateral approach

256. How do posterior antiglide plate outcomes compare with those of lateral fibular plates?

256. Equivalent

257. What complication occurs more frequently with posterior antiglide plating?

257. Peroneal nerve irritation

258. What is the preferred treatment of medial malleolar fracture above the plafond?

258. Open reduction with internal fixation (ORIF)

259. How long after ankle ORIF does functional improvement continue?

259. 2 years

260. How long after ORIF has normal braking ability returned?

260. 9 weeks

Osteochondral Injuries (OCD)

261. What is the most common injury mechanism resulting in talar OCD lesions?

261. Inversion injury

262. In general, what are the three characteristics of lateral talar lesions?

262. Traumatic
Shallow
Anterior

263. What are the three typical characteristics of medial lesions?

263. Atraumatic
Deeper
More posterior

264. Wafer procedures are generally performed for OCD lesions in which location?

264. Lateral

265. A cup procedure is best for OCD lesions in which location?

265. Medial

266. What finding is a poor prognostic factor for response to drilling?

266. Presence of cysts

Talar Injuries and Management

Talar Neck Fracture

267. What radiographic study is particularly useful for identifying a talar neck fracture?

267. Canale view

268. What is the Hawkins classification system?

268. I: nondisplaced
II: with associated subtalar dislocation
III: with subtalar and ankle dislocation
IV: with subtalar, ankle, and talonavicular dislocation

269. What are the reported rates of AVN for each Hawkins stage?

269. I: 13%
II: 30%
III: 100%
IV: 100%

270. Is a talar neck fracture still considered a surgical emergency?

270. Controversial
Some have reported higher AVN rates with earlier surgery

271. What screw direction is best biomechanically?

271. Posterior to anterior

272. What is the reported rate of tibiotalar arthritis after talar neck fracture?

272. 33%

273. What is the reported rate of subtalar arthritis after talar neck fracture?

273. 50%

274. What is the preferred surgical treatment for varus malunion of the talar neck?

274. Triple arthrodesis

Talar Body Fracture

275. What is the classic history of a missed talar body fracture?

275. Ankle sprain that does not recover despite prolonged conservative management

276. What is the test of choice to identify talar body fracture?

276. Computed tomography (CT)

277. What is the indication for ORIF?

277. >2 mm displacement

278. What is the preferred surgical approach?

278. Medial malleolar osteotomy

279. With this approach, what structure must be carefully preserved?

279. Deltoid ligament

280. What is the most common complication associated with talar body fracture?

280. Avascular necrosis (AVN)

281. At what joint is posttraumatic arthritis most likely to develop?

281. Ankle

282. What joint is most often arthritic after talar neck fracture?

282. Subtalar joint

Posterior Process Fracture and Associated Conditions

283. What structure attaches to the talar posteromedial tubercle? To the posterolateral tubercle?

283. Posterior talotibial ligament attaches to posteromedial tubercle
Posterior talofibular ligament attaches to posterolateral tubercle

284. A posterior process fracture must be differentiated from what other clinical condition?

284. Os trigonum and associated FHL tenosynovitis

285. What is the position of the os relative to the FHL tendon?

285. Os is lateral to tendon

286. What patient population is particularly at risk for FHL tenosynovitis/os trigonum syndrome?

286. Dancers

287. What are the two symptoms of FHL tenosynovitis?

287. Posterior ankle pain with plantar flexion
Triggering of the IP joint of the great toe

288. What two studies best differentiate between os trigonum and fracture?

288. Bone scan
MRI

289. What is the preferred treatment for nondisplaced fracture of the posterior process?

289. Weight bearing as tolerated (WBAT) in cast

290. What is the preferred treatment for displaced fracture with subtalar involvement?

290. ORIF

291. What is the preferred treatment for vertical fracture of the posterior process?

291. ORIF

292. What is the preferred treatment for os trigonum refractory to conservative management?

292. Excision

293. What is the preferred treatment for associated medial sided pain?

293. Must exclude FHL entrapment within the tunnel under sustentaculum tali

294. What is the preferred treatment for laceration of the FHL?

294. Repair if lacerated proximal to the MTP and FHB is also disrupted

295. When repairing an FHL laceration, which structure must be identified and protected?

295. Medial plantar nerve

296. An FHL laceration repair should not be attempted at what location?

296. Within the MTP pulley system

Snowboarder's Fracture

297. What is a snowboarder's fracture?

297. Fracture of the lateral process of the talus

298. What two ligaments attach to the lateral talar process?

298. Lateral talocalcaneal ligament
ATFL

299. Snowboarder's fracture mechanism of injury involves what four components?

299. Dorsiflexion
Axial load
Inversion
External rotation

Talar Crush Injuries

300. If an ORIF is performed for talar crush injury, what is critical in the acute postoperative phase?

300. Initiate ROM early

301. What is an alternative to ORIF for a talar crush injury?

301. Tibiocalcaneal fusion

302. What is the most common cause for poor outcome after any crush injury of the foot?

302. Persistent neuritis

Subtalar Injuries and Management

303. What radiographic view is particularly useful for evaluating the subtalar joint?

303. Broden's view

304. Subtalar dislocations in what direction are generally high energy and have poorer outcomes?

304. Lateral

305. If a medial subtalar dislocation is irreducible, which structure is likely responsible?

305. EDB

306. Quick review: What structure is responsible for an irreducible medial tibiotalar dislocation?

306. Peroneus brevis

307. If a lateral subtalar dislocation is irreducible, what structure is likely responsible?

307. Posterior tibialis tendon

308. Subtalar dislocations are often associated with dislocation at what other joint?

308. Talonavicular

Subtalar Arthroscopy

309. What is the preferred location of the anterior arthroscopy portal?

309. 2 cm anterior, 1 cm distal to fibula

310. What is the preferred location of the middle portal?

310. Just anterior to the tip of the fibula

311. What is the preferred location of the posterior portal?

311. Between Achilles tendon and fibula

Calcaneal Injuries and Management

Calcaneus Body Fracture

312. What is the orientation of the primary calcaneal fracture line?

312. Anterolateral (superolateral) to posteromedial (inferomedial)

313. What does Bohler's angle effectively measure?

313. Posterior facet height

314. What is the range of normal Bohler's angle?

314. 25 to 40 degrees

315. On which imaging study is the Sanders classification based?

315. Coronal CT

316. What is the relationship between the number of visualized fracture lines and Sanders class?

316. One fracture line: type II
Two fracture lines: type III
Three fracture lines: type IV

317. Do calcaneus fractures tend to fall into varus or valgus?

317. Varus

318. What percentage of calcaneus fracture patients develop a compartment syndrome?

318. 10%

319. How do the outcomes of surgical and nonsurgical calcaneus fracture treatments compare?

319. Overall, operative outcomes = nonoperative outcomes

320. But patients with what characteristics are especially likely to benefit from ORIF: age?

320. Younger

321. Gender?

321. Female

322. Workman's compensation status?

322. Injury unrelated to work

323. If treating a calcaneus fracture nonoperatively, should a cast be applied? Why?

323. No
Casting is associated with increased rates of reflex sympathetic dystrophy (RSD) and stiffness

324. In general, ORIF is indicated if displacement is greater than?

324. 2 mm

325. How do fracture blisters affect the timing of surgery?

325. Blisters must absorb and reepithelialize before surgery

326. What is the major arterial supply to the calcaneal skin flap?

326. Lateral calcaneal artery

327. How is this artery classically injured during surgery?

327. Horizontal limb of the flap is made too high

328. What structure is at risk if the screws from lateral to medial are too long?

328. FHL

329. What percentage of type II fractures result in reported good or excellent outcome after ORIF?

329. 70%

330. What percentage of type III fractures result in reported good or excellent outcomes?

330. 70%

331. What percentage of type IV fractures result in reported good or excellent outcomes?

331. 10%

332. Therefore, what alternative to ORIF should be considered with type IV fracture?

332. Primary subtalar fusion

333. In what two situations has primary subtalar fusion been shown to be especially helpful?

333. Patient is a laborer
Bohler's angle <0 degrees

334. With bilateral calcaneal fractures, how do operative and nonoperative outcomes compare?

334. Operative outcomes are worse than those for unilateral calcaneal fracture
But better than nonoperative bilateral fracture outcomes

335. What is the preferred treatment for a neglected calcaneus fracture with talar impaction and anterior impingement?

335. Subtalar arthrodesis with bone blocks for height restoration

Fractures of the Anterior Calcaneal Process

336. What ligament is often affected with anterior calcaneal process fractures?

336. Bifurcate ligament

337. This ligament runs between the calcaneus and what two structures?

337. Cuboid
Navicular

338. Nonoperative treatment is acceptable if what percentage of the articular surface is involved?

338. <25%

339. What does nonoperative treatment generally consist of?

339. WBAT in boot or cast

340. If >25% of the articular surface is involved, what are the two treatment options?

340. ORIF
Excision

Fractures of the Tarsal Bones and Associated Conditions

Cuboid Fracture and Subluxation

341. What is the ideal radiographic view for visualizing the cuboid?

341. 30-degree medial oblique view

342. For fractures of the cuboid, what is the goal of ORIF?

342. To restore at least 60% of the articular surface

343. What are the two components of the treatment for a crush injury to the cuboid?

343. Lateral plate
Bone graft

344. Crush injuries are often associated with what other traumatic condition?

344. Homolateral dislocation

345. What population is particularly at risk for cuboid subluxation?

345. Dancers with hypermobile joints

Navicular Avulsion Injuries

346. What is unique about the vascular supply to the navicular? Therefore?

346. Tenuous blood supply (especially central third)
Therefore, all periods of non-weight-bearing (NWB) are longer than would otherwise be expected

347. What is the preferred treatment for a nondisplaced fracture of the tuberosity?

347. 8 to 12 weeks of NWB

348. What are the two indications for operative treatment of navicular tuberosity injuries?

348. Posterior tibial tendon (PTT) avulsion
Displaced

349. What is a common postoperative complication?

349. Posttraumatic flatfoot

350. What is the nonoperative treatment for dorsal ligamentous avulsion?

350. 8 to 12 weeks of NWB immobilization

351. What is the goal of ORIF?

351. Restoration of at least 60% of the articular surface

352. For how long should a nondisplaced stress fracture be immobilized?

352. 6 weeks NWB immobilization

353. What is the preferred treatment of a displaced navicular stress fracture?

353. ORIF

354. Quick review: What is the treatment for Kohler's disease?

354. 6 weeks WBAT in a short leg cast

Accessory Navicular

355. What are the two components of the first-line treatment for a painful accessory navicular?

355. Nonsteroidal antiinflammatory drugs (NSAIDs)
Medial arch support

356. If refractory to these interventions, then what is the next step?

356. Trial of casting

357. If casting is unsuccessful, then what is the next step?

357. Excision of accessory navicular

358. In what patients should the posterior tibial tendon be advanced at the time of surgery?

358. Patients with flat feet

Lisfranc Injuries and Compartment Syndrome

359. What two structures does the Lisfranc ligament connect?

359. Medial cuneiform
Second metatarsal

360. Is the ligament stronger plantarly or dorsally?

360. Plantarly

361. What is a classic clinical sign of a potential Lisfranc injury?

361. Plantar ecchymoses

362. For what length of displacement is nonoperative treatment acceptable?

362. <2 mm

363. What does nonoperative treatment consist of?

363. NWB immobilization for 6 weeks

364. What are the two components of the classic pattern of screw fixation for a Lisfranc injury?

364. Retrograde screw from the first metatarsal into the medial cuneiform
Antegrade screw from medial cuneiform into the second metatarsal

365. With larger displacements, contact area decreases; subluxation in which direction is particularly problematic?

365. Dorsolateral

366. Are outcomes generally better if the injury is ligamentous or bony?

366. Bony

367. In general, screws can be safely removed at what point?

367. 5 months postoperatively

368. What percentage of Lisfranc injury patients develop posttraumatic arthrosis?

368. 25%

369. What is the treatment for posttraumatic arthrosis?

369. Lisfranc arthrodesis

370. What is the treatment for a chronic (missed acute) Lisfranc injury?

370. Lisfranc arthrodesis

Compartment Syndrome of the Foot

371. How many compartments are there in the foot?

371. Nine

372. What are the five major compartments?

372. Medial
Lateral
Central
Interosseous
Calcaneal

373. In what three areas should incisions be placed to release the compartments of the foot?

373. Longitudinal incision medially (to release abductor hallucis/deep compartment)
Between metatarsals 2 and 3
Between metatarsals 4 and 5

Fractures of the Metatarsals

374. What are the two operative indications for first metatarsal stress fractures?

374. Intraarticular displacement
Fracture opens on stress view

375. What does nonoperative treatment of first metatarsal fracture consist of?

375. 6 weeks in a short leg cast

376. What patient population is particularly at risk for metatarsal stress fractures?

376. Female runners

377. What metatarsals are most likely to sustain injury?

377. Second and third

378. In ballet dancers, where do stress fractures classically occur?

378. Base of the second metatarsal

379. With trauma, which structure can avulse from the base of the fifth metatarsal?

379. Lateral band of plantar fascia

380. What is the treatment of choice in that situation?

380. WBAT in cast

381. If a painful nonunion develops, what is a reasonable next step?

381. Pulsed electromagnetic field (PEMF) treatment

382. What is the treatment of choice for a nondisplaced Jones fracture?

382. NWB in a cast

383. In general, how successful is the nonoperative treatment of Jones fractures?

383. 50% succeed and 50% fail

384. How does the treatment differ for high-level athletes?

384. Early ORIF is preferred

385. What is the ideal intramedullary screw size for the treatment of a Jones fracture?

385. 4.5 mm

386. What factor contributes to the failure of operative treatment in athletes?

386. Return to activity too early

387. What is the preferred treatment for an acute diaphyseal stress fracture of the fifth metatarsal?

387. NWB in a cast

388. In which population is nonoperative treatment NOT recommended?

388. High-level athletes
Again, consider early ORIF

389. If sclerosis is noted on x-ray during nonoperative treatment, what is the treatment of choice?

389. ORIF and bone graft

Turf Toe and Sand Toe

390. What is the difference between turf toe and sand toe?

390. Turf toe is a metatarsophalangeal (MTP) joint dorsiflexion injury
Sand toe is a plantar flexion injury

391. If a dorsal MTP dislocation is easily reducible, what does it suggest?

391. The plantar plate has been damaged
MP joint is likely unstable

392. What radiographic finding is suggestive of plantar plate injury?

392. Proximal shift of the sesamoids

General Turf Toe Treatment Algorithm

393. What is the preferred treatment for turf toe with mild sprain?

393. Immediate return to play

394. What is the preferred treatment for turf toe with partial tear?

394. 2 weeks off from play
Tape in extension

395. What is the preferred treatment for turf toe with complete plantar plate injury?

395. Operative treatment

396. What are two additional operative indications for either turf toe or sand toe?

396. Associated intra-articular fracture
Significant instability

■ Arthritic and Prearthritic Conditions

Posterior Tibial Tendon (PTT) Insufficiency and Management

397. The PTT attaches to the midfoot and all of the metatarsals except?

397. First metatarsal

398. Where is the watershed area of blood supply within the PTT?

398. 2 to 3 cm distal to the tip of the medial malleolus

399. As the tibial tendon becomes insufficient, into which position does the forefoot fall?

399. Supinated

400. Into which position does the hindfoot fall?

400. Valgus

401. What other major structure may become tight?

401. Achilles tendon

402. What ligament becomes attenuated?

402. Spring ligament (also called plantar calcaneonavicular ligament)

403. What ligament becomes attenuated with rheumatoid arthritis involving the foot?

403. Talocalcaneal interosseous ligament

404. What are the clinical findings of stage I PTT dysfunction on attempted single leg rise?

404. Painful but possible

405. At this stage, what are the two nonoperative treatment options?

405. Walking boot
NSAIDs

406. If nonoperative treatment is unsuccessful, what is the operative treatment for stage I?

406. Tenosynovectomy

407. What is the clinical definition of stage II posterior tibial tendonitis?

407. Single leg rise is impossible
Flexible deformity of foot

408. What are the two treatment options for stage II?

408. Brace
FDL transfer with calcaneal osteotomy or lateral column lengthening

409. Calcaneal osteotomy versus lateral column lengthening: which is more effective? What has a higher nonunion rate?

409. Lateral column lengthening is more effective
Also has higher rates of nonunion

410. What are the four contraindications to FDL transfer for stage II PTT dysfunction?

410. Hypermobile patient
Neuromuscular disorder (e.g., Charcot-Marie-Tooth)
Obesity
Age >70 years

411. What is the key clinical finding of stage III PTT dysfunction?

411. Fixed deformity

412. What is the key clinical finding of stage IV?

412. Fixed deformity with arthritis

413. What is the preferred surgical treatment for stages III and IV?

413. Triple arthrodesis

414. If surgery is not possible, which braces may be helpful in stage III and IV dysfunction?

414. Ankle–foot orthosis (AFO) (stage III)
Arizona brace (stage IV)

415. What are the two components of the treatment for adolescent supple planovalgus unresponsive to conservative management?

415. Medial tightening
Lateral column lengthening

416. Rigid congenital pes planus is often secondary to what?

416. Middle facet coalition

417. If rigid congenital pes planus is recognized in adolescence, what is the first-line treatment?

417. Bracing

418. If bracing is unsuccessful, what does operative treatment consist of?

418. Resection of coalition or middle facet fusion

419. If these measures fail, then what is the next step?

419. Triple arthrodesis

420. In the adult patient, first-line treatment consists of what?

420. Bracing

421. If bracing is unsuccessful, operative treatment consists of?

421. Subtalar arthrodesis Or triple arthrodesis

Surgical Management of Ankle Osteoarthritis

Ankle Arthrodesis

422. What is the preferred position for ankle fusion?

422. 0 degrees dorsiflexion
5 degrees external rotation
5 degrees hindfoot valgus

423. What is the reported advantage of arthroscopic ankle fusion?

423. Decreased time to union

424. What is the disadvantage of arthroscopic ankle fusion?

424. Limited ability to correct deformity

425. In long-term outcomes after arthrodesis, what is the incidence of hindfoot arthritis?

425. Nearly all patients develop hindfoot arthritis

426. What is the incidence of knee arthritis?

426. No significant increase in knee arthritis rates

427. What is the satisfaction rate?

427. 80% at 7.5 years

Total Ankle Arthroplasty

428. The best ankle arthroplasty results have been reported in what three patient populations?

428. >60 years old
Rheumatoid arthritis
No prior surgery

429. Satisfaction is particularly poor if an arthrodesis is converted to a total ankle in what patient population?

429. Those with a painless arthrodesis

430. What is the rate of hindfoot arthritis development after total ankle arthroplasty?

430. <50%

Supramalleolar Osteotomy

431. What are the two indications for supramalleolar osteotomy?

431. Distal tibial malunion
Primary ankle arthritis

432. On follow-up arthroscopy, what histologic tissue type is noted?

432. Repair-type fibrocartilage

Subtalar Joint Arthritis

433. On tests, what key words indicate subtalar joint pain?

433. Sinus tarsi pain

434. What process must be excluded when evaluating subtalar joint symptoms?

434. Tarsal tunnel syndrome

435. What is the preferred treatment for subtalar arthritis with a flexible hindfoot?

435. Brace

436. What are two surgical options to address subtalar pathology?

436. Subtalar fusion
Triple arthrodesis

437. What are the six general indications for subtalar fusion?

437. Primary osteoarthritis of the subtalar joint
Calcaneus fracture
Stage II posterior tibial tendon dysfunction
Talocalcaneal coalition
Charcot-Marie-Tooth
Rheumatoid arthritis

438. What is the principal advantage of subtalar fusion over triple arthrodesis?

438. Decreased mechanical stress on the ankle

439. At which joint is the greatest loss of motion observed after subtalar fusion: calcaneocuboid or talonavicular?

439. Calcaneocuboid

440. Therefore, which joint must *not* be fused in association with a subtalar fusion?

440. Talonavicular joint

441. What are the six general indications for triple arthrodesis?

441. Osteoarthritis of multiple hindfoot joints
Posttraumatic osteoarthritis
Stage III posterior tibial tendon dysfunction
Fixed hindfoot deformity (as with late treatment for coalition or clubfoot)
Hindfoot instability
Rheumatoid arthritis

442. When performing a triple arthrodesis, what is the desired hindfoot position? Why?

442. 5 degrees valgus
Because unlocks the hindfoot

443. What is the desired forefoot position?

443. Plantigrade

444. What is the desired midfoot position?

444. 0 degrees abduction

445. How often does ankle arthritis develop after triple arthrodesis?

445. 100%

446. Is radiographic adjacent-joint degenerative joint disease (DJD) associated with clinical dissatisfaction after either procedure?

446. No

447. What is the most important factor in determining satisfaction after hindfoot fusion?

447. Postoperative alignment

448. What effect does hindfoot fusion have upon the knee?

448. May lead to increased rates of knee degeneration

449. Quick review: What fusion has not been shown to adversely affect the knee?

449. Tibiotalar

Osteoarthritis of the Foot

450. What four joints of the foot are most commonly affected by osteoarthritis?

450. First MTP joint
Naviculocuneiform joint
MT-cuneiform joint
Intercuneiform joints

451. Arthritic involvement at these joints may lead to what global change in the shape of the foot?

451. Collapsed arch

452. When treating osteoarthritis, what joints should *not* be arthrodesed?

452. Fourth and fifth metatarso-cuboid joints

453. Instead, what is the preferred treatment at those locations?

453. Partial resection with or without a spacer

Hallux Rigidus

454. What two metatarsal head shapes are particularly at risk for the development of hallux rigidus?

454. Flat
Chevron shape

455. What are the indications for cheilectomy on clinical exam and intraoperatively?

455. Negative axial grind test
>50% cartilage surface intact

456. What are the indications for MP arthrodesis on clinical exam and intraoperatively?

456. Positive axial grind test
<50% cartilage surface intact

457. What is the most stable construct for fusion?

457. Plate and compression screw

458. What is the Moberg cheilectomy variant?

458. Dorsal closing wedge osteotomy at the base of the proximal phalanx

Rheumatoid Arthritis and the Inflammatory Arthropathies

459. What joints of the foot are most commonly affected by rheumatoid arthritis?

459. MP joints

460. What are the three components of the sequence of progressive MP joint deterioration?

460. Dorsal subluxation
Claw toe deformity
Bursae develop under MT heads

461. What is the preferred position for first MTP arthrodesis?

461. 15 degrees valgus
10 degrees extension
Neutral rotation

462. What are the two components of the treatment if the hallux IP joint is unstable?

462. Resect the base of the proximal phalanx
Fuse the IP joint

463. What is the preferred position for IP joint arthrodesis?

463. 5 to 10 degrees plantar flexion

464. What are the two surgical options for rheumatoid MP disease of the lesser toes?

464. Weil osteotomy
Resection of proximal phalangeal head and neck

465. Does the hindfoot fall into varus or valgus with rheumatoid arthritis?

465. Valgus

466. Which ligament becomes attenuated?

466. Talocalcaneal interosseous ligament

467. Once the hindfoot deformity becomes rigid and degenerative, what are the two components of the necessary surgical treatment?

467. Triple arthrodesis
Lengthening of the Achilles tendon

Inflammatory Arthropathies and Associated Conditions

468. What two clinical findings are suggestive of psoriatic arthropathy?

468. Sausage toe
Nail pitting

469. What joint is most commonly involved? What is the associated radiographic appearance?

469. DIP joint most commonly involved
X-ray appearance: pencil-in-cup deformity

470. What are three examples of medications that may be helpful in the treatment of psoriatic arthritis?

470. NSAIDs
Sulfasalazine
Methotrexate (if severe)

471. With what three other foot and ankle conditions might such patients also present?

471. Anterior tibial tendon (ATT) tenosynovitis
Plantar fasciitis
Enthesopathies about the Achilles tendon

472. What population is most at risk for ATT tenosynovitis related to inflammatory arthritis?

472. Young males

473. What population is most at risk for ATT rupture?

473. Elderly

474. In general, what are the two components of the treatment for acute ATT rupture?

474. Walking cast for 6 weeks
AFO thereafter if necessary

475. If a significant functional deficit persists, consider which possible transfer?

475. EHL transfer

■ The Diabetic Foot

Ulcers and Osteomyelitis

476. What is the appearance of a Wagner stage 0 diabetic ulcer?

476. Erythema

477. What is the appearance of a Wagner stage I ulcer?

477. Superficial with subcutaneous tissue exposed

478. What is the appearance of a Wagner stage II ulcer?

478. Deeper structures exposed, but not bone

479. What is the appearance of a Wagner stage III ulcer?

479. Exposed bone with periosteal reaction

480. What is the appearance of a Wagner stages IV/V ulcers?

480. Gangrene

481. In general, what is the preferred treatment of Wagner stage 0, I, and II ulcers?

481. Total contact casting

482. What is the general treatment for Wagner stage III, IV, and V ulcers?

482. Surgical debridement and antibiotics

483. Parameters predictive of successful diabetic ulcer healing include which values of ankle-brachial index (ABI)?

483. Greater than 0.6

484. … of ankle pressure?

484. Greater than 70 mm Hg

485. … of toe pressure?

485. Greater than 40 mm Hg

486. … of transcutaneous oxygen pressure?

486. Greater than 40

487. For a diabetic with calcaneal osteomyelitis, is a below-knee amputation (BKA) necessary?

487. Partial calcanectomy is generally sufficient

Charcot

488. What are the two components of the clinical appearance of the acute phase of Charcot in a diabetic foot?

488. Red
Swollen

489. In what two ways can acute Charcot be differentiated from osteomyelitis?

489. Technetium and indium bone scans
Elevation test

490. What is the bone scan appearance of acute Charcot?

490. Cold (does not light up)

491. What is the preferred treatment for the acute phase of Charcot?

491. NWB total contact casting

492. What additional medical treatment might be considered?

492. Bisphosphonates (to minimize bone loss)

493. What must generally be avoided in the acute phase?

493. Do *not* operate in the acute phase

494. When should total contact casting be discontinued?

494. When the skin temperature is symmetric bilaterally

495. Is arthroplasty an option for treatment of Charcot joint?

495. No, it is contraindicated

6

Shoulder and Humerus

■ General Knowledge

Anatomy

Acromion

1. What are the four acromial centers of ossification?

    1. Basiacromion
       Mesoacromion
       Metaacromion
       Preacromion

2. How can you remember the order from the base to the tip?

    2. Alphabetical from base to tip

3. What is the most common location of an os acromiale?

    3. At the junction of meso- and meta-acromion

4. If an os acromiale is present, how often is it bilateral?

    4. 60% of the time

5. What is the indication for surgical treatment of os acromiale? How is it treated? What complication may develop despite treatment?

    5. Only if symptomatic
       If small: excise
       If large: open reduction and internal fixation (ORIF)
       Risk of nonunion with ORIF

6. How is acromial morphology classified?

    6. I: flat
       II: curved
       III: hooked

7. What radiographic study best visualizes acromial morphology?

    7. Supraspinatus outlet view

8. What type is associated with best outcomes for nonoperative treatment of impingement?

    8. I (flat)

9. What artery runs with the coracoacromial ligament?

    9. Acromial branch of thoracoacromial artery

10. Where is the glenoid blood supply the poorest?

    10. Anterosuperiorly

Shoulder

11. What are the borders of the quadrangular space?

   11. Superior: teres minor
       Inferior: teres major
       Medial: triceps
       Lateral: surgical neck of the humerus

12. What are the two contents of the quadrangular space?

   12. Posterior humeral circumflex artery
       Axillary nerve

13. What are the three borders of the triangular space?

   13. Teres minor
       Teres major
       Long head of triceps

14. What are the contents of the triangular space?

   14. Circumflex scapular vessels

15. What are the three borders of the triangular interval?

   15. Long head of triceps
       Teres major
       Humerus

16. What are the two contents of the triangular interval?

   16. Profunda brachii artery
       Radial nerve

17. Relative to the transverse scapular ligament, where does the suprascapular artery run?

   17. Above the ligament

18. Relative to the transverse scapular ligament, where does the suprascapular nerve run?

   18. Below the ligament

19. What is the innervation of the teres major?

   19. Axillary nerve

20. What is the innervation of the supraspinatus?

   20. Suprascapular nerve

21. What is the innervation of the deltoid?

   21. Axillary nerve

22. What is the innervation of the subscapularis?

   22. Upper and lower subscapular nerves

23. What is the innervation of the teres minor?

   23. Lower subscapular nerve

24. Relative to the humeral intertubercular groove, what is the position of the pectoralis major?

   24. Posterior

25. … of the latissimus dorsi?

   25. Floor of groove

26. … of the teres major?

   26. Anterior

27. What is the primary function of the latissimus dorsi?

   27. Shoulder extension

Capsular Ligaments

28. What is the origin of the superior glenohumeral ligament (SGHL)? What is the insertion?

   28. Origin: anterosuperior labrum
       Insertion: lesser tuberosity

29. In which arm position is the SGHL the primary restraint against external rotation and inferior translation?

   29. Adducted

30. What is the origin of the coracohumeral ligament? What are the two sites of the insertion? What is its function? What does the coracohumeral ligament provide restraint against?

30. Origin: lateral base of coracoid process
    Insertions: greater and lesser tuberosities
    Reinforces the capsule of the rotator interval
    Inferior translation and external rotation in adduction (same as SGHL)

31. What is the origin of the middle glenohumeral ligament (MGHL)? What is the insertion? Where is the MGHL seen arthroscopically?

31. Origin: inferior to SGHL
    Insertion: lesser tuberosity
    Crosses subscapularis from superomedial to inferolateral

32. The MGHL is the primary static restraint against external rotation in what arm position?

32. 45 to 60 degrees of abduction

33. What is the origin of the inferior glenohumeral ligament complex (IGHLC)? What is the insertion?

33. Origin: inferior labrum
    Insertion: anatomic neck of humerus

34. What are the three components of the IGHLC?

34. Anterior band
    Posterior band
    Axillary pouch

35. The IGHLC is the primary anterior stabilizer of the shoulder in what arm position?

35. 90 degrees of abduction
    Also provides resistance against inferior translation in this position

36. What band of the IGHLC resists humeral translation in abduction and external rotation?

36. Anterior

37. What band resists humeral translation in abduction and internal rotation?

37. Posterior

Humerus

38. When plating the humerus, the radial nerve is a key consideration. What is the safe distance vertically from the lateral epicondyle?

38. 14 cm

39. ... from the medial epicondyle?

39. 20 cm

40. ... from trochlea to spiral groove?

40. 13 cm

41. ... from trochlea to the site where radial nerve pierces intermuscular septum?

41. 7.5 cm

Surgical Approaches: Key Points

Shoulder

42. With shoulder arthroscopy, what is a common reason of interscalene block failure?

42. Inadequate anesthesia of T2 dermatome

43. What surgical site does this correspond to?

43. Posterior arthroscopy portal

44. An interscalene block administered at the time of surgery may also lead to palsy of what nerve?

44. Phrenic nerve

45. What is the lateral approach to the shoulder?

45. Deltoid splitting approach

46. How far distal to the acromion can the deltoid be safely split? Why?

46. No more than 5 cm
With further split, axillary nerve at risk

47. What is the interval for the posterior shoulder approach?

47. Infraspinatus
Teres minor

48. With the posterior approach, what should be avoided? Why?

48. Avoid dissecting below teres minor (within quadrangular space)
Axillary nerve and posterior humeral circumflex arteries at risk

49. With the deltopectoral approach, which vein is at risk?

49. Cephalic

50. Excessive medial retraction for exposure may injure what structure?

50. Musculocutaneous nerve

51. What two structures should be protected at inferior edge of subscapularis?

51. Axillary nerve
Anterior circumflex artery and veins

Humerus

52. For the anterolateral approach, what is the proximal interval?

52. Deltoid
Pectoralis major

53. What is the distal interval?

53. Brachialis split

54. Why does the distal approach work? What nerves supply the brachialis?

54. Brachialis is duly innervated
Musculocutaneous and radial nerves

55. For the posterior approach, what is the proximal interval?

55. Deltoid
Triceps

56. How much of the humerus can be accessed proximally?

56. Up to 8 cm

Distal Humerus

57. For the anterolateral approach to the distal humerus, what is the interval?

57. Brachialis
Brachioradialis

58. What structure is at risk?

58. Radial nerve

59. For the lateral approach to the distal humerus, what is the interval?

59. Brachioradialis
Triceps

60. Then how does the deeper dissection proceed?

60. Lift extensor carpi radialis longus and brevis (ECRL and ECRB) off
Work anterior to epicondyle and lateral collateral ligament (LCL)

Key Pitching Concepts

61. What are the five phases of throwing?

61. Windup
Cocking
Acceleration
Deceleration
Follow through

62. The highest shoulder rotatory torque, varus torque, compressive force, and shear force occur at what position? What phase does this correspond to?

62. Point of maximum shoulder external rotation
Between cocking and acceleration phases

63. During the acceleration phase, what two things happen at the shoulder in terms of kinetics?

63. Increase in shear force
Increase in flexion torque

64. The highest elbow compressive forces occur at what phase of throwing?

64. Deceleration

65. Maximum elbow valgus stress occurs at what phase?

65. Acceleration

66. What muscle has the greatest increase in electromyograph (EMG) activity during the early cocking phase?

66. Deltoid

67. What three muscles have the greatest increase in EMG activity during the late cocking phase?

67. Subscapularis
Infraspinatus
Teres minor

68. What four muscles have the greatest increase in EMG activity during the acceleration phase?

68. Pectoralis major
Latissimus dorsi
Serratus anterior
Lower extremity musculature

69. What two muscles have the greatest increase in EMG activity during the follow through?

69. Rotator cuff
Biceps

70. At the elbow, what function does the pronator serve during throwing?

70. Protects medial collateral ligament (MCL) from excessive valgus stress

71. With an insufficient MCL, what changes are seen in muscle activity during throwing: laterally versus medially?

71. Increased lateral activity
Decreased medial activity

Clinical Evaluation

Physical Examination: Special Tests

72. O'Brien's test is also called what? In which position is it performed? What is the key finding? What does it suggest?

72. Active compression test
10 degrees adduction, 90 degrees forward flexion, maximum pronation
Pain with resistance that is decreased when the arm is supinated back to neutral is suggestive of superior labrum from anterior to posterior (SLAP) tear

73. How is Speed's test performed? What can Speed's test help diagnose?

73. Resisted forward flexion in scapular plane
Pain suggests biceps pathology

74. How is the Yerguson test performed? What does a positive Yerguson test suggest?

74. Resisted supination
Pain suggests biceps pathology

75. How is the drop arm test performed? The shoulder position is similar to what other test? What does a positive drop arm test suggest?

76. How can the lower and upper subscapularis be tested relatively independently?

75. Maintain forward flexion in scapular plane
Like Speed's
Inability = supraspinatus lesion

76. Lower: lift off test
Upper: belly press test

Radiographic Evaluation

77. What is a Zanca view used for? What view should also be obtained in conjunction?

78. What is a West Point view used for?

79. What is a Stryker view used for? What view should also be obtained in conjunction?

77. Acromioclavicular (AC) joint pathology
Axillary view too

78. Bankart lesion

79. Hill-Sachs lesion
Also anteroposterior (AP) internal rotation view

■ Shoulder: Pathologic States

Shoulder Dislocation, Instability, and Management

Anterior Shoulder Dislocation

80. If a manual reduction of an anterior shoulder dislocation is required, one should also evaluate for what associated injury?

81. What are the two components of the ideal position for shoulder immobilization after reduction?

82. What is an important consideration when deciding duration of immobilization in an adult?

83. What is the most common complication associated with dislocation in a patient <20 years old?

84. What are the three most common complications in patients >40 years old?

85. Among adolescents, recurrent instability is likely a consequence of what two associated injuries?

86. Among adults, what is the likely cause of recurrent instability after dislocation?

87. Among the elderly, what is the likely cause of recurrent instability?

80. Bankart lesion

81. Adduction
External rotation

82. Shoulder stiffness

83. Recurrence

84. 35% associated rotator cuff tear
10 to 15% recurrence
8% axillary nerve palsy

85. Bankart lesion
Disrupted anterior band of inferior glenohumeral ligament complex (IGHLC)

86. Humeral avulsion of glenohumeral ligament (HAGL) lesion

87. Rotator cuff tear

Dislocation Associated with Greater Tuberosity Fracture (Two-Part Proximal Humerus Fracture)

88. With this fracture-dislocation, what post-reduction view should be obtained?

88. Axillary view

89. What are the indications for operative treatment of greater tuberosity fracture in the general population and in the overhead athlete?

89. General population: >5 mm displacement
Overhead athlete: consider surgery if >3 mm because of impingement risk

90. If the greater tuberosity is too osteopenic for screw fixation, what is the preferred alternative?

90. Nonabsorbable sutures passed through fracture fragment and rotator cuff tendon

91. If greater tuberosity is displaced >1 cm, what injury may also be present?

91. Rotator cuff tear

92. At what location does this injury generally occur?

92. Near the rotator interval

93. What are the two clinical consequences of an incompetent rotator interval?

93. Isolated rotator interval tear: posteroinferior instability
Large rotator interval tear with another cuff tear: superior head migration

94. What is the preferred treatment for rotator interval injury with greater tuberosity fracture?

94. Suture closure at the time of surgery
One to three sutures placed from lateral to medial

95. What are the two clinical consequences of a tight rotator interval?

95. Decreased inferior translation
Decreased posterior translation

96. What is the most commonly reported complication of operative treatment of a greater tuberosity fracture associated with shoulder dislocation?

96. Subacromial scarring

Surgery for Anterior Instability

97. What are the four reported advantages of arthroscopic treatment over open surgical techniques?

97. Increased postoperative external rotation
Decreased postoperative pain
Decreased morbidity
Improved cosmesis

98. What has been the classic advantage of open treatment?

98. Decreased recurrence
Recent work suggests techniques approaching equivalence

99. What are the two possible late complications of open treatment?

99. Subscapularis detachment
Bicipital subluxation

Chronic or Recurrent Anterior Dislocation

100. A closed reduction is very unlikely to be successful after how many weeks of dislocation?

100. 3

101. What is the treatment of Hill-Sachs lesion involving <25% articular surface at the time of open reduction?

101. Often do not require treatment
If shoulder remains unstable after reduction, perform infraspinatus transfer

102. What are the three options for a Hill-Sachs lesion involving 25 to 50% of the articular surface?

102. Disimpaction with bone grafting (injury <3 weeks old, good bone stock)
Allograft reconstruction (injury 3 or more weeks old, good bone stock)
Arthroplasty (poor bone stock or cartilage wear)

103. What is the option for a Hill-Sachs lesion if over 50% of the articular cartilage is involved?

103. Arthroplasty

104. Patients with what two anatomic characteristics are particularly likely to benefit from open and/or nonanatomic repair?

104. Engaging Hill-Sachs lesion
Inverted-pear–shaped glenoid

Posterior Instability

105. What are the two major components of the differential diagnosis for posterior shoulder pain?

105. Posterior instability
Internal impingement

106. How can internal rotation be used to help differentiate between the two conditions?

106. Increased internal rotation: posterior instability
Decreased internal rotation: posterior (internal) impingement

107. What two patient populations are classically at risk for posterior instability?

107. Football linemen
Patients with seizure disorders

108. What is the characteristic intraarticular finding in these patients?

108. Posterior labral detachment

Missed (Chronic) Posterior Dislocation

109. A closed reduction is very unlikely to be successful after how many weeks?

109. 4

110. What is the treatment of a reverse Hill-Sachs lesion involving <20% articular surface?

110. Often does not require treatment
If treatment necessary, consider subscapularis tendon transfer

111. What are the two components of the treatment of a reverse Hill-Sachs lesion involving 20 to 40% of the articular surface?

111. Lesser tuberosity transfer
Disimpaction grafting may be an option if injury <3 weeks and good bone stock

112. What is the treatment of a reverse Hill-Sachs lesion involving 40–50% of articular surface?

112. Allograft reconstruction

113. What is the treatment of a reverse Hill-Sachs lesion involving >50% articular surface?

113. Hemiarthoplasty or total shoulder if glenoid degenerative changes are present

114. What is the preferred position for postoperative immobilization? Why?

114. Slight external rotation/extension Relieves posterior capsular tension

115. What is the preferred rehabilitation approach for multidirectional instability or scapular dyskinesis?

115. Closed kinetic chain strengthening

116. What are the effects of thermal capsulorraphy on cell number?

116. Decreased

117. What are the effects of thermal capsulorraphy on tissue length?

117. Shortened

118. What are the effects of thermal capsulorraphy on stiffness?

118. Decreased

119. What are the effects of thermal capsulorraphy after 1 month?

119. Scar and new collagen form

120. How has this affected treatment?

120. Thermal capsulorraphy is no longer routinely used in the treatment of instability

Impingement Syndromes: Key Points

121. With subacromial impingement syndrome, what blood flow changes are seen in the critical zone?

121. Increased vascularity

Internal Impingement

122. What patient population is classically at risk for internal impingement?

122. Overhead athlete

123. What is the characteristic change seen in internal rotation with internal impingement?

123. Decreased

124. What are the other characteristic exam findings?

124. Posterior shoulder pain with external rotation and abduction

125. What are the two characteristic intraarticular findings of internal impingement?

125. Posterior superior labrum frayed Partial thickness articular-sided tear of infraspinatus

126. What is the first-line treatment of internal impingement?

126. Nonoperative rehabilitation

127. If nonoperative treatment is unsuccessful, what are the next two steps?

127. Arthroscopic repair of torn labrum or cuff Release posterior capsule to increase internal rotation

128. What nerve is at risk with a posterior capsular release?

128. Infraspinatus motor branch

129. If all else fails, what is the treatment of last resort? Goal?

129. Humeral derotation osteotomy Goal: decrease retroversion to approximately 30 degrees

130. What patients are particularly at risk for infraspinatus atrophy in the absence of a cyst?

130. Volleyball and baseball players

131. What is the treatment of choice for this condition?

131. Rehabilitation (nonoperative)

Rotator Cuff (RTC) Tear and Repair

132. What are the two classic radiographic findings suggestive of a cuff tear?

132. Greater tuberosity degenerative changes
Greater tuberosity osteolysis

133. Under what conditions does a rotator cuff tear affect shoulder joint reactive force (JRF)? How?

133. If tear extends beyond supraspinatus
Decreases JRF

134. As a rotator cuff deficient shoulder is abducted beyond 30 degrees, what change occurs in the relationship of the humerus to the glenoid?

134. Superior translation

135. Compare with shoulder with rotator cuff intact.

135. Contact area increases with increasing abduction

136. What is the natural history of untreated full-thickness tears?

136. 28% have increased in size after 5 years

137. What is the reported advantage of margin convergence?

137. Decreased strain in free margin of fixed rotator cuff

138. Co-planing the clavicle without resection may lead to what complication?

138. Increased postoperative acromioclavicular joint symptoms

139. When repairing a massive tear, what structure should also be repaired or preserved?

139. Coracoacromial ligament

140. What is the minimum rotator cuff repair healing time?

140. 8 to 12 weeks

141. Patients are generally released to unrestricted activity at what time period?

141. 6 months

142. What four factors are the primary preoperative determinants of tendon healing success after rotator cuff repair?

142. Size and retraction
Tissue quality
Chronicity
Degree of muscle atrophy

143. What organism has been implicated as one of the primary causes of infection after RTC repair?

143. *Propionibacterium acnes*

144. What is the primary goal of revision RTC surgery? What is not the goal?

144. Decreased pain
Not for regaining strength

Labral and Bicipital Pathology

145. What are the intraarticular features of a Buford complex?

145. Middle glenohumeral ligament complex (MGHLC) is cordlike and attached to superior labrum anterior to the biceps
Absent superoanterior labrum

146. Should an attempt be made to repair a Buford complex? Why?

147. What happens if a Buford complex "repair" is attempted?

148. How are SLAP lesions classified?

149. If conservative treatment fails, what is the operative treatment for each type?

150. Superior glenohumeral instability may be associated with what type of SLAP lesion?

151. If superior glenohumeral instability is present, what is the operative treatment of choice?

152. What muscle activity is seen within the long head of biceps when the elbow is immobilized?

153. What is bicipital subluxation generally indicative of?

154. What is the treatment of an isolated acute rupture of the proximal long head of the biceps tendon?

155. Compare the preferred treatment of chronically ruptured or degenerative biceps at time of rotator cuff surgery in younger versus older patient populations.

156. What are the two reported benefits of tenodesis?

Scapular Winging

157. What muscle is affected with a long thoracic nerve injury?

158. What is the characteristic mechanism of injury?

159. Does medial or lateral winging result from a long thoracic nerve injury?

160. What is the initial treatment?

---

146. No
It is a normal anatomic variant

147. Decreased shoulder external rotation

148. I: frayed
II: detached biceps anchor
III: bucket handle, biceps intact
IV: bucket handle into biceps tendon
V: SLAP and labral tear
VI: flap tear
VII: SLAP and capsule tear

149. I: debride
II: reattach biceps anchor
III: debride
IV: repair/tenodesis
V: repair
VI: debride
VII: repair

150. II

151. Fix SLAP lesion only

152. None

153. Subscapularis tear

154. Physical therapy is generally first-line treatment

155. Younger: tenodesis
Older: tenotomy

156. Improved cosmesis
Decreased cramping

157. Serratus anterior

158. Most are traction injuries

159. Medial

160. Observation for up to 18 months

161. If no recovery of function is seen, what is the surgical procedure of choice?

162. What muscle is affected with spinal accessory nerve injury?

163. What other nerve and muscle groups are commonly injured in association?

164. Does medial or lateral winging result from spinal accessory nerve injury?

165. If no recovery of function is seen, what is the surgical procedure of choice?

Winging as a Complication of Node Biopsy

166. Cervical node biopsy may result in injury to what nerve? What type of winging results?

167. Axillary node biopsy may result in injury to what nerve? What type of winging results?

Other Causes of a Stiff and Painful Shoulder

Internal Rotation Contractures

168. What is the likely etiology of decreased shoulder external rotation (ER) in adducted arm?

169. What is the likely etiology of decreased shoulder ER in abducted arm?

170. What is the operative treatment for either of the above conditions?

171. What is the likely etiology for decreased shoulder ER after anterior stabilization?

172. What is the operative treatment for this condition?

173. If the subscapularis ruptures after an anterior stabilization procedure and is irreparable, what is the next surgical intervention?

Adhesive Capsulitis

174. What is the expected long-term outcome of nonoperative treatment on pain?

175. What is the expected long-term outcome of nonoperative treatment on motion?

176. What patient population is particularly resistant to nonoperative treatment?

---

161. Pectoralis major transfer

162. Trapezius

163. Dorsal scapular nerve
     Rhomboids

164. Lateral

165. Levator scapulae and rhomboid transfer

166. Accessory nerve
     Lateral winging

167. Long thoracic nerve
     Medial winging

168. Rotator interval contracture

169. Anteroinferior contracture

170. Arthroscopic release

171. Overtightening of the subscapularis

172. Z-lengthening of subscapularis

173. Pectoralis transfer

174. Pain decreases

175. Motion remains limited relative to unaffected subjects

176. Diabetics

177. When should surgery be undertaken?

177. At 12 to 16 weeks if no improvement with conservative therapy

Calcific Tendonitis

178. What population is most likely to be affected by calcific tendonitis?

178. Females

179. What are the two phases of disease?

179. I: formative phase
II: resorptive phase

180. What is the characteristic appearance of phase I?

180. Homogeneous mass

181. What are the three characteristics of phase II?

181. Diffuse mass
Bursal rupture
Increased pain

182. What is the mainstay of calcific tendonitis treatment?

182. Nonoperative management

183. If no response is noted with nonoperative treatment, then what?

183. Excision

Pectoralis Major Disruption

184. In a young patient, what is the preferred treatment of a pectoralis major muscle belly tear?

184. Nonoperative, as fixation likely to be difficult

185. ... of a tendon avulsion?

185. Repair

■ Fractures and Other Disorders of Bone

Clavicle

186. What are the two poorly prognostic factors for nonoperative treatment of midshaft clavicle fractures?

186. Shortening >2 cm
Comminution

187. What is the Neer classification of lateral third clavicle fractures?

187. I: conoid, trapezoid ligaments intact
II: trapezoid intact to lateral fragment, conoid out to medial fragment
III: extension into AC joint

188. Of these, which type is least stable and has highest risk of nonunion?

188. II

189. When does the medial clavicular physis close? What is the clinical significance?

189. At 24 years of age
Prior to closure, apparent dislocation may actually be a physeal injury

190. A posterior sternoclavicular (SC) dislocation may be associated with what additional injury?

190. Tracheal compression

191. How should an acute posterior SC dislocation be treated?

191. Closed reduction if acute (<10 days) regardless of symptoms
Perform in operating room with chest prepped and draped and vascular support available

192. How is sternoclavicular arthritis refractory to nonoperative management treated?

192. Medial clavicular excision

193. What structures must be identified and protected during this procedure? Why?

193. Leave costoclavicular ligaments (especially posterior) Necessary for stability

Distal Clavicular Osteolysis

194. What are the two components of the initial treatment of distal clavicular osteolysis?

194. Sling and antiinflammatories Injections

195. If unresponsive to conservative management, then what is the operative treatment?

195. Distal clavicle resection

196. What structure must be identified and protected during this procedure? Why?

196. Posterosuperior AC joint capsule If injured, AP instability of the clavicle may result

197. If osteolysis is present bilaterally, what condition must be considered?

197. Hyperparathyroidism

Scapula and Glenoid

198. What are the two operative indications for scapular neck fractures (Ideberg types 3, 4, and 5)?

198. >1 cm displacement >40 degrees angulation

199. What is the preferred surgical approach?

199. Posterior (Judet) approach

200. How do reported operative and nonoperative outcomes of floating shoulder injury compare?

200. Equivalent, assuming individual injuries meet criteria for nonoperative treatment

201. What is the radiographic characteristic of a scapulothoracic dissociation?

201. Medial scapular border displaced laterally from spine

202. What structure is often injured in association?

202. Subclavian artery

203. What is the etiology of a snapping scapula?

203. Scapulothoracic crepitus

204. What are the two operative indications for glenoid fracture without scapular involvement?

204. Involvement of >25% articular surface Glenohumeral joint subluxation or instability

205. What is the preferred surgical approach?

205. Deltopectoral

206. What is the operative indication for a coracoid fracture?

206. >1 cm displacement

Proximal Humerus

207. What treatment for minimally displaced proximal humerus fracture results in the best outcome?

207. Early physical therapy and motion

208. Outcomes have been shown to be significantly worse if what associated injury is present?

208. Rotator cuff tear

209. What are the two components of the general treatment algorithm for a two-part surgical neck fracture?

209. Reduce
Assess stability

210. If unstable after reduction, what are the three treatment options?

210. Closed reduction and percutaneous pinning (CRPP)
Intramedullary (IM) nailing
Open reduction and internal fixation (ORIF)

211. What two structures are especially at risk with CRPP?

211. Axillary nerve
Posterior humeral circumflex artery

212. What condition is a relative contraindication to use of an IM nail?

212. Osteoporosis

213. For a four-part proximal humerus fracture, which structure must be protected with ORIF?

213. Anterior humeral circumflex artery

214. Why?

214. Minimize risk of avascular necrosis

215. What is the treatment for avascular necrosis with collapse?

215. Hemiarthroplasty

216. If treating a four-part fracture with a hemiarthroplasty, should cement be used or not?

216. Yes

217. What two factors have been shown to be associated with good surgical outcomes?

217. Early surgery (<14 days)
Anatomic reduction of tuberosity (10 mm below superior surface of head)

218. What salvage option exists if tuberosity nonunion develops?

218. Reverse shoulder prosthesis

Humeral Trauma: Surgical Approaches and Management

219. After open reduction and internal fixation of the humeral shaft, what is the weight-bearing status?

219. Weight bearing as tolerated (WBAT)

Antegrade Nailing of the Humeral Shaft

220. With proximal locking screws, what is the preferred trajectory?

220. Lateral to medial

221. What structure is at risk with this trajectory?

221. Axillary nerve

222. What structure would be at risk with an anteroposterior (AP) trajectory proximally?

222. Also axillary nerve

223. With distal locking screws, what is the preferred trajectory?

223. Anteroposterior

224. What structure is at risk with this trajectory?

224. Musculocutaneous nerve

225. What two structures would be at risk with a lateral-to-medial trajectory?

225. Lateral antebrachial cutaneous nerve
Radial nerve

226. When treating a humeral shaft nonunion, what is the preferred surgical approach?

226. Anterior

227. What are the two components of the surgical treatment of choice?

227. ORIF with compression plate
Extensive radial nerve release if necessary

■ Arthroplasty of the Shoulder

Preoperative Decision Making

228. When considering a total shoulder arthroplasty, it is critical to assess the glenoid. What is the best plain radiographic view for glenoid assessment?

228. Axillary view

229. What pattern of glenoid wear is typical of rheumatoid arthritis?

229. Central

230. What pattern of glenoid wear is typical of osteoarthritis?

230. Posterior

231. What effect does osteoarthritis have upon glenoid version?

231. Glenoid becomes retroverted

232. In what two ways can glenoid retroversion be corrected?

232. Anterior reaming
Posterior augmentation

233. What are two contraindications to glenoid resurfacing?

233. Cuff arthropathy
Glenoid worn to coracoid process

234. What percentage of osteoarthritic patients have true cuff arthropathy?

234. Only 5%

235. What is the clinical appearance of a "Milwaukee shoulder"?

235. Similar to that of rotator cuff arthropathy

236. What is the proposed etiology?

236. Hydroxyapatite and calcium phosphate deposition

237. In patients in whom glenoid resurfacing is contraindicated, what three options are available?

237. Hemiarthroplasty
Reverse prosthesis
Superior advancement of subscapularis and teres (close defect)

238. What is the optimal position for shoulder arthrodesis?

238. 30 degrees abduction
30 degrees flexion
30 degrees internal rotation

Key Concepts

239. What type of glenoid component has the best reported outcomes?

239. All-polyethylene

240. In what degree of version should the stem generally be placed?

240. 20 to 30 degrees retroversion

241. What intraoperative landmark can be used to approximate the correct version?

242. The stem should be placed into less retroversion if what occurs?

243. If a small supraspinatus tear is identified intraoperatively, is a total shoulder contraindicated?

244. Why is it important to dry the taper before placing the head on the neck?

245. During a total shoulder revision, should the glenoid component be removed or replaced?

246. What is a common asymptomatic finding at the glenoid on long-term radiographic followup?

241. Place fin of prosthesis just posterior to bicipital groove

242. The glenoid is left in retroversion

243. No
Total shoulder OK if only small supraspinatus tears

244. A wet head/neck taper decreases interface strength by 50%

245. Replaced

246. Increased lucency at the glenoid–cement interface

7

Elbow

■ General Knowledge

Anatomy

1. What is the normal elbow carrying angle for males? Females?
2. Through what two anatomic landmarks does the elbow center of rotation pass?
3. Relative to the coronoid, how far distal does the elbow capsule extend?
4. … does the brachialis insert?
5. … does the anterior branch of the medial collateral ligament (MCL) insert?
6. What is the relative distribution of load between the radius and ulna at the wrist?
7. … at the elbow?

8. Why is there a difference?
9. What are the three components of the clinical significance of the anconeus muscle?

Surgical Approaches to the Elbow

10. For the medial approach to the elbow, what is the proximal interval?
11. What is the distal interval?

12. For the anterior approach, what is the interval?
13. For what clinical situation is the anterior approach most commonly used?

1. Males: 7 degrees valgus
   Females: 13 degrees valgus
2. Centers of trochlea and capitellum
   Anteroinferior medial epicondyle

3. 6 mm distal

4. 11 mm distal
5. 18 mm distal

6. 80% radius
   20% ulna

7. 60% radius
   40% ulna
8. Interosseous membrane
9. Kocher approach
   Ulnar nerve compression
   Posterolateral rotatory instability

10. Brachialis
    Triceps
11. Brachialis
    Pronator teres
12. Brachialis
    Pronator teres
13. Pulseless type III supracondylar fracture

14. For the anterolateral approach, what is the proximal interval?

14. Brachialis
    Brachioradialis

15. What is the distal interval?

15. Brachioradialis
    Pronator teres

16. With this approach, how can the posterior interosseous nerve (PIN) be best protected?

16. Supinate the forearm

17. For the posterolateral approach, what is the interval?

17. Anconeus
    Extensor carpi ulnaris (ECU)

18. How can the PIN be protected with this approach?

18. Pronate the forearm

19. What approach is best for addressing a capitellar shear fracture?

19. Kocher

■ Trauma and Instability

Elbow Dislocation and Instability

Elbow Dislocation

20. To reduce a dislocated elbow, in what position should the forearm be held?

20. Supination

21. To maintain postreduction stability, in what position should the forearm be placed?

21. Pronated

22. For how long should the reduced elbow be immobilized?

22. Several days

23. What is the most common complication of a simple elbow dislocation?

23. Loss of terminal extension

Posterolateral Rotatory Instability (PLRI)

24. To test for PLRI, in what position should the elbow be held?

24. Hold the elbow supinated

25. What two loads should be applied?

25. Axial
    Valgus

26. In an unstable elbow, what happens with extension? With flexion?

26. Extension dislocates
    Flexion reduces

27. What muscle provides a secondary restraint against PLRI?

27. Anconeus

Complications of Dislocation

28. What percent of simple dislocations develop heterotopic ossification (HO)?

28. 3%

29. What percent of fracture dislocations develop HO?

29. 20%

30. Maximal recovery of motion is expected by what time?

30. 6 months

31. What is the functional elbow flexion-extension range of motion (ROM)?

31. 30 to 130 degrees

32. Indications for elbow contracture release include an elbow ROM of less than ____.

32. 40 to 105 degrees

33. What structure is at risk with contracture release?

33. Ulnar nerve

34. What is the recommended timing of elbow HO resection?

34. Within 6 months of fracture

35. What is the radiographic marker indicating when it is acceptable to excise the HO?

35. HO appears mature on plain radiographs

36. Are additional tests necessary?

36. No

Hinged Elbow Fixators for Instability

37. What are the three indications for applying a hinged fixator to an unstable elbow?

37. Persistently unstable despite ligamentous repair
Delayed treatment of stiff/dislocated elbow
Protect bony open reduction with internal fixation (ORIF) of coronoid, radial head, capitellum

Elbow Fractures

Distal Humerus

38. In ORIF for diaphyseal distal humeral fractures, in what two ways can the construct torsional stiffness be increased?

38. Longer plates and screws
Bicortical fixation

39. What is the treatment for a nondisplaced lateral column distal humerus fracture?

39. Cast in supination

40. What is the treatment for a nondisplaced medial column distal humerus fracture?

40. Cast in pronation

41. If the distal triceps is taken down for dissection, how should it be repaired?

41. Suture through transosseous tunnels

42. What are the two most common complications associated with distal humeral ORIF?

42. Decreased elbow ROM
Ulnar nerve injury

Radial Head

43. What ligamentous structure is commonly injured with radial head fracture?

43. MCL

44. What nerve is most commonly injured?

44. Posterior interosseous nerve

45. When planning treatment for a radial head fracture, patients with what distal injury must be excluded? Why?

45. Essex-Lopresti lesion
Contraindication to radial head excision without prosthetic replacement

46. Must also check for what associated bony injury? Why?

46. Coronoid fracture
Component of "terrible triad" injury
Contraindication to radial head excision without prosthetic replacement

47. If there are no contraindications to excision, can a partial excision of the radial head be performed?

47. No
Radial head excision must be "all or none"

Olecranon

48. To maintain the stability of the elbow, what percent of the olecranon must be intact?

48. 30%

49. What is the ideal fracture pattern for use of a tension band?

49 Transverse

50. What are the three indications for plate fixation?

50. Comminuted
Distal to coronoid
Oblique fracture pattern

Coronoid

51. To maintain elbow stability, what percent of the coronoid must be intact?

51. 50%

52. Therefore, what is the indication for coronoid ORIF?

52. >50% coronoid involved

53. A coronoid fracture may be a marker of what condition?

53. Posteromedial rotatory instability (PMRI)

54. What is the preferred surgical approach to address coronoid fracture?

54. Dissect between two heads of the flexor carpi ulnaris (FCU)

Capitellum

55. What is a Hahn-Steinthal injury?

55. Capitellar fracture fragment consists of bone and cartilage

56. How is it treated?

56. ORIF

57. What is a Kocher-Lorenz injury?

57. Capitellar fracture fragment consists of cartilage

58. How is it treated?

58. Excision

Monteggia Fracture

59. What is the definition of a type I Monteggia fracture?

59. Fracture apex anterior
Anterior radial head dislocation

60. What is the definition of a type II Monteggia fracture?

60. Fracture apex posterior
Posterior radial head dislocation

61. What is the definition of a type III Monteggia fracture?

62. What is the definition of a type IV Monteggia fracture?

63. In what position should the elbow be casted after ORIF of Monteggia type I?

64. … type II?

65. How can a Monteggia fracture be differentiated from a transolecranon fracture/dislocation?

66. What is the primary stabilizer of the PRUJ?

61. Metaphyseal fracture
    Lateral dislocation

62. Radius and ulna fractures
    Anterior dislocation

63. 110 degrees of flexion

64. 70 degrees flexion

65. In a transolecranon fracture, proximal radioulnar joint (PRUJ) remains intact

66. Annular ligament

Distal Biceps Pathology

67. What is the long-term outcome of an unrepaired distal biceps rupture on flexion strength?

68. Supination strength?

69. What two nerves are at risk with distal biceps repair?

70. What is the theoretical advantage of a one-incision repair?

71. What is the theoretical advantage of a two-incision repair?

72. What is the main disadvantage of a two-incision repair? Especially if what?

73. How can a two-incision repair be modified to minimize risk of HO?

74. What is a positive prognostic factor for postoperative return to function after distal biceps repair?

75. What is a general rule of thumb concerning restoration of strength with a distal biceps repair of the dominant arm?

67. Flexion strength nearly restored

68. Remains significantly diminished
    Patients complain particularly of supination fatigue

69. Lateral antebrachial cutaneous nerve
    Radial nerve

70. Less dissection, so lower risk of heterotopic ossification (HO)

71. Less risk of injury to the posterior interosseous nerve

72. Increased risk of HO
    Especially if the ulna is exposed subperiosteally

73. Avoid subperiosteal dissection at ulna
    Use a muscle splitting approach for the second incision

74. Dominant arm involvement

75. Can restore strength to that of the nondominant arm

Overuse Syndromes

76. What group of patients is classically at risk for capitellar osteochondritis dissecans (OCD)?

77. What is the principal determinant of how an OCD lesion is treated?

78. Besides the capitellum, OCD can also affect what bony structure?

76. Adolescent athletes

77. Stage of the lesion

78. Radial head

79. What is the definition of Panner's disease?

79. Capitellar osteochondrosis

80. What age group is at risk for Panner's disease?

80. Young

81. Are outcomes of Panner's disease generally good or poor?

81. Good

82. What is Little Leaguer's elbow?

82. Medial epicondyle stress fracture

83. What is the first-line treatment for this condition?

83. No throwing for 3 months

84. What are the three operative indications?

84. >10 mm displacement
Medial epicondyle displaced into elbow joint
Failure of nonoperative treatment

85. Is excision of the medial epicondyle an acceptable treatment?

85. No!

Medial Collateral Ligament Injury

86. In what position should the elbow be held to test the integrity of the MCL?

86. 20 degrees flexion

87. If an MCL rupture is left untreated in an overhead athlete, where does arthritis often develop?

87. Radiocapitellar joint

88. Where does the olecranon impinge?

88. Posteromedially

89. Therefore, what are the two observed degenerative changes?

89. Posteromedial olecranon osteophyte
Medial olecranon fossa wear

Epicondylitis

90. What is the provocative test for golfer's elbow (medial epicondylitis)?

90. Increased pain with resisted wrist flexion and pronation

91. What is the provocative test for tennis elbow (lateral epicondylitis)?

91. Cozen's test
Pain at lateral epicondyle with resisted wrist dorsiflexion

92. With golf, the lead arm usually suffers from what condition?

92. Lateral epicondylitis

93. The trailing arm suffers from what condition?

93. Medial epicondylitis

94. What is the characteristic pathologic change seen with lateral epicondylitis?

94. Angiofibroblastic hyperplasia

95. What pathology is characteristic of Morton's neuroma?

95. Perineural fibrosis with nerve degeneration (Renaut bodies)

■ Elbow Arthroscopy

96. What arthroscopy portal should be made first?

96. Anterolateral

97. How can iatrogenic injury best be prevented?

97. Distend joint with fluid prior to portal creation

98. What are the traditional anterolateral portal landmarks?

99. What two structures are at risk with this portal?

100. What are the landmarks for the anteromedial portal?

101. What two structures are at risk with this portal?

102. What are the landmarks for the posterolateral portal?

103. What structure is inadequately visualized from inside the joint?

104. Where do most MCL tears occur?

105. What are the two most common complications of elbow arthroscopy?

98. 1 cm anterior
3 cm distal to lateral epicondyle

99. Radial nerve
Lateral antebrachial cutaneous nerve

100. 2 cm distal
2 cm anterior to medial epicondyle

101. Medial antebrachial cutaneous nerve
Median nerve

102. 3 cm proximal to olecranon
Just lateral to triceps

103. MCL

104. Distally

105. Persistent drainage from portals
Transient ulnar nerve neuropraxia

Elbow Arthroplasty

106. What is the procedure of choice for primary osteoarthritis?

107. What is the procedure of choice for rheumatoid arthritis and posttraumatic arthritis in a young patient? What about arthrodesis?

108. What is the procedure of choice for the elderly rheumatoid or posttraumatic patient?

109. What is another common indication for total elbow arthroplasty? Why?

106. Outerbridge Kashiwagi (ulnohumeral arthroplasty)

107. Interposition arthroplasty
Arthrodesis is not generally a good option

108. Total elbow arthroplasty

109. Elderly patients with comminuted elbow fractures
ORIF is not a great option because of osteopenia, limited distal fixation

Ulnohumeral Arthroplasty (Outerbridge-Kashiwagi)

110. What two steps does the Outerbridge-Kashiwagi procedure consist of?

111. What are the two classic indications?

112. Of these, which is most important?

113. If ROM is severely limited, what procedure should be performed concurrently?

110. Excise olecranon tip
Drill out olecranon fossa

111. Degenerative arthritis
Pain on terminal extension and flexion

112. Degenerative arthritis

113. Ulnar nerve decompression

Total Elbow Arthroplasty

114. Successful use of an unlinked elbow prosthesis requires what clinical situation?

115. What is the principal complication of unlinked prostheses?

114. Bone and ligaments are in good condition

115. Instability

116. What complication is associated with a lateral approach?

117. What is the principal complication of a linked total elbow?

118. What are the overall outcomes of linked versus unlinked total elbow arthroplasties?

116. Increased risk of ulnar nerve dysfunction

117. Mechanical failure

118. Equivalent

8

Hand, Wrist, and Forearm

■ Surgical Anatomy: Key Points

Hand Anatomy

1. Where are the two ossification centers of the second through fifth metacarpals located?

   1. Body (ossifies at 8 weeks)
      Neck (ossifies at 3 years)

2. How is the first metacarpal ossification center unique?

   2. Ossification center at the base (like phalanx)

3. What two intrinsic muscles are responsible for flexion at the metacarpophalangeal (MCP) joints?

   3. Interossei (IO)
      Lumbricals

4. What two muscles are responsible for flexion of the proximal interphalangeal (PIP) joints?

   4. Flexor digitorum superficialis (FDS)
      Flexor digitorum profundus (FDP)

5. What muscle is responsible for flexion of the distal interphalangeal (DIP) joints?

   5. FDP

6. What intrinsic muscles are innervated by the ulnar nerve?

   6. Third and fourth lumbricals
      All volar interosseous muscles
      All dorsal interosseous muscles
      Adductor pollicis
      Deep head flexor pollicis brevis
      All four hypothenar muscles

7. What structures are responsible for extension at the MCP joints?

   7. The extensor digitorum communis (EDC)

8. What structures are responsible for extension at the PIP joints?

   8. Intrinsic muscles (through the lateral bands)
      Central slip of the EDC

9. What structures are responsible for extension at the DIP joints?

   9. Terminal tendon of the EDC

10. What structures span between extensor tendons?

    10. Juncturae tendinum

11. What is the origin of the opponens digit quinti? What is the insertion? What is the function?

    11. Origin: hook of hamate
        Insertion: ulnar fifth metacarpal
        Function: adduct and flex the fifth metacarpal

12. How many dorsal interossei are there?
13. On which digits are they located?

14. What dorsal interosseous muscle does not have two muscle bellies?
15. Do dorsal interossei abduct or adduct?
16. How many palmar interossei are there?
17. On which digits are they located?

12. Four
13. Radial aspect of index finger
    Radial and ulnar aspects of long finger
    Ulnar aspect of ring finger
14. Third dorsal IO

15. Abduct
16. Three

17. Situated toward the midline on:
    Index finger—ulnar aspect
    Ring finger—radial aspect
    Small finger—radial aspect

Lumbricals

18. How many lumbricals are there?
19. Origin?
20. Insertion?
21. Innervation?

18. Four
19. FDP tendon
20. Radial lateral band
21. Ulnar nerve (two): bipennate
       lumbricals
    Median nerve (two): unipennate
       lumbricals

22. What is the relationship of the lumbricals to the transverse intermetacarpal (IM) ligaments?
23. In what hand deformity do lumbricals play a key role?
24. What is the classic symptomatic description of this syndrome?
25. Why does paradoxical extension occur?

22. Lumbricals pass volar to transverse IM ligament
23. Lumbrical plus hand

24. Paradoxical extension of the PIP with actual digital flexion
25. A transected FDP tendon retracts with active flexion
    Lumbrical is drawn proximally by retracting FDP
    Lumbrical pulls on the lateral band
    PIP extension results

26. What is the preferred treatment of chronic lumbrical plus hand?
27. What two structures form the lateral bands?

26. Lumbrical release from FDP origin
27. (Dorsal/volar) interosseous muscles
    Lumbricals (attached to the radial lateral bands)

Relationships Between Structures in the Hand

28. Is Cleland's ligament dorsal or volar relative to Grayson's?

28. Cleland: dorsal
    Grayson: volar

29. What is the relationship of the digital nerves to the digital arteries in the digit?

29. Nerve volar to artery in digit

30. What is the relationship of the digital nerves to the digital arteries in the palm?

30. Nerve dorsal to artery in palm

Deep Arch of the Hand

31. What artery provides the principal supply to the deep palmar arch?

31. Radial

32. Is the deep arch relatively proximal or distal to the superficial palmar arch?

32. Proximal

33. The deep arch is codominant with the superficial arch in what percentage of patients?

33. 21.5%

34. Between which two bones does the radial artery course to pass from the dorsal to the volar hand?

34. Between the base of the first and second metacarpals

35. The deep arch is complete in what percentage of patients?

35. 98.5%

36. The superficial arch is complete in what percentage of patients?

36. 78.5%

Wrist Anatomy

37. What carpal bone is the first to ossify?

37. Capitate

38. What are the next to ossify (in order)?

38. Hamate
Triquetrum
Lunate
Scaphoid

39. What is the last carpal bone to ossify?

39. Pisiform

40. At what age?

40. Around 9 years

41. At which articulation does the majority of wrist flexion occur?

41. Radiocarpal joint (two thirds)

42. Where does the remainder of wrist flexion occur?

42. Intercarpal joint (one third)

43. Are the radiocarpal ligaments stronger volarly or dorsally?

43. Volarly

44. Are the scapholunate ligaments stronger volarly or dorsally?

44. Dorsally

45. Are the lunotriquetral ligaments stronger volarly or dorsally?

45. Volarly

46. What is the importance of the radioscapholunate (RSL) ligament (ligament of Testut)?

46. Serves as a vascular conduit supplying the SL ligament

47. What are the contents of each of the six compartments of the wrist?

47. First: APL, EPB (abductor pollicis longus, extensor pollicis brevis)
Second: ECRL, ECRB (extensor carpi radialis longus and brevis)
Third: EPL (extensor pollicis longus)
Fourth: EDC, EIP (extensor digitorum communis, extensor indicis proprius)
Fifth: EDM (extensor digiti minimi)
Sixth: ECU (extensor carpi ulnaris)

48. What structure in the first compartment may have multiple slips (important if release needed)?

48. APL

49. In which compartment is the PIN (posterior interosseous nerve) located?

49. Floor of the fourth compartment

Relationships Between Structures at the Wrist

50. What is the relationship between the EIP and EDC of the index finger?

50. EIP is ulnar to EDC of the index finger

51. What is the relationship between the EDM and EDC of the small finger?

51. EDM is ulnar to EDC of the small finger

52. What is the relationship between EPL and EPB?

52. EPL ulnar to EPB

53. What is the relationship between ECRB and ECRL?

53. ECRB is ulnar to ECRL

Forearm Anatomy

54. What are the compartments of the forearm?

54. Volar
Dorsal
Mobile wad

55. With a compartment syndrome, the greatest degree of injury occurs where?

55. Deep

Vascular Supply

56. The brachial artery contributes to what distal arteries?

56. Radial and ulnar arteries

57. What artery (radial/ulnar) is the origin of the interosseous arteries?

57. Ulnar artery

58. What percentage of the population has a persistent median artery?

58. 10%

Surgical Approaches to the Radius

59. The proximal volar Henry approach is between what two muscle groups?

59. PT (pronator teres)
BR (brachioradialis)

60. The distal volar Henry approach is between what two muscle groups?

60. BR
Flexor carpi radialis (FCR)

61. The proximal dorsal approach is between what muscle groups?

61. EDC
ECRB

62. The distal dorsal approach is between what muscle groups?

62. ECRB
EPL

■ Flexor and Extensor Tendon Anatomy, Injury, and Repair

Acute Flexor Tendon Injury

Relevant Anatomy

63. Flexor tendon blood supply is via vincula entering (dorsally or volarly?

63. Dorsally

64. By what methods are tendons nourished?

64. Synovial nutrition
Longitudinal intertendinous vessels
Vessel branches in vincula

65. This process of synovial nutrition is also known as what?

65. Imbibition

66. The two terminal slips of FDS join at what location?

66. Camper's chiasm

67. What structure passes over this point?

67. FDP

68. What is the relationship of the FDP to the FDS at all locations except at Camper's chiasm?

68. FDP deep to FDS in the palm and digits except at Camper's chiasm

69. What pulleys are considered critical to normal finger function? Why?

69. A2
A4
These are the most critical for preventing flexor tendon bow-stringing

70. What pulleys are located over the joints of the digits?

70. A1
A3
A5

71. When exposing the PIP volar plate, what pulleys can be sacrificed safely?

71. Distal part of C1
Entire A3
Proximal part of C2

72. What are the zones of flexor tendon injury?

72. I: distal to FDS insertion (FDP only)
II: from A1 pulley (both FDP and FDS, "no-man's land") to FDS insertion
III: proximal to A1 pulley distal to carpal tunnel
IV: within carpal tunnel
V: wrist/forearm

Management of Acute Injury

73. What is the treatment for flexor tendon injury involving <25% tendon diameter?

73. Trim torn fragment

74. What is the treatment for injury involving 25 to 50% of tendon diameter?

74. Epitenon repair

75. What is the treatment for injury involving over 50% of tendon diameter?

76. Clinically obvious bow-stringing suggests what associated injuries?

77. What are the three flexor tendon healing phases, and characteristics of each?

78. At which time point is the repair weakest?

79. The majority of the repaired tendon strength returns by what time?

80. When is the maximum strength of the repair achieved?

81. What is the most important factor in determining strength of repair?

82. The addition of epitendinous suture increases repair strength by how much?

83. Is there a reported advantage to pulley release at the time of flexor tendon repair?

84. Rehabilitation protocols emphasize what type of motion?

85. If an active motion rehabilitation program is planned, how many crossing suture strands are necessary?

86. What are the two general types of rehabilitation protocols?

87. What is the classic position for hand and wrist splinting after flexor tendon repair?

88. What is the advantage of a continuous passive motion (CPM) device postoperatively?

89. What is the frequency of symptomatic flexor tendon adhesions at 3 months after repair?

90. What clinical exam findings are suggestive of postoperative tendon adhesions?

91. What is the reported advantage of antiadhesion gel application?

75. Core and epitenon repair

76. Flexor tendon sheath disruption likely involving A2 and A4 pulleys

77. Inflammatory (days, 0 to 5): minimal strength, suture imparts tendon repair strength
Fibroblastic (day 5 to 3–6 weeks): increasing strength, fibroblasts proliferate
Remodeling (>day 28): collagen cross-linking

78. Days 6 to 12 (end of inflammatory phase)

79. 28 days (end of fibroblastic phase)

80. 6 months (end of remodeling phase)

81. Number of crossing core suture strands

82. 50%

83. Increased tendon excursion

84. Patient-controlled passive motion

85. At least six strands

86. Duran (active extension, patient flexes passively)
Kleinert (active extension, dynamic splint flexes passively)

87. Wrist flexed 30 degrees
Metaphalangeals (MCPs) flexed 70 degrees

88. Decreased rate of adhesions
Maintains joint motion

89. 50% of patients require tenolysis at 3 months

90. Full passive range of motion (ROM)
Decreased active ROM

91. Improved active PIP motion

92. Has polyvinyl alcohol been shown to be effective against adhesions?

92. No, increases risk of rupture

93. Repairs rupture most commonly at what location?

93. Knot

94. Rupture is most often secondary to what?

94. Gap formation

Flexor Pollicis Longus Injury

95. What two pulleys are most important?

95. Oblique
A1

96. Is early motion advocated after flexor pollicis longus (FPL) repairs?

96. No

97. Why not?

97. Because FPL rupture rate is up to 20% (versus 2 to 5% for other digits)

Rugger Jersey Finger (FDP Avulsion)

98. What is the most commonly affected finger?

98. Ring finger

99. If the avulsed FDP remains attached to a bony fragment, to what location does it commonly retract?

99. A4 pulley

100. What is the treatment method of choice for an FDP avulsion with an attached fracture fragment?

100. Open reduction with internal fixation (ORIF) of fragment

101. If no fracture fragment is attached, what is the most important consideration in planning tendon repair and why?

101. Location of the retracted tendon
Dictates the timing of the repair

102. What is the timing for repair of an avulsed FDP retracted all the way to the palm? Why?

102. Repair within 7 to 10 days
Because vascular supply to retracted tendon is poor

103. If FDP retracts only to the PIP joint, what is the recommended timing of repair? Why?

103. Within 3 months (does not need to be as acute)
Because vincula are intact

Chronic Flexor Tendon Rupture

104. If a patient has a chronic FDP rupture but the FDS is intact, what are the three general treatment options?

104. No treatment
Fusion of the DIP joint
Flexor tendon grafting

105. If a flexor tendon reconstruction is necessary for chronic rupture, what are the three general tendon graft options?

105. Palmaris longus (PL)
Plantaris tendon
Toe extensor

106. If a Hunter rod is used in the first stage of reconstruction, when is the definitive repair to be performed?

106. ≥3 months after 1st stage

Trigger Finger

107. What tendon is involved in the development of trigger thumb?

107. FPL

108. At what pulley does triggering occur?

108. A1 pulley

109. What percentage of patients respond to initial steroid injection?

109. 60%

Infantile Trigger Thumb

110. How often is the condition bilateral?

110. 25 to 33%

111. What percentage of cases with infantile trigger thumb will spontaneously resolve with observation?

111. 30%

112. What is the preferred treatment if it fails to resolve by age of 1?

112. Surgical release

113. How does infantile trigger finger surgery differ from that of the adult?

113. Must release and explore beyond the A1 pulley

114. What is the preferred direction of incision?

114. Transverse

115. What is the greatest risk of infantile trigger thumb surgery?

115. Radial digital nerve injury at the thumb

Extensor Tendon Pathology

116. Odd-numbered extensor tendon zones lie over what anatomic structures?

116. Joints

117. Even-numbered extensor tendon zones lie over what anatomic structures?

117. Bony shafts

118. What is the preferred rehabilitation for injuries between MCP (zone 5) and forearm (zone 9)?

118. Early motion on postoperative day (POD) 3 in a dynamic splint

Mallet Finger

119. How is mallet finger treated?

119. Volar extension splint (e.g., Stack splint)

120. Despite immobilization of the DIP, what should rehabilitation include?

120. Emphasize motion of PIP

121. A chronically untreated mallet finger may lead to what clinical condition?

121. Swan-neck deformity

122. What subset of mallet finger injuries requires surgery?

122. Bony mallet avulsion fractures with volar subluxation of the DIP joint
Relative surgical indication is a surgeon with a mallet finger who wants to return to work

Sagittal Band Injuries

123. What is the role of the sagittal band?

123. Facilitates extension of the MP joint

124. What is the most common mechanism of sagittal band rupture?

124. Resisted flexion injury

125. What digit is most commonly affected?

125. Long finger

126. What is the classic presenting complaint?

126. Cannot actively extend
Can maintain active extension

127. If sagittal band rupture is <2 weeks old, how is it generally treated?

127. Extension splint of metacarpophalangeal joint (MCP) with interphalangeal (IP) joints free

128. If more than 2 weeks old, how is it generally treated?

128. Extensor centralization procedure

■ Fractures and Dislocations of the Hand and Digits

Carpometacarpal Joint

Thumb

129. With thumb pinch, where are the greatest forces experienced?

129. Carpometacarpal (CMC) joint

130. What four ligamentous structures contribute to CMC joint stability?

130. Anterior oblique ligament (AOL)
Dorsoradial capsule
Posterior oblique ligament
Intermetacarpal ligament

131. Of these, which is considered the most important for CMC stability?

131. AOL

132. How can a radiographic stress view be obtained to evaluate stability?

132. Anteroposterior (AP) view with both thumbs radially abducting against each other

133. With chronic AOL disruption, what happens at the CMC joint?

133. Metacarpal base subluxates dorsally

134. Dorsal CMC subluxation may be associated with what process at the MP joint?

134. Compensatory hyperextension at the MP joint

135. If MP hyperextension is present, what is the preferred intervention at the MP joint?

135. Capsulodesis or arthrodesis to correct

136. In what direction do degenerative changes occur at the CMC joint?

136. Volar to dorsal

137. Degeneration at what other site is a contraindication to CMC arthrodesis?

137. Scaphoid-trapezium-trapezoid (STT) arthritis

138. In older patients, what is the most common procedure for diffuse CMC arthritis?

138. Trapezium excision with or without ligament interposition

139. What are the disadvantages of resection arthroplasty for CMC arthritis?

139. Weakness with pinch
Thumb shortening
Decreased ability to adduct thumb

140. Quick review: in what fracture does the deep anterior oblique ligament (palmar beak ligament) also play a key role?

140. Anterior oblique ligament is the primary restraint in a Bennett's fracture
Anterior oblique ligament anchors volar lip of metacarpal to tubercle of the trapezium; small volar lip fragment remains attached to anterior oblique ligament, which is attached to trapezium

141. What tendon provides the primary displacing force with a Bennett's fracture?

141. Abductor pollicis longus

Other Digits

142. What is the ideal radiographic view for identifying fourth/fifth carpometacarpal dislocations?

142. 30 degree pronated view

Metacarpophalangeal and Interphalangeal Joints

Thumb Metaphalangeal Ulnar Collateral Ligament Injuries

143. Does the ulnar collateral ligament (UCL) generally avulse proximally or distally?

143. Distally

144. What two clinical findings are suggestive of thumb UCL ligament injury?

144. Over 45 degrees opening on stress of UCL
Over 15 degrees of side-to-side difference

145. How is the accessory UCL tested in isolation?

145. Stress in full extension

146. How is the proper UCL tested in isolation?

146. Stress in 30 degrees of flexion

147. What is a Stener lesion?

147. The distal edge of the ulnar collateral ligament displaces superficial and proximal to the adductor aponeurosis. It becomes lodged between the adductor pollicis aponeurosis and its normal position. It is clinically significant because it will have persistent instability due to lack of healing. It is an indication for surgery.

148. What structure is interposed in a Stener lesion and prevents the UCL from healing?

148. Adductor pollicis aponeurosis

Metacarpophalangeal Arthrodesis

149. The greatest MCP wear occurs with what hand motion?

149. Grasping

150. What is the optimal position for thumb MP joint arthrodesis in flexion, pronation, and abduction?

150. 10 degrees flexion
10 degrees pronation
 0 degrees abduction

Collateral Ligament Injury Metacarpophalangeal Joint

151. What is the preferred treatment for simple (partial) tear?

151. Buddy tape to adjacent digit for 3 weeks

152. What is the preferred treatment for complete tear?

152. Buddy tape to adjacent digit for 6 weeks

153. Operative intervention is indicated for what situation? Why?

153. Complete tear of radial collateral ligament (RCL) of index PIP joint
Surgery restores stability in pinch

154. What is the most likely diagnosis in a patient with acute loss of active and passive MCP motion but with a PIP that remains mobile?

154. Catching and locking of the collateral ligament on an osteophyte

155. What is the preferred initial treatment if reducible?

155. Reduce and observe

156. What is the preferred treatment if irreducible?

156. Surgical excision of the cause of collateral ligament catching (e.g., osteophyte, joint debridement)

Dorsal Dislocation of the Proximal Interphalangeal Joint without Fracture

157. Interposition of what structure may result in an incomplete reduction?

157. Volar plate

158. With dorsal dislocations, does the volar plate generally avulse proximally or distally?

158. Distally

159. What is the treatment if a stable reduction is achieved?

159. Early active motion

160. What if the reduction remains unstable?

160. Extension block splint

161. If untreated, what long-term complication may develop?

161. Swan-neck deformity, PIP hyperextension

Volar Dislocation of the Proximal Interphalangeal Joint Without Fracture

162. With a volar dislocation, the head of the phalanx is often entrapped between what two structures?

162. Lateral band
Central slip (straight volar dislocation = central slip only)

163. How can the intrinsics best be relaxed to facilitate reduction?

163. Flex finger at MP joint

164. What structure is commonly injured with a volar dislocation? What is the resultant deformity?

164. Central slip commonly injured (also in rotatory dislocation)
Acute boutonniere deformity

Fracture-Dislocation at the Proximal Interphalangeal Joint (Pilon-Type Injury)

165. What is the preferred treatment if fracture fragments are nondisplaced?

165. Extension block splint

166. What is the preferred treatment if fracture fragments are displaced and comminuted?

166. Traction device

167. What is the preferred treatment if fracture is a single displaced fragment?

167. ORIF if >25% but <40% articular surface involved

168. What is the salvage procedure if treatments are unsuccessful?

168. Volar plate arthroplasty

Posttraumatic and Osteoarthritic Changes at the Proximal Interphalangeal and Distal Interphalangeal Joints

169. With what pathologic process is a mucous cyst associated?

169. Arthritic DIP joint

170. What is the natural history of mucous cysts?

170. 20 to 60% spontaneously resolve

171. What is the indication for operative treatment of a mucous cyst?

171. Persistent drainage due to increased risk of infection

172. In general, what is the preferred treatment for posttraumatic arthrosis of PIP and DIP joints?

172. Fusion

173. What type of fixation is generally best for IP joint fusion? What is the preferred position?

173. Screws are best for DIP joints, can use Kirschner (K) wires or screws for PIP joint
DIP joint 0 to 5 degrees, PIP (index = 40, middle = 45, long = 50, small = 55)

Quick Review and Clarification of Key Points: For each of the following injured structures, is the avulsion generally distal or proximal?

174. Volar plate at PIP.

174. Distal

175. UCL (thumb MCP).

175. Distal

176. MCL at the elbow.

176. Distal

Posttraumatic Hand Deformity

Swan-Neck Deformity

177. What are the four possible causes of a swan-neck deformity?

177. Lax PIP volar plate
Mallet finger
Volarly subluxed MCP joint (as with rheumatoid arthritis)
Chronic FDS laceration

178. What is the resultant PIP position?

178. Hyperextended

179. What is the DIP position?

179. Flexed

180. What are three treatment options for swan-neck deformity?

180. Silver ring splint/figure-8 splint
Central slip tenotomy
Oblique retinacular ligament reconstruction

Boutonniere Deformity

181. Boutonniere deformity results from an injury to what two structures?

181. Central slip
Triangular ligament

182. Then what happens?

182. Lateral bands sublux volarly

183. What is the resultant PIP position?

183. Flexion

184. What is the DIP position?

184. Hyperextension

185. What test is used for evaluation of a boutonniere finger?

185. Elson test: bend PIP to 90 degrees; if resisted PIP extension sends DIP into rigid extension, then positive

186. In what situation is acute operative intervention for boutonniere deformity required?

186. A displaced avulsion fracture fragment is present

187. What is the nonoperative treatment of acute boutonniere?

187. Six weeks of PIP extension splint wear
Active flexion of the DIP (pulls lateral bands dorsally)

188. What are two operative treatments for chronic boutonniere deformity?

188. Terminal tendon tenotomy (Fowler)
Central slip reconstruction

Intrinsic Minus (Claw) Hand

189. What nerves are involved in an intrinsic minus hand?

189. Median (lumbrical muscles)
Ulnar (lumbricals and IO)

190. With claw hand, what is the position of the MCPs and IPs?

190. MPs hyperextended
IPs flexed

191. What two clinical problems are associated with intrinsic minus hand?

191. Decreased grip strength
Decreased pinch strength

192. What is the goal of operative intervention?

192. Correct MCP hyperextension
Facilitate IP extension

193. What role do the intrinsics have on the thumb?

193. Increase pinch

Intrinsic Plus Hand

194. With intrinsic plus hand, what is the position the MCPs and IPs?

194. MCPs flexed
IPs extended

195. What clinical test is most relevant?

195. Bunnell test

196. How does the Bunnell test work?

196. Differentiates extrinsic tightness from intrinsic tightness
If intrinsics are tight, when MCP is extended (relaxes EDC), cannot flex the PIP joints
If extrinsics are tight, when MCP is flexed (tensions EDC), cannot flex PIP joints

197. What does nonoperative treatment involve?

197. Intrinsic stretch (MP extension/IPs flexed)

■ Wrist Trauma and Associated Disorders

Scaphoid Fracture

198. In general, if you see a fracture of the scaphoid, you should also exclude what two injuries?

198. Perilunate dislocation
Capitate fracture

199. For nondisplaced fractures of the scaphoid, what is the preferred time of immobilization for distal pole fracture?

199. 6 weeks

200. What is the preferred time of immobilization for scaphoid waist fracture?

200. 12 weeks

201. What is the preferred time of immobilization for proximal pole fracture? Thus, what should be considered?

201. 5 months
Consider surgery for proximal pole fractures even if nondisplaced

202. Is it generally necessary to include the thumb in the cast?

202. No proven benefit to including the thumb (controversial)

203. What is the reported advantage of a long arm cast over a short arm cast?

203. Decreased time to union

204. What radiographic findings are suggestive of an unstable scaphoid fracture?

204. Humpback deformity (flexed and shortened)
Displacement >1 mm
Scapholunate angle >60 degrees
Capitolunate angle >15 degrees

205. What is the treatment of choice for unstable scaphoid fractures?

205. ORIF

206. ORIF remains an option for a missed fracture for how long?

206. Until arthritic changes are seen
Generally up to 5 years after injury

207. What is the blood supply to the scaphoid?

207. Major: dorsal scaphoid branch of the radial artery in a retrograde fashion (supplies 70 to 80%, including entire proximal pole)
Volar scaphoid branch of the superficial branch of the radial artery in a retrograde fashion (supplies 20 to 30% distal of scaphoid)

208. What is the avascular necrosis (AVN) rate for a proximal 1/5 fracture?

208. 100%

209. What is the AVN rate for proximal 1/3 fracture?

209. 33%

210. In terms of vascular supply, which approach to the scaphoid is generally safer?

210. Volar approach, because blood supply enters distally and dorsally

211. At what anatomic location is the dorsal approach considered safe from a vascular standpoint?

211. Dorsal approach is safe proximal to the ridge on the waist

212. What is the plane of dissection for the volar scaphoid approach?

212. Between FCR and radial artery

213. What two structures should be repaired once volar surgery is complete?

213. Long radiolunate ligament
Radioscaphocapitate

214. The dorsal approach is generally used for what type of scaphoid fracture?

214. Proximal pole fractures

215. What two structures must one be careful to avoid?

215. Superficial radial nerve
Radial artery (deep)

216. At the time of surgery, the proximal pole is known to be vascularized in what situation?

216. If it is observed to bleed

217. If the scaphoid fractures goes on to nonunion, what are the available graft types?

217. Inlay: if no associated collapse (92% union rate)
Interposition: if associated collapse or scaphoid deformity present (70 to 90% union rate)

218. A vascularized graft should be used for?

218. Scaphoid nonunion with AVN

219. On what artery is the vascularized graft based?

219. 1,2 intercompartmental supraretinacular artery

Disorders of the Other Carpal Bones

Preiser's Disease

220. What is Preiser's disease?

220. AVN of the scaphoid without fracture

221. What is the first-line treatment of Preiser's disease?

221. Trial of immobilization

222. In what percentage of patients is immobilization alone successful?

222. 20%

223. If nonoperative treatment fails, what are the options?

223. Vascularized graft
Scaphoid excision and four-corner fusion

Avascular Necrosis of the Capitate

224. What is the first-line treatment of capitate AVN?

224. Trial of immobilization

225. If immobilization fails, what are the surgical treatments?

225. Vascularized bone graft
Capitate head resection arthroplasty with fascial anchovy interposition
Midcarpal arthrodesis

Trapezium Fractures

226. How are trapezium fractures classified?

226. I: base of trapezial ridge
II: tip of trapezial ridge
III: body fracture

227. What is the preferred treatment for each type?

227. I: immobilization
II: increased risk of nonunion with immobilization, excise for symptomatic nonunions
III: ORIF if displaced/immobilization for nondisplaced

Distal Forearm Fractures

228. What radiograph exaggerates ulnar variance?

228. Pronated grip view

229. What happens to ulnar variance with pronation?

229. More positive ulnar variance

230. Overdistraction with external fixation may lead to increased risk of what complication?

230. Complex regional pain syndrome

231. What are the four radiographic criteria suggestive of distal radioulnar joint (DRUJ) instability?

231. Ulnar styloid fracture
Wide DRUJ
>5 mm shortening
Dislocation

232. What are the criteria for nonoperative treatment of a simple transverse ulna shaft fracture?

232. <50% displacement
<10 degrees angulation

233. What is the preferred treatment for a Monteggia fracture?

233. ORIF of the ulna

234. After ORIF of the ulna in a Monteggia fracture, if the radial head is not reduced what is the next step in management?

234. Reassess the ulna and revise ORIF (will correct the radial head)

Acute Triangular Fibrocartilage Complex (TFCC) Injuries and Management

235. What structures comprise the TFCC?

235. Dorsal radioulnar ligament
Volar radioulnar ligament
Articular disk
Meniscus homologue
Ulnar collateral ligament
Extensor carpi ulnaris subsheath
Ulnolunate ligaments

236. What is the difference between Palmer class I and class II lesions of the TFCC?

236. Class I injuries are traumatic
Class II injuries are degenerative

237. What are Palmer class I TFCC injury types A to D?

237. A: central tear
B: ulnar avulsion with or without ulnar styloid fracture
C: ulnolunate, ulnotriquetral avulsion (distal avulsion)
D: radial avulsion

238. What is the preferred treatment for class 1A TFCC injury that has failed nonoperative treatment?

238. Arthroscopic debridement

239. What is the preferred treatment for class 1B, 1C, and 1D?

239. 1B: repair
1C: type 1B repair and ulnar extrinsic ligament capsulodesis or repair
1D: reattach to sigmoid notch

240. Of the TFCC injuries, which is the best vascularized (most amenable to acute repair): central or peripheral?

240. Peripheral tear (better blood supply)

Ganglion Cysts

241. Are ganglion cysts more commonly dorsal or volar at the wrist?

241. Dorsal (70 to 80%)
Volar (20 to 30%)

242. With what site of injury are dorsal ganglion cysts most commonly associated?

242. Scapholunate ligament disruption

243. With what sites of injury are volar ganglion cysts most commonly associated?

243. Radiocarpal
STT joints

244. What percentage of dorsal cysts recur after excision?

244. 10%

245. What percentage of volar cysts recur after excision?

245. 20%

■ Wrist Instability, Arthritis, and Management

General Concepts

246. What changes occur in the proximal carpal row with radial deviation?

246. Scaphoid, lunate, and triquetrum flex

247. What changes with ulnar deviation?

247. Scaphoid, lunate, and triquetrum extend

248. What should the scapholunate (SL) angle be on a lateral wrist x-ray?

248. <60 degrees and >30 degrees

249. What is the definition of carpal instability dissociative (CID)?

249. Intercarpal ligament (within a given carpal row) disrupted

250. What are the three types of CID?

250. Dorsal intercalated segmental instability (DISI)
Volar intercalated segmental instability (VISI)
Axial instability (carpal collapse)

251. What are the definition and mechanism of carpal instability nondissociative (CIND)?

251. Malposition or abnormal movement of the entire proximal or distal carpal row with normal relationships within the row (for example, midcarpal instability, STT instability, distal radius malunion)

252. What is the definition of carpal instability complex (CIC)?

252. Carpal instability within and between carpal rows
Combination of dissociative and nondissociative

Dissociative Carpal Instability: Dorsal Intercalated Segmental Instability

253. What conditions can lead to the development of DISI?

253. Scapholunate dissociation
Unstable scaphoid fracture
Kienböck disease (carpal collapse + scaphoid flexes)

Scapholunate Dissociation

254. DISI results from the disruption of what two ligaments?

254. Scapholunate (SL) ligament (DISI does not occur with isolated SL tear, chronic strain of other ligaments that causes DISI)
Volar radiocarpal ligaments

255. What are the components of the SL ligament?

255. Dorsal
Palmar
Proximal (membranous)

256. Of these, which is the strongest?

256. Dorsal SL ligament

257. Are the volar or dorsal radiocarpal ligaments stronger?

257. Volar generally stronger

258. Where is the weak spot in the volar ligaments?

258. Space of Poirier

259. What are five radiographic findings consistent with SL dissociation (SLD)?

259. SL gap >3 mm
A break in Gilula's arc
Cortical ring sign
SL angle >60 degrees
Radiolunate angle >15 degrees

260. What is the preferred treatment for acute SLD?

260. Ligamentous repair

261. In general, this can be accomplished until the injury is how old?

261. 6 weeks

262. What are the treatment options for chronic SLD?

262. Scaphoid-trapezium-trapezoid (STT) fusion
Blatt dorsal capsulodesis
Ligament reconstruction
Internal fixation with SL screw
Scaphoid-lunate-capitate (SLC) fusion

263. What is the potential long-term consequence of untreated scapholunate dissociation?

263. Scapholunate advanced collapse (SLAC) wrist deformity

Scapholunate Advanced Collapse and Scaphoid Nonunion Advanced Collapse Wrists

264. What are the three Watson stages of arthritic change with a SLAC wrist?

264. I: scaphoid-styloid arthritis
II: radioscaphoid arthritis
III: capitolunate arthritis (radiolunate joint usually spared)

265. How is the progression of arthritis different with scaphoid nonunion advanced collapse (SNAC)?

265. SNAC exhibits radioscaphoid sparing because proximal pole not loaded

266. What is the surgical treatment for stage I SLAC?

266. Debridement
Styloidectomy

267. What is the surgical treatment for stage II SLAC?

267. Scaphoid excision and four-corner fusion
Proximal row carpectomy

268. What is an alternative option available for stage II SNAC, but not for stage II SLAC?

268. Excision of distal pole of scaphoid if no scaphocapitate arthritis is present

269. What is the surgical treatment for stage III SLAC?

269. Scaphoid excision and four-corner fusion
Wrist fusion for pancarpal arthritis

270. If performing a styloidectomy for a stage I SNAC wrist, what else must be done?

270. ORIF and graft scaphoid

Kienböck Disease

271. What is Kienböck disease?

271. Avascular necrosis of the lunate

272. What population is particularly at risk and why?

272. Ulnar negative variance
Because load on the lunate is increased
Decreased radial inclination
Most common in young men ages 20 to 40

273. What are the radiographic stages of Kienböck disease (Lichtman)?

273. I: positive magnetic resonance imaging (MRI), plain films negative
II: sclerosis on x-ray, no collapse
IIIA: articular collapse/no carpal collapse
IIIB: articular collapse/carpal collapse + DISI
IV: carpal degenerative joint disease (DJD)

274. What is the preferred initial treatment for stage I disease?

274. Immobilization
Nonsteroidal antiinflammatory drugs (NSAIDs)

275. What is the preferred surgical treatment for stage II?

275. Radial shortening and consider revascularization

276. What is the preferred surgical treatment for stage IIIA?

276. Radial shortening and consider revascularization

277. What is the preferred surgical treatment for stage IIIB?

277. STT fusion, capitate shortening, or proximal row carpectomy depending on stage of DISI

278. What is the preferred surgical treatment for stage IV?

278. Wrist arthrodesis

279. Shortening the radius by 4 mm leads to what percentage decrease in radial load?

279. 45%

280. If a patient is ulnar positive and has Kienböck disease, what is the preferred treatment?

280. Capitate shortening with or without vascularized bone graft

Dissociative Carpal Instability: Volar Intercalated Segmental Instability

281. What is VISI?

281. Volar flexion of the lunate relative to the long axis of the radius and capitate

282. What two structures are necessarily disrupted with VISI?

282. Lunotriquetral (LT) ligament
Dorsal radiotriquetral ligament

283. What are four radiographic features consistent with VISI?

283. Broken Gilula's arc
Radiolunate angle >15 degrees
Capitolunate angle >15 degrees
Scapholunate angle <30 degrees

284. What is the preferred treatment for an acute LT disruption?

284. LT pinning

285. What is the preferred treatment for chronic LT disruption?

285. LT fusion

286. If the patient has an ulnar positive wrist, and the LT is unstable, what should be done?

286. Ulnar shortening osteotomy with or without LT pinning may be effective in restoring stability because of tightening extrinsic ligaments

Carpal Instability Nondissociative

287. What is the typical clinical presentation of CIND?

287. Clunking wrist with radial and ulnar deviation

288. What is the characteristic radiographic finding?

288. Sudden shift of proximal carpal row with radial and ulnar deviation
Midcarpal instability

289. What joints can be affected with CIND?

289. Midcarpal
Radiocarpal

290. What is the general treatment approach to midcarpal nondissociative instability?

290. Nonoperative treatment first (immobilization and activity modification)
Arthroscopic heat shrinkage capsulodesis
Dorsal wrist ligament repair/reconstruction
If unsuccessful, then fusion across the midcarpal joint

291. What is the most common cause leading to the development of radiocarpal instability?

291. Malunion of distal radius fracture

Combined Carpal Instability

292. What are the most common causes leading to combined carpal instability?

293. What is scaphocapitate syndrome?

294. What is the treatment of choice for scaphocapitate syndrome?

Perilunate Dislocation

295. What are the four Mayfield stages of perilunate dislocation?

296. What mechanism reproduced Mayfield stages of perilunate dislocation in a cadaver model? What is the position of the wrist and forearm?

297. Based on cadaver modeling, what position of the wrist and forearm is required for a perilunate dislocation to result?

298. What radiographic marker predicts poor outcome after ORIF for perilunate dislocation?

Chronic TFCC Injuries

299. With what radius/ulna relationship are class II TFCC injuries generally associated?

300. What are the five types of Palmer's class II (degenerative) TFCC injury?

301. In general, what are the initial forms of treatment for class II tears?

302. What is the condition of the TFCC with IIA and IIB tears?

---

292. Scaphocapitate syndrome
Perilunate dislocation

293. A unique injury: a force causes proximal capitate and scaphoid waist fractures, which can lead to perilunate dislocation

294. ORIF if displaced fractures or instability

295. I: scapholunate
II: scapholunate, lunocapitate
III: scapholunate, capitolunate, lunotriquetral
IV: volar lunate dislocation

296. Pronation + ulnar deviation on a hyperextended wrist

297. ORIF followed by 8 to 12 weeks casting

298. Persistent scapholunate gap

299. Ulnar positive

300. A: TFCC wear without perforation or chondromalacia
B: lunate/ulna chondromalacia
C: TFCC perforation with lunate chondromalacia
D: lunate and/or ulnar chondromalacia, and lunotriquetral ligament perforation
E: TFCC perforation with generalized arthritic changes involving the lunate and ulna, and perforation of the lunatotriquetral ligament

301. Immobilization
NSAIDs

302. TFCC is intact

303. What does operative treatment for IIA, IIB injuries entail?

303. Open ulnar shortening
Arthroscopic evaluation

304. What is the maximum resection allowed for the wafer resection (partial resection of the ulnar dome)

304. 4 mm

305. In IIC injuries, the TFCC is perforated, so operative treatment generally includes what two procedures?

305. Arthroscopic debridement of perforation and water resection of distal ulna through perforation

306. What is a key contraindication to a wafer procedure?

306. If >2 mm of shortening is required

307. What is the difference between D and E class II injuries?

307. IID: LT ligament disrupted, no VISI
IIE: LT ligament disrupted and VISI and generalized arthritis

308. What operative procedures are appropriate for type IID, IIE degeneration?

308. Arthroscopic debridement of TFCC and LT ligament
Ulnar shortening

309. What is an indirect benefit of ulnar shortening?

309. Lunotriquetral stability improves

310. If the LT articulation remains unstable after ulnar shortening, what is the next step?

310. Pin across lunate and triquetrum

Chronic Conditions of the Distal Radioulnar Joint

Caput Ulnae

311. In general, which condition begins the process leading to eventual caput ulnae?

311. DRUJ synovitis
May be caused by such disorders as rheumatoid arthritis

312. What is caput ulnae syndrome?

312. Results from synovitis and stretching of ulnar carpal ligaments
Progresses to dorsal dislocation of the ulna, supination of the carpus, and subluxation of the extensor carpi ulnaris tendon
If untreated, ulnar translocation can occur

313. In which direction does the ECU sublux?

313. Volar
Ulnar

314. What is the operative treatment for ECU subluxation if nonoperative treatment fails?

314. Extensor retinacular flap used for ECU sheath reconstruction

315. What events classically follow ECU subluxation?

315. Volar ECU subluxation causes loss of ulnar deviation and extension, which radially deviates the wrist and brings the ulnar extensor tendons directly over the distal ulna
Vaughn-Jackson syndrome develops (attritional extensor tendon rupture)

316. How can Vaughn-Jackson syndrome be clinically differentiated from PIN palsy?

316. Tenodesis test: tendons are intact in PIN palsy

317. What is the preferred surgical treatment for early DRUJ synovitis?

317. Synovectomy

318. Once caput ulnae develop, what treatment options are available?

318. Darrach resection of the ulna (stabilized by volar capsule) and ECU relocation with retinacular flap
Suave-Kapandji

319. After Suave-Kapandji, why can pain develop with resisted elbow flexion?

319. Instability of the proximal ulna

Distal Radioulnar Joint Arthritis

320. What operative options are available for DRUJ arthritis?

320. Ulnar head resection (hemiresection arthroplasty)
Darrach procedure
Suave-Kapandji
DRUJ prosthetic replacement

■ Hand and Wrist Reconstruction After Tissue Loss

General Concepts

321. Is there a general rule of thumb about timing of coverage in an injury with tissue loss?

321. In general, <7 days is preferred

322. In general, vascularized flap coverage is required for what clinical situation?

322. Soft tissue loss with exposed bone, nerve, or tendon

323. What are the two general types of flaps and examples of each?

323. Random-pattern: not associated with a named vessel, but from many minute vessels from the subdermal or subcutaneous plexus
Axial-pattern flap: associated with a named vessel that serves as an arterial pedicle

324. With a random-pattern (e.g., transpositional) flap, what is the ideal length/base ratio?

324. 1:1

Specific Commonly Tested Axial Flaps of the Extremities

325. What vessel is associated with a radial arm flap?

325. Radial artery

326. If using a radial arm flap, what must be included on preoperative examination?

326. Allen test
Arteriogram in the setting of significant trauma

327. What vessel is associated with a lateral arm flap?

327. Posterior radial collateral artery from profunda brachii

328. What vessel is associated with a scapular free flap?

328. Circumflex scapular artery

329. What vessel is associated with a serratus flap?

329. Thoracodorsal artery (branch of the subscapular artery)

330. What postoperative complication may be associated with the use of a serratus flap?

330. Scapular medial winging (injury to the long thoracic nerve)

331. In general, what two flaps provide the best coverage for a full thickness shoulder deficit?

331. Latissimus dorsi flap
Pectoralis major flap

332. What vessel is associated with a latissimus dorsi flap?

332. Thoracodorsal artery

333. What vessel is associated with a groin flap?

333. Superficial circumflex iliac artery

334. What vessel is associated with a medial gastrocnemius flap? In what clinical situation is this vessel potentially not viable?

334. Medial sural artery
If patient has had a knee dislocation, be careful, because this artery is a branch of the popliteal

335. What vessel is associated with a free fibula transfer?

335. Peroneal artery

336. What is the general indication for a free fibula transfer?

336. Diaphyseal reconstruction with bone defects >6 cm

337. What complications may occur if too much fibula is harvested?

337. Valgus hindfoot deformity
Syndesmotic injury

338. What vessel is associated with a free iliac crest transfer?

338. Deep circumflex iliac artery

339. What is the general indication for a free iliac crest transfer?

339. Metaphyseal reconstruction

Z-plasty

340. What is the general rule regarding Z-plasty limb lengths?

340. Limb lengths are always the same regardless of angle

341. In general, more lengthening is achieved if the angle is?

341. Smaller

342. What is the optimal angle?

342. 60 degrees

343. What is the risk with smaller angles between limbs of the Z-plasty?

343. Necrosis of the tip of the flap

344. A 60-degree angle cut between limbs of the Z-plasty gives a lengthening of approximately what percentage?

344. 75%

345. A 30-degree angle between limbs of the Z-plasty optimizes which parameter?

345. Length

Specific Clinical Situations that May Require Coverage

346. What is the preferred treatment for a fingertip amputation injury that is less than 1 cm^2 without exposed bone?

346. Allow to heal by secondary intention

347. What is the preferred treatment for a fingertip amputation injury that is greater than or equal to 1 cm²?

347. Hypothenar full thickness skin graft

348. What is the preferred treatment if bone exposed?

348. Rongeur the bone back first, but take care to maintain adequate nailbed support

349. Is there a patient population in whom healing by secondary intention may be appropriate, even with exposed bone?

349. The very young (less than 2 to 3 years old)

350. In what patients can a composite flap (essentially a biologic bandage) be used?

350. Appropriate for patients up to 3 years old with fingertip amputations

351. What are the treatment options for more extensive volar digital tissue loss (volar oblique injury) with exposed bone?

351. Cross finger flap
Thenar flaps

352. For what two fingers can a thenar flap be used?

352. Index finger
Long finger

353. At what time should the thenar flap be divided?

353. 2 to 3 weeks

354. What is the principal complication of a thenar flap in a patient over 40 years old?

354. PIP joint contracture

355. What are other options for proximal volar digital coverage?

355. Axial flag flap
Vascular island flap

356. What are the treatment options for transverse amputation or dorsal oblique amputation with exposed bone?

356. Volar V-Y flap
Double lateral V-Y flap

357. What are the three treatment options for volar oblique or transverse tissue loss in the thumb?

357. Moberg flap (if <2 cm²)
Heterodigital island flap
Cross finger flap (if 2 to 3 cm²)

358. What is the preferred treatment for dorsal tissue loss in the thumb?

358. Dorsal first metacarpal artery island flap

359. For coverage of the dorsal hand when underlying soft tissue bed is adequate, what type of graft is best?

359. Meshed split-thickness skin graft (not a full-thickness graft)

Ring Avulsion Injury

360. What are two indications for amputation?

360. Complete degloving
Bony injury with associated nerve or vessel injury

High-Pressure Injection Injury

361. What is the most important factor in determining outcome?

361. The type and amount of material injected

362. What are three negative prognostic factors?

362. Presentation >10 hours after injury
>7000 psi injection pressure
Oil-based paints and industrial solvents

363. What is the amputation rate after a high-pressure injection injury?

363. 50%

364. What is the preferred treatment?

364. Aggressive surgical management with prompt incision and drainage (I&D) and wide mechanical debridement

Replantation

365. What are the warm ischemia time limits for replantation for the digit and forearm?

365. Less than 12 hours for digit
Less than 6 hours for forearm

366. What are the cool ischemia time limits?

366. Less than 24 hours for digit
Less than 12 hours for forearm

367. What factor principally determines whether a replant will be technically possible and successful?

367. Mechanism of injury

368. Under what conditions might digital replantation be preferred?

368. Thumb
Multiple digits
Partial hand amputation
Any upper extremity part in children
Above the wrist
Individual digits amputated distal to FDS (zone 1)

369. What is the Mangled Extremity Severity Scale (MESS) score used for, and what are its components?

369. To predict the outcome of a limb salvage attempt; it consists of injury, ischemia, shock, age (Hansen, J Trauma 1990)

370. What is the significance of a MESS score >7?

370. Poor limb viability prognosis

371. What is the significance of a MESS score <4?

371. Relatively good prognosis for limb viability

372. What is the fastest technique to address multiple digital amputations? In what order?

372. Structure-by-structure approach results in a higher viability rate
Order of structures: bone, extensors, flexors, artery, nerve, vein (acronym BEFANV)

373. In what order should structures be attached for a forearm replant?

373. Artery first
Inclusion of a fasciotomy is mandatory

374. In what order should digits be reattached?

374. Thumb
Long
Ring
Small
Index

375. What form of postoperative monitoring is most reliable?

375. Doppler

376. What is the most common cause of early replant failure (within 12 hours of surgery)?

376. Thrombosis secondary to vasospasm

377. What is the most common cause of late replant failure (after 12 hours)?

377. Venous congestion (most common cause of loss)

378. What are the two most common complications after replant surgery?

378. Infection (No. 1)
Cold intolerance

Thumb Reconstruction

379. What is the most important requirement when considering thumb reconstruction for traumatic amputation or congenital deficiency?

379. A stable CMC joint is required for reconstruction
Otherwise, must perform pollicization of another digit

380. What flap best duplicates thumb appearance and size in an adult with an amputation distal to the MP joint?

380. Wraparound flap

381. What is an alternative to pollicization of another digit if a stable CMC joint is present?

381. Toe-to-thumb transfer

382. What are the general benefits of a toe-to-thumb transfer for reconstruction?

382. Good function, and acceptable appearance and sensibility
Growth potential

383. What is the advantage of transferring the great toe rather than the second toe?

383. Offers better stability
Better functional and aesthetic result

384. What is the disadvantage of using the great toe?

384. Cannot take the great toe MTP (metatarsophalangeal) joint
Can take the MP joint if use the second toe

385. What vascular pedicle is associated with a great toe transfer?

385. First dorsal metatarsal artery (branch of the dorsalis pedis)

■ Neuropathies and Neural Disorders of the Upper Extremity

Neural Anatomy and Physiology

386. What is the principal component of myelin?

386. Lipid

387. The nerve axon and myelin sheath together form what structure?

387. Peripheral nerve fiber

388. Peripheral nerve fibers are covered by what?

388. Endoneurium

389. What are bundles of nerve fibers referred to as?

389. Fascicles

390. What is the layer that covers the fascicles called?

390. Perineurium

391. What are the functions of the perineurium?

391. Provide tensile strength
Acts as blood–brain barrier protecting against infection

392. A collection of fascicles together form what macroscopic structure?

392. Peripheral nerve

393. What is the outermost layer covering a peripheral nerve?

393. Epineurium

394. What is the general function of the epineurium?

394. Protect the nerve against external pressure

395. An action potential triggers what chemical sequence at the neuromuscular junction?

395. Calcium influx and acetylcholine (ACh) release

396. What then occurs at the motor endplate?

396. ACh leads to an influx of sodium and results in depolarization of the cell

397. What is the normal resting potential of the cell?

397. –70 mV

Corpuscles

398. What quality of sensation corresponds to each of the following corpuscle types: Meissner?

398. Light touch (tactile corpuscles) type of mechanoreceptor (only present in glabrous skin)
Moving two point discrimination/ quickly adapting

399. Merkel?

399. Light pressure and texture
Static two point discrimination/slow adapting

400. Pacini?

400. Deep pressure touch and high-frequency vibration
Quickly adapting

401. Ruffini?

401. Skin stretch/slow adapting mechanoreceptor (exist only in the glabrous dermis)
Temperature

402. What is the best clinical test of Meissner corpuscle function?

402. Moving two-point discrimination

403. What is the best clinical test of Merkel corpuscle function?

403. Static two-point discrimination

404. Are most reflex arcs monosynaptic or polysynaptic?

404. Polysynaptic

405. Pain fibers are principally of which type?

405. C

406. Are pain fibers generally myelinated?

406. No, generally unmyelinated

Neural Pathology

Peripheral Nerve Injury

407. Describe neuropraxia.

407. Conduction block (injury to the myelin) without wallerian degeneration
Axons intact

408. Describe axonotmesis.

408. Conduction block (injury to axons and myelin) with wallerian degeneration (distal)
Axon, myelin degenerate
Endoneural tubes remain

409. Describe neurotmesis.

409. All layers disrupted
Wallerian degeneration occurs
Requires surgery

410. What degree of nerve injury has the most variable extent of recovery?

410. Axonotmesis

411. What microstructural change occurs when a nerve is elongated by at least 8%?

411. Decreased microcirculation

412. At what degree of stretch do nerve ischemia and axonal loss occur?

412. 15% stretch

413. What electromyograph (EMG) findings are consistent with denervation?

413. Fibrillations

414. How long after injury are they generally seen?

414. 2 to 4 weeks

415. What EMG finding is consistent with reinnervation?

415. Polyphasic potentials

Recovery After Injury

416. What is the most important prognostic factor for recovery after peripheral nerve injury?

416. Degree of injury
Distance of injury from motor endplates

417. What is the general rule for the rate of nerve regeneration in children?

417. 3 to 5 mm/day

418. What is the rate of regeneration in adults?

418. 1 mm/day

419. What is the best clinical indication of nerve regeneration?

419. Advancing Tinel's sign

420. Are distal or proximal peripheral nerve injuries generally better prognostically?

420. Distal injuries have better prognoses than proximal

Key General Points Regarding Nerve Repair and Surgery

421. What key consideration must be kept in mind during attempted nerve repair?

421. Avoid tension

422. What is the time limit beyond which delayed repair is unlikely to be successful?

422. 18 months, because of irreversible motor endplate demise

Compressive Neuropathies

423. With chronic compression, is sensory or motor function affected first?

423. Sensory function is lost first

424. What electrodiagnostic study demonstrates changes first: EMG or nerve conduction velocity (NCV)?

424. NCV (sensory latency) changes seen before EMG

425. What is the order of sensory functional loss with chronic compression?

425. Threshold functions are lost first
Then static two-point discrimination
Moving two-point discrimination
Moving touch
Pain
Pressure
Total anesthesia results

426. What tests are most sensitive for the presence of compressive neuropathy?

426. Threshold tests

427. What are some examples of threshold tests?

427. Semmes monofilament (slow adapting fibers)
Vibration (quick adapting)

428. What is the key Semmes monofilament number for the hand?

428. 2.83 mm

429. What is the key Semmes monofilament number for the foot?

429. 5.07 mm

430. What are some examples of density tests?

430. Static two-point discrimination (slow adapting fibers)
Moving two-point discrimination (quick adapting)

Brachial Plexopathy

Anatomy of the Brachial Plexus and Adjacent Structures

431. The brachial plexus and subclavian artery lie between what two structures in the neck?

431. Anterior scalene muscle
Middle scalene muscle

432. Axillary artery branches are categorized in relation to the pectoralis minor. What branches are in zone 1?

432. Superior thoracic artery

433. What branches are in zone 2?

433. Thoracoacromial artery
Lateral thoracic artery

434. What branches are in zone 3?

434. Subscapular artery (which gives rise to the circumflex scapular artery)
Anterior humeral circumflex artery
Posterior humeral circumflex artery

Clinical Features: General

Supraclavicular injuries can be preganglionic or postganglionic. For preganglionic injuries, clinical effects are dependent on location.

435. What is the clinical feature if the injury is at C5 to C7?

435. Medial winging (long thoracic nerve palsy)

436. What are the two clinical features if the injury is at C8-T1?

436. Horner's syndrome (inferior ganglion)
Positive histamine response

437. In general, how do the outcomes of pre- and postganglionic injuries compare?

437. Postganglionic injury outcomes are generally better

438. In general, how do the outcomes of supra- and infraclavicular injuries compare?

438. Infraclavicular outcomes are generally better

Obstetric Plexopathies

439. What risk factors are associated with obstetric brachial plexus palsy (BPP)?

439. Large baby
Long labor
Shoulder dystocia
Breech
Forceps delivery
Previous birth with shoulder dystocia or BPP

440. When considering brachial plexus microsurgery, what are the indications for surgery at 1 month?

440. Global palsy

441. What is the significance of the 2-month mark in a child with obstetric BPP?

441. If deltoid and biceps are firing, complete recovery is possible

442. If biceps recovery is present by 3 months, what is the next treatment?

442. Continue to observe for recovery

443. What is Horner's syndrome?

443. Ptosis (drooping eyelid), meiosis (constricted pupil), anhydrosis (lack of sweating); clinical syndrome caused by damage to the sympathetic nervous system

444. If no biceps recovery is present by 5 to 6 months, what is the next treatment?

444. Brachial plexus microsurgery

445. What is Erb's point?

445. Junction of the C5 and C6 nerve roots

446. An injury at Erb's point can be identified by sparing of the function of which nerve?

446. Dorsal scapular nerve (already branched off of C5)

447. What roots are affected with Erb-Duchenne palsy?

447. C5-C6

448. What is the position of the arm classically referred to as?

448. Waiter's tip (shoulder internally rotated, elbow extended, wrist flexed)

449. What palsy has the best prognosis?

449. Erb Duchenne palsy (C5-C6)

450. What roots are affected with Klumpke paralysis?

450. C8-T1

451. What are the resultant clinical features in Klumpke paralysis?

451. No intrinsic function (median or ulnar intrinsics)
No long finger flexors
No flexor pollicis longus or flexor digitorum profundus

452. What is the prognosis for Klumpke paralysis?

452. Poor

453. In general, what are the goals of treatment while waiting for plexus recovery to take place?

453. Prevent contractures (with passive ROM)
Prevent skeletal changes and joint deformity

454. If a chronic obstetric BPP is untreated, what is the resulting position of the shoulder?

454. Adduction and internal rotation deformity

455. What are the secondary joint deformities that develop in the shoulder?

455. Glenoid retroversion
Posterior subluxation
Medial flattening of the humeral head

456. What musculoskeletal procedures can be performed if no recovery occurs?

456. Anterior releases
Latissimus dorsi and teres major transfers to the cuff (posterior augmentation)

457. What procedure can be performed for late presentation or fixed shoulder internal rotation deformity?

457. Rotational humeral osteotomy (to gain more external rotation)

Brachial Plexus Injuries in the Adult

458. In general, what are the indications for immediate brachial plexus exploration?

458. Penetrating trauma
Iatrogenic injury

459. What are the indications for early exploration (before 3 months)?

459. High-energy injury
Global brachial plexus palsy

460. What are the indications for delayed exploration (3 to 6 months)?

460. Gunshot wound
Low-energy injury
Partial brachial plexus palsy

461. Clinical features suggestive of root avulsion include what pain distribution?

461. Severe pain in anesthetized limb

462. ... paralysis of what involuntary musculature?

462. Diaphragmatic paralysis

463. ... associated injuries that may make one suspicious for possible avulsion include?

463. Transverse process fractures
Scapulothoracic dissocation

464. MRI findings consistent with root avulsion include?

464. Empty root sleeves
Pseudomeningocele (high T2 signal)
Cord shift away from the midline

465. A normal NCV in an anesthetic portion of the upper extremity implies what injury pattern?

465. Avulsion injury (the dorsal root ganglion remains in continuity with the peripheral nerve)

Quick Review

466. What is the general prognosis for avulsion injuries and why?

466. Poor
Because roots are components of central (not peripheral) nervous system
Irreparable damage

467. C8, T1 avulsions are associated with what clinical sign?

467. Horner's syndrome

468. Brachial plexus priorities of repair: in what order should function be restored?

468. Elbow flexion
Shoulder stability
Wrist extension

469. What is a Steindler flexorplasty?

469. Move flexor pronator mass proximally to serve as a flexor of the elbow

470. What is the indication for a flexorplasty?

470. Lack of elbow flexion

Carpal Tunnel Syndrome

Anatomy of the Carpal Tunnel

471. What are the borders of the carpal tunnel?

471. Scaphoid tubercle
Hamate

472. What are the contents of the carpal tunnel?

472. Nine flexor tendons (FDP, four; FDS, four; FPL, one)
Median nerve

473. What is the relative orientation of the flexor tendon slips?

473. Slips to third and fourth digits are volar to second and fifth

474. What is the most common anatomic variation of the recurrent motor branch of the median nerve?

474. Extraligamentous recurrent course distal to carpal tunnel

475. What side of the median nerve does the palmar cutaneous branch come off of?

475. Radial

476. The palmar cutaneous branch of median nerve lies between what two structures?

476 Palmaris longus
Flexor carpi radialis

Clinical Features

477. How effective is a steroid injection at providing short-term relief of symptoms?

477. 80% of patients report acute relief

478. What percentage of patients have continued relief of symptoms at 1 year after steroid injection?

478. 22%

479. What is the preferred wrist position for a carpal tunnel splint?

479. Neutral

480. What is the advantage of endoscopic carpal tunnel release over the open procedure?

480. Possible accelerated early postoperative rehabilitation
Possible less pillar pain

481. What are the possible disadvantages of endoscopic surgery?

481. Incomplete division of the transverse carpal ligament
Cut the recurrent motor branch of the median nerve

482. Is there any difference in long-term outcomes?

482. No

483. The highest rates of incomplete transverse carpal ligament division are seen with what types of carpal tunnel procedures?

483. Mini-incision or endoscopic Transverse incision (avoid)

484. What is the only indication for repair of the transverse carpal ligament after division?

484. Simultaneous flexor tendon repair

485. Postoperatively, when does pinch strength return to baseline?

485. 6 weeks

486. Postoperatively, when does grip strength return to baseline?

486. 12 weeks

Pronator Syndrome

487. What nerve is involved with pronator syndrome?

487. Median nerve

488. In the forearm, what is the course of the median nerve?

488. Between the two pronator heads
Between the FDS and FDP

489. What are the possible sites of compression?

489. Supracondylar process—ligament of Struthers (seen in 1% of patients)
Lacertus fibrosus
Heads of pronator teres
Origin of FDS

490. In what percentage of the population is a supracondylar process present?

490. 1%

491. What ligament is associated with a supracondylar process?

491. Ligament of Struthers

492. What structures may be compressed by a supracondylar process?

492. Median nerve
Ulnar nerve
Brachial artery (forearm claudication symptoms)

493. How can pronator syndrome be differentiated from carpel tunnel syndrome (CTS)?

493. Pronator syndrome also affects the palmar cutaneous branch of the median nerve resulting in numbness in palm (spared with CTS)

494. Are the superficial flexors or deep flexors affected by pronator syndrome?

494. Superficial flexors (except flexor carpi ulnaris [FCU])

Anterior Interosseous Nerve Syndrome

495. What is anterior interosseous nerve (AIN) syndrome?

495. Anterior interosseous nerve compression
Mostly motor
Presents with pain

496. In the forearm, what is the course of the AIN?

496. Between the FDP and FPL

497. What are the possible sites of compression?

497. Pronator teres (PT)
FDP
Gantzer's muscle (accessory head of FPL) rare

498. Are the superficial flexors or deep flexors affected with AIN syndrome?

498. Deep flexors

499. What muscles are innervated by the AIN?

499. FDP index and long
FPL
Pronator quadratus (PQ)

500. How can the FDP and FPL be tested?

500. Ask patient to make the "OK" sign with index finger and thumb
Flex thumb IP joint and flex DIP joint of index finger

501. How can the PQ be tested?

501. Resisted pronation with the elbow flexed (eliminates contribution of pronator teres)

502. If the FPL is the only muscle affected, what diagnosis must be considered?

502. FPL rupture (Mannerfelt-Noonan syndrome)

503. If bilateral involvement, what diagnosis must be considered?

503. Parsonage-Turner syndrome

504. What is the classic clinical presentation of this syndrome?

504. Preceding shoulder pain followed by weakness

505. What is the presumed etiology?

505. Viral

506. What study is helpful in the diagnosis of Parsonage- Turner syndrome?

506. EMG

Neuropathies Associated with the Ulnar Nerve

Cubital Tunnel Syndrome

507. What are the possible sites of compression resulting in ulnar neuropathy at the elbow?

507. Between FCU heads
Arcade of Struthers (IM septum)
Tunnel (ligament)
Anconeus epitrochlearis

508. What is Froment's sign?

508. Intrinsic weakness due to ulnar nerve injury
Tests pinch strength
FPL compensates for weakness of adductor pollicis

509. How can one test for Froment's sign?

509. Sheet of paper between thumb and index, key pinch grip
Thumb flexes at IP because no adductor function

510. What is Jeanne's sign?

510. Thumb MP hyperextension during attempted active thumb flexion

511. What is a positive Pollock test?

511. Ulnar two FDPs weak

512. What is a poorly prognostic factor for cubital tunnel syndrome?

512. Intrinsic atrophy

513. What is the preferred method for ulnar nerve transposition?

513. Better to transpose submuscularly with muscuolofascial lengthening technique

514. What is the ideal position for splinting the elbow for cubital tunnel?

514. Elbow at 30 to 45 degrees of extension
Forearm neutral (to relax FCU)

Guyon's Canal

515. What are the walls of Guyon's canal?

515. Floor: transverse carpal and pisohamate ligament
Roof: volar carpal ligament
Ulnar: pisiform
Radial: hamate

516. What are the three zones? What is a common cause of compression in each zone?

516. I: motor and sensory deficits (ganglia—80% nontraumatic, hook of hamate fracture)
II: motor deficit only (same as zone I)
III: sensory deficit only (ulnar artery thrombus)

517. If thrombosis leads to embolus, what is the resulting clinical effect?

517. Sympathetic nerve response
Further limitation of flow to ring finger, due to takeoff angle of common digital arteries at 3–4 webspace

518. What is the treatment for embolus?

518. Resection of thrombotic segment, with or without arterial repair or vein graft
Sympathectomy

519. How does a hook of hamate fracture classically present?

519. Stick-handling sports (e.g., baseball, golf)

520. What complication is associated with hook of hamate fracture?

520. Irritation or attritional rupture of ulnar sided flexor

Ulnar Nerve Distal to Guyon's

521. The superficial branch of the ulnar nerve supplies what structures?

521. Dorsal and volar aspect of ulnar side of ring

522. What structures does the deep branch supply?

522. Hypothenar muscles
Intrinsics, except first two lumbricals
Adductor pollicis

523. The deep branch courses with what structure?

523. Deep (palmar) branch of ulnar artery

524. What is the most important secondary adductor (non-ulnar)?

524. EPL

525. What is the relationship of the ulnar nerve and artery in forearm and Guyon's canal?

525. Ulnar nerve is ulnar to artery in forearm and Guyon's canal

526. What is the blood supply to the ulnar nerve?

526. Superior ulnar collateral artery (major)
Inferior ulnar collateral artery (minor)
Post-ulnar recurrent artery (major)

527. What is the Martin-Gruber anastomosis?

527. Motor connection in forearm between median and ulnar nerves

528. Where does the anastomosis originate?

528. Median nerve proper or AIN

529. At which location does the intrinsic innervation revert to the ulnar nerve?

529. Elbow

530. If an anastomosis is present, and the median nerve is cut in the arm, then what?

530. Intrinsics are also lost

531. If the ulnar nerve is cut, then what?

531. Intrinsics are spared

532. The nerve of Henle is a branch of what nerve?

532. Ulnar nerve

533. To which location does it provide sensation?

533. Distal forearm

534. To what structure does the nerve of Henle also provide sympathetic innervation?

534. Ulnar artery

535. What structures are principally at risk with ulnar nerve transposition?

535. Median antebrachial cutaneous nerve
Medial brachial cutaneous nerve

Posterior Interosseous Nerve Syndrome

536. The posterior interosseous nerve (PIN) innervates what structures?

536. ECRB
Supinator
EIP
ECU
EDC
EDM
EPL
EPB
APL

537. What are the symptoms of PIN syndrome?

537. Pain
Weakness in PIN-innervated muscle groups

538. What is the classic finding with wrist extension in PIN syndrome and why?

538. Radial drift with wrist extension
ECRL remains functional and is unopposed by the extensor carpi ulnaris muscle

539. If the radial nerve were compressed above the level of the PIN, what would the clinical findings be that would help in the diagnosis?

539. PIN muscle groups weak, and Mobile wad also (BR/ECRL)

540. What structures may potentially contribute to such proximal radial nerve compression?

540. Triceps
Holstein-Lewis fracture

541. What are the potential sites of compression with PIN syndrome?

541. FREAS.
Fibrous bands
Radial artery recurrent leash of Henry
ECRB
Arcade of Frohse
Supinator

542. In rheumatoid arthritis, one must consider what other condition with similar clinical findings?

542. Extensor tendon rupture

543. How can rupture be excluded?

543. Tenodesis test: Lack of passive digital extension when wrist flexed

544. In general, is an EMG helpful in the diagnosis of PIN syndrome?

544. Yes

545. Following a radial nerve injury, what is the general order of muscle recovery?

545. Proximal to distal
Thus, BR/ECRL (mobile wad) is first to recover
Then the supinator
ECRB
ECU
EDC/EIP
EPL (third compartment)
APL/EPB (first compartment)

546. What are the symptoms of radial tunnel syndrome?

546. Pain only, no motor or sensory deficits

547. What other clinical condition must be excluded?

547. Lateral epicondylitis

548. Is an EMG generally helpful in the diagnosis of radial tunnel syndrome?

548. No

549. Wartenberg syndrome involves compression of what nerve?

549. Superficial branch of the radial nerve

Key Tendon Transfers for Peripheral Nerve Injuries

550. In general, what is the effect on strength of a muscle transfer?

550. Lose 1 grade of strength

Radial Nerve Injury

To restore function after radial nerve injury, there are three key tendon transfers to know:

551. Transfer 1: palmaris longus (PL) to what?

551. EPL

552. Transfer 2: pronator teres to what?

552. ECRB

553. Transfer 3: (1 of 3) to what structure?

553. (FCU or FCR or FDS) to EDC

Low Median Nerve Injury

554. What is the most important function to restore?

554. Thumb opposition

555. What transfer is generally the best in this situation?

555. FDS (four) to APB

556. In general, APB function is a good marker of what?

556. Median nerve innervation

High Median Nerve Injury

557. What is the most important function to restore?

557. Thumb flexion (FPL)

558. What transfer is generally the best in this situation?

558. BR to FPL

Ulnar Nerve Injury

559. What tendon is generally transferred to the APL?

559. ECRB

560. To restore intrinsic function, tendons are also generally transferred to what structures?

560. FDS to lateral bands

Other Commonly Tested Neurologic Conditions

Reflex Symphathetic Dystrophy

561. What is the timing and what are the clinical findings of the acute phase of reflex sympathetic dystrophy (RSD)?

561. 0 to 3 months after onset
Painful
Warm, red, sweaty skin

562. What is the timing and what are the clinical findings of the subacute phase of RSD?

562. 3 to 12 months
Painful
Brawny edema, trophic changes
Osteopenic bone

563. What is the timing and what are the clinical findings of the chronic phase of RSD?

563. >12 months
Glossy, cool skin
Contractures

564. What is the triple-phase bone scan appearance of RSD?

564. Stage 1: increased uptake
Stage 2: diffuse uptake at MP joints and juxtaarticular areas of digits
Stage 3: diffuse asymmetric uptake in the IP, MP, IC (intercarpal) and RC (radiocarpal) joints of affected limb

565. What is the primary mode of therapy used for RSD patients?

565. Pain-free active ROM

Hand–Arm Vibration Syndrome

566. What are the characteristic clinical features?

566. Caused by the use of vibrating tools or machinery
Increased vibration and temperature thresholds
Cold intolerance

Suprascapular Nerve

567. What symptom is associated with compression?

567. Posterolateral shoulder pain

568. At which site is the suprascapular nerve generally compressed?

568. Suprascapular notch by the transverse scapular ligament

569. What muscle groups are affected?

569. Supraspinatus
Infraspinatus

570. What other condition also affects periscapular muscles? How is it different?

570. Spinoglenoid notch cyst
This condition affects only infraspinatus muscle

571. Is an EMG generally helpful in the diagnosis of suprascapular nerve compression?

571. Yes

Thoracic Outlet Syndrome

572. What are the two basic types of thoracic outlet syndrome?

572. Vascular
Neurogenic

573. What artery is generally responsible for vascular thoracic outlet syndrome?

573. Subclavian artery

574. What are some potential causes of neurogenic thoracic outlet syndrome?

574. Cervical rib
Pancoast tumor
Compression by anterior scalene muscle or anomalous scalene insertion
Cervical transverse process
Clavicle or first rib malunion

575. What does operative treatment include?

575. First rib resection, or
Cervical rib resection, or
Scalenotomy, or
Scalenectomy

■ Other Pathologic States of the Hand and Upper Extremity

Vascular Disorders

576. Side-to-side upper extremity pressure differences in excess of ___ mm are abnormal.

576. 20 mm side-to-side difference

577. Describe the cold stimulation test.

577. Used to demonstrate autonomic vascular dysfunction in vasospastic patients
Normal patient: takes 10 minutes to return to baseline after cold stimulus
>20 minutes to return to baseline is abnormal
Can help predict result of surgical sympathectomy

Buerger's Disease (Thromboangiitis Obliterans)

578. What patient population is especially at risk for Buerger's disease?

578. Smokers

579. In which direction does the disease progress?

579. Distal to proximal; disease is more severe peripherally

Giant Cell Arteritis (Polymyalgia Rheumatica)

580. What population is especially at risk?

580. Elderly women

581. What are the common diagnostic methods for polymyalgia rheumatica?

581. Temporal artery biopsy
Erythrocyte sedimentation rate (ESR) elevation

582. What other bodily regions may also be affected?

582. Shoulders
Pelvic girdle

583. What is the treatment?

583. High-dose steroids
Arterial reconstruction

Takayasu Arteritis

584. What population is especially at risk?

584. Young females

585. What is the mechanism of disease?

585. Intimal proliferation

Raynaud's Disease (Primary Raynaud's)

586. What population is especially at risk?

586. Middle-aged women

587. What is the angiographic appearance of primary Raynaud's?

587. Generally normal

Raynaud's Phenomenon

588. What are examples of potential causes?

588. Vascular disease
CREST syndrome (calcinosis cutis, Raynaud's phenomenon, esophageal dysfunction, sclerodactyly, and telangiectasia)
Lupus
Dermatomyositis

589. What population is especially at risk for vascular disease?

589. Elderly men

590. What is the angiographic appearance of Raynaud's phenomenon?

590. Abnormal

591. Does atherosclerotic disease more commonly affect the left or the right upper extremity?

591. More commonly affects the left subclavian (may result in subclavian steal syndrome)

Volkmann's Ischemic Contracture

592. What muscles are most often affected with Volkmann's contracture?

592. FDP
FPL

593. It is associated with an intrinsic ___ hand.

593. Minus

594. Only the most severe cases also involve what muscle groups?

594. Extensors

Miscellaneous Vascular Conditions

595. What is the pathologic manifestation of polyarteritis nodosa?

595. Aneurysms of small vessels (e.g., digital arteries)

Rheumatoid Arthritis

The Rheumatoid Wrist

596. For the rheumatoid wrist, what are the early radiocarpal interventions?

596. ECRL to ECU transfer helps correct radial deviation and supination
Synovectomy of DRUJ

597. What are the later intervention options?

597. Radiolunate fusion
Wrist fusion
Total wrist arthroplasty (in the low demand patient only)

Metacarpophalangeal Joint Disease and Ulnar Deviation

598. How is early MCP disease treated?

598. Stage 1: medical management, splinting
Stage 2: synovectomy
Stage 3: centralization of extensor tendon, ulnar intrinsic release

599. Is fusion or arthroplasty preferred for advanced disease: thumb versus other MCP joints?

599. Thumb MCP fusion OK (if CMC not fused)
Other MCP joints: arthroplasty generally preferred

600. In general, successful resurfacing arthroplasty requires what?

600. Intact collateral ligaments

601. When treating advanced rheumatoid arthritis (RA) disease with MCP arthroplasty, what other potential pathology must be addressed first?

601. The wrist

602. What is the treatment for advanced PIP rheumatoid disease?

602. Arthrodesis or arthroplasty

Tendon Rupture in Rheumatoid Arthritis

603. What is the relative frequency of rupture of different tendons (in descending order)?

603. EDM
EDC (ring, small)
EPL

604. What tendon is generally transferred to a ruptured EDM?

604. EIP

605. What tendon is generally transferred to a ruptured EDC (small)?

605. EIP

606. What tendon is generally transferred to a ruptured EPL?

606. EIP

607. What is Mannerfelt-Noonan syndrome? What is its significance?

607. FPL rupture in rheumatoid arthritis
Most common flexor tendon rupture in RA

608. What is the preferred treatment for Mannerfelt-Noonan?

608. FDS transfer

609. Bottom line: what tendons are generally most useful for transfers in RA ruptures?

609. EIP
FDS (ring)

Key review point: rheumatoid arthritis may lead to intrinsic tightness; may need release.

Dupuytren's Disease

610. What geographic populations are at the highest risk?

610. Northern Europeans

611. Inheritance pattern?

611. Autosomal dominant
Sporadic (majority)

612. Penetrance?

612. Variable

613. What gender is most at risk of developing Dupuytren's disease?

613. Male

614. What are the three stages of Dupuytren's disease?

614. Proliferative
Involutional
Residual

615. What are the proliferative phase features: Key cells? Matrix? Gap junctions? Vascularity?

615. Large myofibroblasts
Minimal extracellular matrix
High number of gap junctions
High vascularity

616. What are the features of the involutional stage: Key cells? Collagen types?

616. Dense myofibroblasts
High ratio of type III to type I collagen

617. What are the features of the residual phase?

617. Fibrosis
Acellular
No nodules

618. Is Dupuytren's generally a volar or dorsal process?

618. Volar

619. What ligamentous structure is generally spared: Cleland's or Grayson's?

619. Cleland

620. What structures are generally involved?

620. Pretendinous bands
Spiral bands (at the MCP joint)
Natatory ligament
Grayson's
Lateral digital sheath

621. What are the components of the spiral cord?

621. Pretendinous bands
Spiral band
Grayson's
Lateral digital sheath

622. What commonly tested structure is not a component of the spiral cord?

622. Natatory ligament

623. What is the position of the spiral cords in relation to the neurovascular bundles?

623. Spiral cords are deep to the neurovascular bundles

624. What is the significance of this anatomic relationship?

624. Neurovascular bundles are pushed volarly and toward the midline
At increased risk with surgical intervention

625. What is the best predictor of the degree of neurovascular bundle displacement?

625. Magnitude of PIP contracture

626. Corticosteroid injections are proven effective for what Dupuytren's structures?

626. Nodules not associated with cords

627. What are the surgical indications for Dupuytren's disease?

627. MCP joint contracture >30 degrees
PIP joint contracture

628. What is the preferred surgical intervention?

628. Regional palmar fasciotomy of the affected digit

629. What about total palmar fasciotomy? Why not?

629. No longer favored procedure
Palm sensitivity

630. Should carpal tunnel release be performed with Dupuytren's surgery? Why?

630. No concomitant carpal tunnel release
Increased flare reaction

631. What is the preferred management of the surgical incision?

631. Leave the transverse component of Z-plasty incisions open

632. What if the PIP contracture >40 degrees?

632. 15- to 20-degree flexion contracture favored over PIP instability

633. What are the long-term outcomes of Dupuytren's releases at the MCP joint and the PIP joint?

633. MCP correction tends to be maintained
PIP contracture tends to recur

634. Complications are associated with what clinical conditions?

634. Alcoholism
Seizure disorder
Diabetes mellitus

635. Before any revision Dupuytren's surgery, what test is critical to perform?

635. Allen test

Infections

Flexor Tenosynovitis and Deep Spaces of the Hand

636. The thumb flexor sheath communicates with what bursal space?

636. Radial bursa

637. The thumb flexor sheath communicates with what index finger bursal space?

637. Thenar space

638. The thumb flexor sheath communicates with what long and ring finger space?

638. Midpalmar space

639. The thumb flexor sheath communicates with what small finger space?

639. Ulnar bursa

640. What is the location of the septum dividing the radial and ulnar bursae?

640. Third metacarpal

641. In what percentage of patients do the radial and ulnar bursae communicate?

641. 50 to 80%

642. Parona's space is located where?

642. Deep space at the level of the carpal tunnel
This is defined in the next question

643. What are the borders of this space?

643. PQ (dorsally)
Flexors (volarly)
FCU (ulnarly)
FPL (radially)

644. A distal infection extending proximally to this space is referred to as what?

644. A horseshoe abscess: communication between the radial and ulnar bursae at the space of Parona

645. What is the earliest sign of flexor tenosynovitis?

645. Pain with passive extension

Paronychia

646. What is the most likely causative organism?

646. *Staphylococcus aureus*

647. If no response to standard therapy, then consider which organism?

647. *Candida* (especially common with diabetic patients)

Fight Bite

648. What are the most common organisms associated with fight bites?

648. *S. aureus*
Streptococcus

649. What other organism may be associated with a fight bite?

649. *Eikenella* (7–29% of patients)

650. What organisms are associated with dog and cat bites?

650. *Streptococcus*
Anaerobes
Pasteurella
Staphylococcus

Subcutaneous Fungal Infection

651. How do these infections commonly present?

651. Nodular mass

652. What is the causative organism?

652. *Sporothrix schenckii*

653. From?

653. Rose thorns

654. What is the treatment of choice?

654. Potassium iodide

Atypical Mycobacterium

655. Atypical mycobacteria may also present how?

655. Nodular mass

656. What special stain is used to identify mycobacteria?

656. Ziehl-Neelson stain

657. What medium?

657. Lowenstein-Jensen

Herpetic Whitlow

658. What prep is used to identify herpetic whitlow?

658. Tzanck

659. In cases of whitlow, should an I&D be performed?

659. No

660. What is a common means by which oral secretion may result in herpetic whitlow of the finger?

660. Nail biting

661. What is the treatment for herpetic whitlow?

661. Oral acyclovir

Diagnostic Imaging: Bone Scan

662. Describe the timing and clinical usefulness of each of the three phases of the bone scan: phase I?

663. Phase II timing and features?

664. Phase III timing and features?

662. Within the first 2 minutes after injection
Is an arteriogram

663. 5 to 10 minutes after injection
Areas of cellulitis appear intense

664. 2 to 3 hours after injection
Areas of osteomyelitis appear intense

9

Pediatric Orthopaedic Surgery

■ Embryology: Key Points

Week 3

1. At week 3, mesoderm gives rise to what?
2. Somites are responsible for the ____ skeleton?
3. Somites differentiate into what two parts? What does each form?
4. Dermomyotome differentiates into what two parts? What does each form?
5. Notochordal tissue eventually disappears, but, while present, induces formation of what?
6. What remnant of notochord remains?

1. Somites
2. Axial
3. Dermomyotome (dermis, muscle) Sclerotome (vertebral column)
4. Epimere (dorsal muscle) Hypomere (ventral muscle: abdomen, thorax)
5. The vertebral column

6. Nucleus pulposus

Week 4

7. Ectoderm and mesoderm interact to form what?
8. The apical ectodermal ridge is responsible for the ____ skeleton?
9. What does the apical ectodermal ridge control?
10. This process is inhibited by what pharmacologic agent? What is the associated defect?
11. What two genes regulate limb formation?
12. What does the zone of polarizing activity (ZPA) control?

7. Apical ectodermal ridge
8. Appendicular
9. Proximal to distal development Mediates interdigital necrosis
10. Thalidomide Phocomelia
11. Homeobox Sonic hedgehog
12. Anteroposterior (AP) axis of the limb

13. What does the Wnt (wingless) signaling center control?
14. From what do limb muscles develop?

13. Dorsoventral development of the limb
14. Limb bud mesenchyme

Neural Crest Cells

15. Neural crest cells arise from what?
16. Where do they start? Then what happens?
17. What eight structures do they form?

15. Ectoderm
16. Start at margins of the neural tube
    Then they migrate with neural tube
17. Spinal cord
    Pharyngeal arches
    Dorsal root ganglion (DRG)
    Peripheral sensory nerves
    Adrenal medulla
    Sympathetic chain
    Schwann cells
    Melanocytes

Key Lists of Structures and Origins

18. What three structures does ectoderm form?

19. What does mesoderm form?
20. What are three examples of connective tissue?

21. What three entities does endoderm form?

18. Skin
    Nervous system
    Neural crest cells
19. Connective tissues
20. Bone
    Muscle
    Blood
21. Lung
    Gut lining
    Associated organs

Cervical Spine Development

Atlas Development

22. From how many ossification centers does the atlas form?
23. What are they?

24. When do the two neural arches fuse posteriorly?
25. When does the anterior arch fuse to the posterior arch? at what location?

22. Three

23. Anterior arch
    Two neural arches
24. At age 3 to 4 years

25. At age 7 years
    Neurocentral synchondrosis

Axis Development

26. When does the odontoid process begin forming? From what?

27. These longitudinal centers fuse at __ months to form what?

26. In utero (by 7th month of gestation)
    From two separate ossification
        centers on either side of the midline
27. 3 months to form chondrum
        terminale

28. How many total ossification centers are present in the axis at birth?
29. What are they?

28. Four

29. Odontoid process (from chondrum terminale)
    Body (centrum)
    Two neural arches

30. When do the neural arches fuse posteriorly to each other?
31. When do the neural arches fuse to the body?
32. What separates the body from odontoid process?
33. How long might the dentrocentral synchrosis persist?
34. Chondrum terminale is what?

30. At age 2 to 3 years

31. At age 3 to 6 years

32. Dentocentral synchondrosis

33. May persist until age 11 years
    May be confused with a fracture

34. Secondary ossification center, which appears at the tip of the apex

35. The chondrum terminale ossifies at age 5 to 8 years to become what?
36. When does it generally fuse to the remainder of the odontoid process?

35. Ossiculum (os) terminale

36. At age 10 to 13 years

Remainder of the Cervical Spine

37. How many ossification centers are in each vertebral body?
38. What are they?

37. Three

38. Vertebral body
    Two neural arches

39. The neural arches fuse posteriorly to each other by what age?
40. The vertebral body fuses with the neural arches by what age?
41. What is the significance of this fusion?
42. 95% of canal diameter has been achieved by what age?
43. Secondary ossification centers may resemble fractures at what three locations?

39. 2 to 3 years

40. 8 years

41. Fixes canal diameter

42. 5 years

43. Tip of transverse process
    Tip of spinous process
    Superior/inferior aspects of the vertebral bodies

Congenital Torticollis

44. Congenital torticollis is commonly associated with what two conditions?
45. In these patients, what conditions must be excluded?
46. What is the indication for surgery for congenital torticollis?

44. Hip dysplasia
    Metatarsus adductus

45. Atlanto-occipital abnormalities

46. Persists for over 1 year despite therapy

Other Common Embryology Questions and Review

47. What does lateral plate mesoderm form?

47. Red blood cells

48. Vascular invasion and appearance of primary ossification centers occurs when?

48. At 8 weeks

49. Secondary ossification centers appear when?

49. At 39 weeks

50. What is the first ossification center to appear?

50. Distal femur

What is the tissue of origin for the following glands:

51. Parathyroid gland?

51. Third and fourth pharyngeal pouches

52. Thyroid gland?

52. Foramen cecum

53. Anterior pituitary gland?

53. Rathke's pouch

54. Adrenal medulla?

54. Neural crest

55. Adrenal cortex?

55. Mesoderm

56. What adult structure is a remnant of the notochord?

56. Nucleus pulposus

57. From what do the trunk muscles arise?

57. Myotomes of somite

58. From what do the limb muscles arise?

58. Limb bud mesenchyme

■ Review of Key Genetics Facts

59. Classically, mendelian disorders are associated with how many genes?

59. One

60. What is the difference between triploidy and trisomy?

60. Triploidy means that all chromosomes are in triplicate, totaling 69
Trisomy means that one chromosome is in triplicate (e.g., as in Down syndrome)

61. What are two X-linked dominant disorders?

61. Hypophosphatemic rickets
Pseudohypoparathyroidism

62. What are six X-linked recessive disorders?

62. Spondyloepiphyseal dysplasia tarda
Hemophilia
Hunter's syndrome
Duchenne's muscular dystrophy
Becker's muscular dystrophy
Menkes' syndrome

63. What is the definition of genetic locus?

63. Position of the genes on chromosome

Anticipation

64. What is the definition of anticipation?

64. Increasing severity of disease with each generation

65. What is a disorder that displays anticipation?

65. Myotonic dystrophy

66. What is the mode of inheritance for this disorder?

66. Autosomal dominant (AD)

67. What genetic sequence is repeated?

67. CTG

68. What is the associated clinical problem?

68. Inability to relax muscle

69. What is genomic imprinting?

69. Clinical manifestation of disease depends on which parent has the mutation

70. What is a disorder that displays imprinting?

70. Prader-Willi (father)
Angelman (mother)

71. What is germline mosaicism?

71. Only gonadal cells carry the mutation

■ Disorders of the Growth Plate

Review of Key Bone Formation Facts

72. What three processes involve intramembranous bone formation?

72. Flat bone
Distraction osteogenesis (except if unstable)
Blastema (after amputation)

73. What two processes involve appositional bone formation?

73. Periosteal enlargement
Bone formation with remodeling

74. What process of bony healing is seen with rigid plating?

74. Haversian remodeling

Enchondral Ossification

75. At what relative oxygen tension does enchondral calcification occur?

75. Low oxygen tension

76. Growth plate chondrocytes produce what protein?

76. Indian hedgehog protein

77. What is the function of this protein?

77. Signals release of parathyroid hormone–related peptide (PTHrP) production

78. What is the ultimate effect?

78 Inhibits chondrocyte maturation

79. What disorder results from mutation in PTHrP?

79. Jansen's metaphyseal dysplasia

80. The perichondral ring of Lacroix is continuous with what structure?

80. Groove of Ranvier

81. What are the two functions of the ring?

81. Provides mechanical support to bone–cartilage junction
Contributes chondrocytes to increase bone latitudinal growth

Classification of Enchondral Ossification Disorders by Location

List the key disorders for each location:

82. Epiphyseal dysplasias (three)?

82. Spondyloepiphyseal dysplasia
Chondrodysplasia punctata
Multiple epiphyseal dysplasia

83. Reserve zone (four)?

83. Pseudachondroplasia
Kniest
Diastrophic dysplasia
Gaucher's/Niemann-Pick

84. Proliferative zone (three)?

84. Achondroplasia
Gigantism
Hypochondroplasia

85. Hypertrophic zone?

85. Mucopolysaccharidoses (e.g.,
Morquio's, Hurler's)

86. Zone of provisional calcification
(four)? Exception?

86. Rickets/osteomalacia
SCFE (exception: renal failure SCFE
occurs at spongiosa)
Physeal fracture
Enchondroma

87. Primary spongiosa (two)?

87. Metaphyseal chondrodysplasia (e.g.,
Jansen, Schmid)
Osteomyelitis

88. Secondary spongiosa (three)?

88. Osteopetrosis
Osteogenesis imperfecta
Scurvy

Spondyloepiphyseal Dysplasias

89. What is (are) the two associated
inheritance patterns?

89. Congenita: AD
Tarda: X-linked

90. What is the mutation?

90. Type II collagen

91. What is the gene?

91. *COL2A1*

92. What is the zone?

92. Epiphyseal

93. Does the disorder result in
proportionate or disproportionate
dwarfism?

93. Disproportionate

94. What is the subclassification (short
limb or short trunk)?

94. Short trunk

95. Spondyloepiphyseal dysplasia
must be differentiated from which
disorder?

95. Multiple epiphyseal dysplasia (MED)

Spondyloepiphyseal Dysplasia Congenita

96. What is the relative severity of
congenita?

96. More severe than tarda

97. What is the key feature of the face?

97. Flat

98. What are the two key features of the
hips?

98. Delayed epiphyseal appearance
Coxa vara

99. What are the two key features of the spine?

100. What is the key feature of the knees?

101. What is the key feature of the feet?

Spondyloepiphyseal Dysplasia Tarda

102. Relative severity?

103. What is the key feature of the legs?

104. In all types of spondyloepiphyseal dysplasia, what organ must be checked? For what?

Chondrodysplasia Punctata

105. What are the two inheritance forms?

106. What is the mutation?

107. What is the relative severity of Conradi-Hunermann? What are the key features?

108. What is the relative severity of the AR form? Rhizo, meso, or acro? What is the prognosis?

109. What is the x-ray appearance of either type?

Multiple Epiphyseal Dysplasia

110. What is the inheritance?

111. What are the two mutations?

112. What is the zone?

113. Proportionate or disproportionate?

114. What is the subclassification (short limb or short trunk)?

115. What is the defining feature?

116. What is the key feature of the hips? Rule out?

117. What are the three key features of the knees?

118. What three MED features are not seen in Perthes?

119. If you see bilateral Legg-Calvé-Perthes disease (LCPD) and want to check for dysplasia, what is the test of choice?

---

99. Odontoid hypoplasia
Vertebral beaking

100. Genu valgum

101. Clubfeet

102. Less severe

103. No angular deformity

104. Eyes, for retinal detachment

105. AD, as in Conradi-Hunermann
Autosomal recessive (AR)

106. Peroxisomal enzymatic defect

107. Less severe
Variable features

108. More severe
Rhizomelic dwarfism
Fatal early

109. Multiple punctate calcifications

110. AD

111. Collagen IX
COMP (cartilage oligometric matrix protein)

112. Epiphysis

113. Disproportionate

114. Short limb

115. Irregular delayed ossification at multiple epiphyses

116. Coxa vara
Rule out Perthes

117. Flat femoral condyles
Double-layer patella
Genu valgum

118. Bilateral symmetric involvement
Early acetabular changes
No metaphyseal cysts

119. Skeletal survey

Disorders of the Reserve Zone

Pseudoachondroplasia

120. What is the inheritance?

121. What is the mutation?

122. What is the zone?

123. What is the key feature of the face?

124. What is the key feature of the spine?

125. What are the two key features of the joints?

126. What are the two general characteristics of the x-ray appearance?

120. AD

121. COMP

122. Reserve

123. Normal

124. Cervical instability

125. Flexion contractures
Osteoarthritis

126. Metaphyseal flaring
Delayed epiphyseal ossification

Kniest Dysplasia

127. What is the inheritance?

128. What is the mutation?

129. What is the zone?

130. Proportionate or disproportionate?

131. What is the subclassification?

132. What is the key feature of the joints?

133. What is the femoral appearance?

134. What two clinical problems is it associated with?

127. AD

128. Type II collagen

129. Reserve zone

130. Disproportionate

131. Short trunk

132. Contractures

133. Dumbbell shaped

134. Retinal detachment
Cleft palate

Diastrophic Dysplasia

135. What is the inheritance?

136. What is the mutation?

137. What is the zone?

138. Proportionate or disproportionate?

139. What is the subclassificaion?

140. What are the two key features of the face?

141. What are the two key features of the spine? What is the natural history?

142. What is the key feature of the joints?

143. What is the key feature of the hips?

144. What are the two key features of the feet?

145. What is the key feature of the hands?

135. AR

136. Sulfate transport protein on chromosome 5

137. Reserve

138. Disproportionate

139. Short limb

140. Cleft palate
Cauliflower ears

141. Atlantoaxial instability
Cervical kyphosis: spontaneously resolves

142. Contractures

143. Dysplasia

144. Bilateral skewfoot
Rigid clubfoot

145. Hitchhiker thumbs

Gaucher

146. What is the inheritance?

147. What is the zone?

146. AR

147. Reserve

148. What is the classification?
149. What is accumulated?
150. What population is particularly at risk?
151. What is the key feature of the hips?
152. What is the key feature of the knees?
153. What is the key feature of the organs?
154. What is the key feature of the pain?
155. What is the x-ray appearance of involved bone?

148. Lysosomal storage disease
149. Cerebroside
150. Ashkenazi Jews
151. Femoral head necrosis
152. Erlenmeyer flask shaped distal femur
153. Hepatosplenomegaly (HSM)
154. Bone pain indicates Gaucher crisis
155. Moth-eaten

Niemann-Pick

156. What is the inheritance?
157. What is accumulated?
158. What are the two key features of the bones?

156. AR
157. Sphingomyelin
158. Expanded marrow space
Cortical thinning

Disorder of the Proliferative Zone: Achondroplasia

159. What is the inheritance?
160. What is the mutation?

161. What is the zone?
162. Proportionate or disproportionate?
163. What is the subclassification?
164. What is the parental risk factor?
165. Rhizo, meso, or acro?
166. What is the key feature in general?
167. What are the two key features of the face?
168. What is the key feature of the hands?
169. What are the three key features of the spine?

170. What is the prognosis for an infant with kyphosis? What is the treatment?
171. What is the x-ray feature of the spine?
172. What is the key feature of the pelvis?
173. What are the two key features of the knees?
174. What are two components of thanatophoric dysplasia?

159. AD
160. *FGFR3* on chromosome 4
Defect causes *FGFr3* to be constituently active
161. Proliferative
162. Disproportionate
163. Short limb
164. Advanced paternal age
165. Rhizomelic (proximal involvement)
166. Ligamentous laxity
167. Frontal bossing
Midface hypoplasia
168. Trident
169. Lumbar stenosis (short pedicles)
Foramen magnum stenosis
Kyphosis
170. Usually spontaneously resolves
Extension brace until over 2 years old
171. Decreased interpedicular distance
172. Champagne glass
173. Genu varum
Inverted V distal femoral physis
174. Achondroplasia
Restrictive lung disease

Disorders of the Hypertrophic Zone: Mucopolysaccharidoses

175. What is the zone?

175. Hypertrophic zone

176. Proportionate or disproportionate?

176. Proportionate

177. What is the most common type?

177. Morquio's

178. What type results in the shortest height?

178. Morquio's

179. What type has the worst prognosis?

179. Hurler's, fatal by age 10

180. What is the general feature of the hips?

180. Coxa vara

181. What are the two general features of the spine?

181. Vertebral beaking
Odontoid hypoplasia/instability: may lead to myelopathy

182. What is the general feature of the hands?

182. Bullet metacarpals

183. What is the general feature of the knees?

183. Genu valgum

Hunter

184. What is the inheritance?

184. X linked recessive

185. Intelligence is generally _____?

185. Decreased

186. What is the key feature of the cornea appearance?

186. Clear

187. What is excreted in urine?

187. Dermatan/heparan sulfate

Hurler

188. What is the inheritance?

188. AR

189. What is the mutation?

189. Alpha-L-iduronidase

190. Intelligence is generally _____?

190. Decreased

191. What is the key feature of the cornea appearance?

191. Cloudy

192. What is excreted in urine?

192. Dermatan/heparan sulfate

Morquio

193. What is the inheritance?

193. AR

194. What is the mutation?

194. N-acetylgalactose-6 sulfate

195. Intelligence is generally _____?

195. Normal

196. What is the key feature of the cornea appearance?

196. Cloudy

197. What is excreted in urine?

197. Keratan sulfate

Sanfilippo

198. What is the inheritance?

198. AR

199. Intelligence is generally _____?
200. What is the key feature of the cornea appearance?
201. What is excreted in urine?
202. What feature is unique to Sanfilippo?

199. Decreased
200. Clear
201. Heparan sulfate
202. Development is normal until age 2

Disorders Specific to the Zone of Provisional Calcification

Rickets/Osteomalacia

203. What is the zone?
204. What are the two qualities of affected bone?
205. What is the key feature of the physis?
206. What is the key feature of the skull?
207. What is the key feature of the knees?
208. What is the key feature of the ribs?
209. What is the key feature of the spine?
210. What are the two histologic features of rickets?
211. What is a milkman's fracture?

203. Zone of provisional calcification
204. Brittle
     Bowed long bones
205. Cupped and widened
206. Flat
207. Genu varum
208. Rachitic rosary at costochondral junction
209. Dorsal kyphosis
210. Wide osteoid seams
     Swiss cheese trabeculae
211. Pseudofracture on compression side of bone

Disorders of the Primary Spongiosa: Metaphyseal Chondrodysplasias

212. What is the zone?
213. What is the condition of the epiphysis?
214. Proportionate or disproportionate?
215. What is the subclass?
216. What are the three types of metaphyseal chondrodysplasia?

212. Primary spongiosa
213. Normal
214. Disproportionate
215. Short limb
216. Jansen
     Schmid
     McKusick

Jansen

217. What is the inheritance?
218. What is the mutation?
219. What is the relative severity?
220. What are the two key features?

217. AD
218. PTHrP
219. Most severe
220. Hypercalcemia
     Bulbous metaphyseal expansion

Schmid

221. What is the inheritance?

221. AD

222. What is the mutation?	**222.** Type X collagen
223. What is the relative severity?	**223.** Less severe
224. What disorder must be excluded?	**224.** Rickets
225. What is the key feature of the hips?	**225.** Coxa vara
226. What is the key feature of the knees?	**226.** Genu varum

McKusick

227. What is the inheritance?	**227.** AR
228. What population is particularly at risk?	**228.** Amish
229. What is McKusick also known as?	**229.** Cartilage-hair dysplasia
230. What are the two key features?	**230.** Odontoid hypoplasia and cervical instability Fibular overgrowth

Disorders of the Secondary Spongiosa

Osteopetrosis

231. What are the two forms of the inheritance?	**231.** AD (mild form) AR (malignant form)
232. The autosomal dominant form is also known as what?	**232.** Albers-Schönberg disease
233. What is the mutation?	**233.** Carbonic anhydrase defect Chromosome 11
234. What is the zone?	**234.** Secondary spongiosa
235. Where does the defect manifest itself?	**235.** Thymus
236. This results in failure of what?	**236.** Osteoclastic resorption
237. What is the histologic characteristic?	**237.** Osteoclasts without ruffled border
238. What are the key molecules involved in osteoclast development and bone remodeling?	**238.** RANKL: expressed on osteoblasts RANK: expressed on osteoclasts OPG (osteoprotegrin): produced by osteoblasts RANKL binds to RANK on osteoclast precursors leading to osteoclast differentiation, hence increased bone resorption OPG acts as decoy receptor for RANKL inhibiting osteoclastogenesis Nude mice knockout model: knock out RANKL → osteopetrosis
239. What is the quality of affected bone?	**239.** Dense (marble)
240. What is the key feature of the spine?	**240.** Rugger jersey: looks like stripes on a lateral film
241. What is the key feature of the knee?	**241.** Erlenmeyer flask shaped distal femur

242. What is the three treatments for the malignant form of disease?

242. Bone marrow transplant
Calcitriol with or without steroids
Interferon-gamma-1β

Osteogenesis Imperfecta

243. What is the mutation?

244. What is the gene?

245. What is the zone?

246. By what two means is osteogenesis imperfecta diagnosed?

247. What is the quality of affected bone?

248. What is characteristic about the height?

249. What is the key feature of the ligaments?

250. What is characteristic about the fracture healing?

251. What intervention should be considered when the patient is over 2 years old?

252. What are two possible early interventions?

253. What is the key feature of the spine? When should surgery be considered?

254. What is the key feature of the brainstem?

255. What is the best pharmacologic therapy?

256. What are the three benefits of bisphosphonate therapy?

257. Do bisphosphonates help the scoliosis?

258. Classify the four types by relative severity (from most severe to least)?

243. Type I collagen

244. COL1A2

245. Secondary spongiosa

246. Skull films
Fibroblast culture

247. Brittle

248. Short

249. Lax

250. Normal
But remodeling is increased

251. Consider prophylactic intramedullary (IM) nails

252. Bracing
Sofield osteotomy for bow or fracture

253. Scoliosis
Operate when curve over 50 degrees

254. Basilar invagination

255. Bisphosphonate therapy

256. Improved cortical thickness
Decreased incidence of fracture
Improved height of collapsed vertebral bodies

257. No

258. II
III
I
IV

Type I

259. What is the inheritance?

260. What is the sclera appearance?

261. When do children generally present with disease?

262. How is hearing characteristically affected?

259. AD

260. Blue

261. Preschool age

262. Hearing loss

Type II

263. What is the inheritance?

264. What is the sclera appearance?

265. What is the prognosis?

263. AR

264. Blue

265. Lethal early

Type III

266. What is the inheritance?

267. What is the sclera appearance?

268. How do children with type III generally present?

266. AR

267. White

268. Fractures at birth

Type IV

269. What is the inheritance?

270. What is the sclera appearance?

271. What is the relative severity of type IV in relation to other types?

272. What is the key feature of the hearing?

269. AD

270. White

271. Mild

272. Normal

Scurvy

273. What is the zone?

274. Scurvy results from a deficiency of what?

275. Vitamin C deficiency then leads to a deficiency of what?

276. What is the ultimate effect?

277. What is the key systemic feature?

278. What is the key feature of the gums?

279. What is the key feature of the joints?

280. What are the two key x-ray findings?

281. Why do the clefts develop?

282. What can be seen around the ossification centers?

273. Secondary spongiosa

274. Vitamin C

275. Chondroitin sulfate

276. Impaired collagen growth and hydroxylation

277. Fatigue

278. Bleeding gums

279. Effusions

280. Thin cortices
Metaphyseal clefts

281. From compression fractures

282. Lines

Disorders of Intramembranous Ossification

Cleidocranial Dysostosis

283. What is the inheritance?

284. What is the mutation?

285. What are the two functions of mutant protein?

286. What is the zone?

283. AD

284. *CBFA1* on chromosome 6

285. Osteoblast differentiation
Osteocalcin expression

286. No zone

287. Why?

287. Because intramembranous, not enchondral, ossification affected

288. Proportionate or disproportionate?

288. Proportionate

289. Is it usually unilateral or bilateral?

289. Usually unilateral

290. Is the whole clavicle missing?

290. Usually lateral clavicle absent only But sometimes the whole clavicle is absent (appearance of touching shoulders)

291. What is the key feature of the head?

291. Delayed skull suture closure

292. What is the key feature of the hips?

292. Coxa vara

293. What is the key feature of the pelvis?

293. Widened symphysis pubis

Congenital Pseudarthrosis of the Clavicle

294. What clavicle is most commonly affected with congenital pseudarthrosis?

294. Right

295. Is involvement generally unilateral or bilateral?

295. Unilateral

296. What portion of the clavicle is missing?

296. Center: medial and lateral clavicle not united

297. How are the majority of patients with congenital pseudarthrosis successfully treated?

297. Nonoperatively

298. What is the indication for surgery with this condition?

298. Scapular winging

Review of Key Disorders and Features: Quick Solution Guide

Name the disorders associated with each of the listed features:

299. Short trunk dwarfism (two)?

299. Kniest Spondyloepiphyseal dysplasia

300. Proportional dwarfism (two)?

300. Mucopolysaccharidoses Cleidocranial dysostosis

301. Odontoid hypoplasia/cervical instability (seven)?

301. Pseudachondroplasia SED (spondyloepiphyseal dysplasia) congenita McKusick (metaphyseal chondrodysplasia) Morquio (mucopolysaccharidosis) Diastrophic dysplasia Down syndrome Neurofibromatosis

302. Joint contractures (four)?

302. Kniest Diastrophic dysplasia Arthrogryposis Pseudachondroplasia

303. Joint dislocations (two)?

303. Ehlers-Danlos Larsen's syndrome

304. Other disorders with laxity (three)?

304. Osteogenesis imperfecta
Fragile X
Down syndrome

305. Genu valgum (four)?

305. SED congenita
MED
Ellis–van Creveld
Multiple hereditary exostoses (MHE)

306. Genu varum (four)?

306. Achondroplasia
Schmid (metaphyseal
    chondrodysplasia)
Rickets
Osteogenesis imperfecta (OI)

307. Coxa vara (five)?

307. SED congenita
MED
Schmid (metaphyseal
    chondrodysplasia)
Morquio (mucopolysaccharidosis)
Cleidocranial dysostosis

308. Erlenmeyer flask–shaped distal
femur (two)?

308. Gaucher's
Osteopetrosis

309. Rugger jersey spine (two)?

309. Osteopetrosis
Renal osteodystrophy

310. Obese, decreased IQ (two)?

310. Prader-Willi
Albright's (pseudo-
    hypoparathyroidism)

311. Biconcave vertebrae (two)?

311. Osteoporosis/osteomalacia (due to
    compression fracture)
Sickle cell disease

312. Thymic defect or antibodies versus
thymus (two)?

312. Myasthenia gravis (competitive
    inhibitor)
Osteopetrosis

■ Other Commonly Tested Pediatric Syndromes

List of Syndromes and Features

Laron's Dysplasia

313. What is the inheritance?

313. AR

314. What is the mutation?

314. Deficient growth hormone (GH)
    receptor

315. Laron's dysplasia is also known as
what?

315. Pituitary dwarfism

Progressive Diaphyseal Dysplasia (Camurati-Engelmann)

316. What is the inheritance?

316. AD

317. What is the defining feature?

317. Symmetric cortical thickening of
    long bones

318. What is the usual treatment of this disorder?

318. Nonsteroidal antiinflammatory drugs (NSAIDs)

Dysplasia Epiphysealis Hemimelia (Trevor's)

319. What is the defining feature of Trevor's?

319. Epiphyseal osteochondroma (knee)

Fascioscapulohumeral Dystrophy

320. What is the inheritance?

320. AD

321. What is the creatine phosphokinase (CPK) level in these patients?

321. Normal

322. What are the two key features?

322. Facial weakness
Proximal shoulder weakness bilaterally with winging

323. What is the treatment if weakness is severe?

323. Scapulothoracic fusion

Limb-Girdle Dystrophy

324. What is the inheritance?

324. AR

325. What is the genetic defect?

325. Sarcoglycan defect

326. What is the CPK level?

326. Elevated

327. What two areas are affected?

327. Shoulder
Pelvis

Ellis–van Creveld

328. What is the inheritance?

328. AR

329. What is the gene?

329. *EVC* gene

330. What are the two key features of the digits?

330. Polydactyly
Nail abnormalities

331. What are the two key features of the knees?

331. Genu valgum
Abnormal patellofemoral joints

332. What is the key feature of the heart?

332. Congenital heart disease

Nail-Patella Syndrome

333. What is the inheritance?

333. AD

334. What is the gene?

334. Lim homeobox (*LMX1B*): regulates transcription in limb-patterning and kidney formation

335. What are the two features of the knee?

335. Genu valgum
Absent patellae

336. When does the patella normally ossify?

336. At age 3 to 6 years

337. At which other joint is increased valgus also seen?

337. Elbows

338. What two other conditions must be excluded with nail-patella syndrome?

338. Kidney disease
Glaucoma

339. What radiographic feature is common to both Ellis–van Creveld and nail-patella syndromes?

339. Iliac horns

McCune-Albright Syndrome

340. What is the inheritance?

340. None; sporadic mutation

341. What is the mutation? Activating or deactivating?

341. Gs-α adenylate cyclase coupling
Activating

342. What is the key feature of the bone?

342. Fibrous dysplasia

343. What is the key feature of the skin?

343. Café-au-lait spots

344. What is the timing of puberty?

344. Precocious

Dyschondrosteosis (Lerri-Weill Syndrome)

345. What is the inheritance?

345. AD

346. What is the gene?

346. *SHOX* gene

347. What is the key feature of the height?

347. Short

348. Dyschondrosteosis is associated with what peripheral deformity?

348. Madelung's deformity

Fragile X

349. What sex is affected?

349. Male

350. What is the key feature of the joints?

350. Lax

351. What is the key feature of the feet?

351. Flat

352. What is the key feature of the spine?

352. Scoliosis

353. What is the key feature of the gonads?

353. Macro-orchidism

Down Syndrome

354. What is the mutation?

354. Trisomy 21

355. What are the two key features of the hips?

355. Slipped capital femoral epiphysis (SCFE) (hypothyroidism)
Instability

356. What is the key feature of the feet?

356. Pes planus

357. What is the key feature of the spine?

357. Atlantoaxial instability

358. What is the key feature of the ligaments?

358. Lax

359. What are the two key endocrine features?

359. Hypothyroidism
Diabetes mellitus

360. What is the key cardiovascular feature?

360. Heart disease

361. What is the treatment for an asymptomatic Down syndrome child with atlantoaxial instability?

361. No contact sports
Fusion if ADI >10 mm
(ADI = atlanto-dens interval)

362. Quick review: With what four cervical spine conditions are contact sports contraindicated?

362. Congenital upper cervical fusions or instability (e.g., os odontoideum)
Grade II spondylolisthesis
Atlantoaxial instability (e.g., Down syndrome)
History of diffuse axonal injury

Turner's Syndrome

363. What is the mutation?

363. 45XO

364. What sex is affected?

364. Females

365. What is the key feature of the height?

365. Short

366. What is the key feature of the neck?

366. Webbed

367. What is the key feature of the elbows?

367. Cubita valga

368. Turner's syndrome is associated with what anesthetic complication?

368. Malignant hyperthermia

369. Turner's must be differentiated from what similar syndrome?

369. Noonan's syndrome

370. In what three ways is Noonan's different?

370. Normal gonads
Mental retardation
Severe scoliosis

371. Quick review: What three disorders are also associated with malignant hyperthermia?

371. Duchenne's muscular dystrophy (MD)
Arthrogryposis
Osteogenesis imperfecta

372. How is an individual at risk for malignant hyperthermia diagnosed?

372. Muscle biopsy

373. What is the pharmacologic treatment for malignant hyperthermia?

373. Dantrolene

Prader-Willi

374. Prader-Willi is associated with what genetic concept?

374. Imprinting (parent with mutation determines the disorder)

375. What is the mutation?

375. Partial chromosome 15 deletion (paternal)

376. The same mutation inherited from the mother results in what syndrome?

376. Angelman's syndrome

377. What is the key Prader-Willi feature in the infant?

377. Hypotonic

378. What are the three key Prader-Willi features in the adult?

378. Obesity
Mental retardation
Hypogonadism

Menkes' Syndrome

379. What is the inheritance?

379. X-linked recessive (XLR)

380. What is the mutation?

380. Copper transport protein

381. What is the key feature of the hair?

382. What other disorder has similar features?

Rett's Syndrome

383. What sex is affected?

384. When do symptoms generally present?

385. Is Rett's a static or progressive condition?

386. What is the key feature of the movement disorder?

387. What is the key feature of the spine?

388. Can Rett's scoliosis be braced?

Beckwith-Wiedemann

389. What is the key orthopaedic feature of this disease?

390. What is the triad of other classic features?

391. What two neoplasms are associated with Beckwith-Wiedemann?

392. How are affected patients screened for neoplasm development?

393. What condition is the next most common cause of hemihypertrophy?

394. In that case, what is hemihypertrophy due to?

Marfan Syndrome

395. What is the inheritance?

396. What is the mutation?

397. What is the chromosome?

398. What is the key feature of the eye?

399. What is the key feature of the chest?

400. What are the two key cardiovascular features? What is the preferred pharmacologic treatment?

401. What is the key feature of the spine? What is the usual treatment?

402. What is the key feature of the hips?

---

381. Kinky hair

382. McKusick (metaphyseal chondrodysplasia)

383. Female

384. At age 6 to 18 months

385. Progressive

386. Stereotaxic hand movements

387. Scoliosis

388. Unresponsive to bracing

389. Hemihypertrophy

390. Organomegaly
Omphalocele
Large tongue

391. Wilms' nephroblastoma
Hepatoblastoma

392. Serial abdominal ultrasounds until age 5
Serial α-fetoprotein (AFP) level until age 3

393. Neurofibromatosis

394. Plexiform neurofibroma

395. AD

396. Fibrillin

397. 15

398. Superior dislocation of the lens

399. Pectus deformity

400. Valvular abnormalities
Aortic arch enlargement
Beta-blockers to minimize aortic dissection

401. Scoliosis
Surgery usually necessary (bracing ineffective)

402. Protrusio

Homocystinuria

403.	What is the inheritance?	**403.**	AR
404.	What is the enzyme defect?	**404.**	Cystathionine synthetase
405.	The defective enzyme then results in abnormal metabolism of what?	**405.**	Methionine
406.	And the accumulation of?	**406.**	Homocysteine
407.	How is homocystinuria diagnosed?	**407.**	Elevated urine homocysteine
408.	In what two ways can homocystinuria be differentiated from Marfan's?	**408.**	Inferior lens dislocation Osteoporosis
409.	What are the two components of the treatment of homocystinuria?	**409.**	Vitamin B_6 Low methionine diet
410.	Homogentisic acid oxidase deficiency is associated with what disorder?	**410.**	Alkaptonuria (not the same) AR Also known as ochronosis

Ehlers-Danlos

411.	How is the classic form of Ehlers-Danlos inherited?	**411.**	AD
412.	The mutation affects the production of what key component?	**412.**	Type V collagen
413.	What is the general feature of the skin?	**413.**	Hyperlax
414.	What is the general feature of the joints?	**414.**	Hypermobile
415.	What is the general feature of the spine?	**415.**	Scoliosis
416.	What is the general feature of the feet?	**416.**	Clubfeet
417.	What cardiovascular condition is associated with Ehlers-Danlos?	**417.**	Aortic root dilation

Duchenne Muscular Dystrophy

418.	What is the inheritance?	**418.**	XLR
419.	What is the mutation?	**419.**	Absent dystrophin
420.	What population is affected by Duchenne MD?	**420.**	Young males
421.	What laboratory finding may be indicative of Duchenne's?	**421.**	Elevated CPK
422.	What two other tests are useful for definitive diagnosis?	**422.**	DNA Muscle biopsy
423.	What are two classic exam findings?	**423.**	Calf pseudohypertrophy Gower's sign
424.	What is the first muscle group affected?	**424.**	Hip extensors
425.	At what age do affected patients generally lose ambulation?	**425.**	10 years

426. Posterior tibialis tendon transfer and knee-ankle-foot orthosis (KAFO) offer what benefit to ambulation?

426. Two additional years of ambulation

427. At what age do affected patients generally become wheelchair-bound?

427. 15 years

428. What is the pharmacologic therapy? Why?

428. Steroids
Because they upregulate dystrophin associated proteins, especially utrophin

429. What is the key feature of the foot?

429. Equinovarus

430. What is the key feature of the spine?

430. Neuromuscular scoliosis

431. When should surgery be performed to address the scoliosis?

431. Early (25- to 30-degree curves)

432. Through what approach?

432. Posterior fusion only (no anterior)

433. What is the critical forced vital capacity (FVC) value for surgery?

433. Must be over 40% to optimize operative safety

434. Compare patient satisfaction with multilevel releases versus isolated foot surgery.

434. Isolated posterior tibialis transfer, tendo-Achilles lengthening (TAL), toe flexor tenotomies preferred

Becker Muscular Dystrophy

435. What is the inheritance?

435. XLR

436. What is the mutation?

436. Decreased (not absent) dystrophin

437. What is the relative severity of Becker's?

437. Less severe than Duchenne

438. How can the two disorders be clinically differentiated?

438. Becker patient will survive beyond age 22 without respiratory support

439. Becker MD is also associated with what?

439. Red-green color blindness

Polymyositis/Dermatomyositis

440. What patient population is generally affected?

440. Females

441. What are the two typical laboratory abnormalities?

441. Elevated CPK
Elevated erythrocyte sedimentation rate (ESR)

442. The initial presentation of disease is often preceded by what?

442. Febrile illness

443. What does a muscle biopsy show?

443. Inflammatory changes

Myasthenia Gravis

444. What is the characteristic presenting symptom?

444. Easy fatigability

445. What is the mechanism of disease?

445. Competitive inhibition of acetylcholine (ACh) receptors

446. Due to what?

446. Antibodies in thymus

447. What two medications are commonly used for treatment?

448. What is the operative treatment of myasthenia gravis?

447. Cyclosporine
Anti-acetylcholinesterase

448. Thymectomy

Dejerine-Sottas

449. What is the inheritance?

450. What is the age of onset?

451. What is the severity of disease relative to traditional Charcot-Marie-Tooth (CMT)?

452. Dejerine-Sottas is also known as what variant of CMT?

449. AR

450. Infancy

451. More severe than CMT

452. CMT III

Riley-Day

453. What population is particularly at risk?

454. What is the inheritance?

455. Riley-Day is also known as what?

456. What are three common symptoms?

457. What is the pathognomonic oral finding?

458. What does Riley-Day have in common with Friedrich, CMT, and spinal muscular atrophy (SMA)?

459. As compared with what?

453. Ashkenazi Jews

454. AR

455. Dysautonomia

456. Postural hypotension
Sweating
Sensory loss (decreased pain)

457. No tongue papillae

458. Absent deep tendon reflexes (DTRs)

459. Duchenne muscular dystrophy (DTRs present)

Friedrich Ataxia

460. What is the inheritance?

461. What is the mutation?

462. What is the age of onset?

463. What are the features of the classic triad?

464. What is the feature of the eyes?

465. What is the feature of the heart?

466. What is the feature of the foot?

467. Is motor or sensory function affected?

468. What is the classic electromyograph (EMG) finding?

460. AR

461. Frataxin gene

462. 7 to 15 years

463. Ataxic
Absent DTRs
Extensor Babinski sign

464. Nystagmus

466. Cardiomyopathy

466. Cavus

467. Both

468. Increased polyphasic potentials

Polio

469.	What is the mechanism?	**469.**	Anterior horn cell destruction
470.	Are motor or sensory systems affected?	**470.**	Motor only

Spinal Muscular Atrophy

471.	What is the inheritance?	**471.**	AR
472.	What is the mechanism?	**472.**	Loss of anterior horn cells
473.	What is the mutation?	**473.**	Survival motor neuron gene on chromosome 5
474.	Progressive or static?	**474.**	Progressive
475.	Compare with what entity?	**475.**	Arthrogryposis (nonprogressive)
476.	Classify the three types by decreasing severity?	**476.**	Acute Werdnig-Hoffman Chronic Werdnig-Hoffman Kugelberg-Welander
477.	What muscle groups are involved?	**477.**	Proximal
478.	What extremities are more involved: arms or legs?	**478.**	Legs more than arms
479.	What is the key feature of the lower extremities?	**479.**	Contractures
480.	Is the scoliosis progressive or not?	**480.**	Progressive
481.	Therefore, consider surgery when?	**481.**	Operate early (like muscular dystrophy)
482.	What is the downside of surgical intervention?	**482.**	Short-term decrease in upper extremity function
483.	With spinal muscular atrophy (SMA), are reflexes present or absent?	**483.**	Absent
484.	Compare with muscular dystrophy?	**484.**	MD has reflexes present

Guillain-Barré

485.	Disease onset generally follows what condition?	**485.**	Viral illness
486.	What is the mechanism?	**486.**	Demyelination from distal to proximal
487.	How is Guillain-Barré diagnosed?	**487.**	Elevated cerebrospinal fluid (CSF) protein
488.	The direction of demyelination is similar to what other condition?	**488.**	Polyneuropathy, organomegaly, endocrinopathy, M protein, skin changes (POEMS) (multiple myeloma)
489.	Quick review of EMG findings: SMA?	**489.**	Fasciculations
490.	Friedreich's ataxia?	**490.**	Polyphasic potentials

Proteus Syndrome

491.	What is the key feature of the hands/feet?	**491.**	Overgrown hands/feet

492. What is the key feature of the spine?

492. Scoliosis

493. What is the key feature of the face?

493. Bizarre facial features

494. What are the two key features of the skin abnormalities?

494. Lipomas
Nevi

Klippel-Trenaunay

495. With this condition, what is overgrowth due to?

495. Arteriovenous malformations

Klippel-Feil

496. What is the classic triad of features?

496. Low posterior hairline
Short webbed neck
Decreased cervical range of motion (ROM) (fused segments)

497. With what two musculoskeletal conditions is Klippel-Feil associated?

497. Sprengel's deformity
Cervical stenosis

498. With what systemic condition is Klippel-Feil often associated?

498. Renal disease

499. What is the treatment if asymptomatic?

499. Restrict from contact sports

500. What is the treatment if myelopathic?

500. Operative decompression of cervical spine

Sprengel's Deformity

501. What is Sprengel's deformity?

501. Undescended scapula

502. What is the resultant functional problem?

502. Decreased abduction

503. What are the three musculoskeletal manifestations of Sprengel's?

503. Winging
Hypoplasia
Omovertebral bar (30%)

504. What two disorders may be associated?

504. Klippel-Feil
Renal disease

505. At what age should surgery be performed if necessary?

505. 3 to 8 years

506. Operative procedures: what is the Woodward procedure?

506. Distal advancement of scapula and muscle (detach from spine)

507. What is the Green procedure?

507. Distal advancement of scapula and muscle (detach from scapula)

508. What adjunctive procedure should also be performed?

508. Clavicle osteotomy

509. If a clavicle osteotomy is not performed, there is an increased risk of what complication?

509. Brachial plexus injury

510. Sprengel's deformity must be differentiated from what?

510. Fibrotic deltoid bands

Idiopathic Juvenile Osteoporosis

511. What age group is at risk?

511. 8 to 14 years

512. What are the two defining features?

512. Osteopenia
Bone pain

513. What is the ultimate outcome?

513. Self-resolving

Caffey's Disease

514. What age group is at risk?

514. Infant

515. What is the clinical feature?

515. Jaw or ulna thickening after febrile illness

Review of Key Features and Differential Diagnoses

List the disorders associated with each of the following descriptions:

516. Four disorders associated with scapular winging?

516. Fascioscapulohumeral dystrophy (AD, normal CPK, facial weakness)
Limb-girdle dystrophy (AR, elevated CPK, affects shoulder and pelvis)
Klippel-Feil (Sprengel and triad)
Pseudarthrosis of the clavicle

517. In Erb's plexus palsy, is winging good or bad prognostically?

517. Bad, because indicates injury proximal to Erb's point (preganglionic problem)

518. Three anterior horn cell disorders?

518. Arthrogryposis (nonprogressive)
Polio (motors only)
Spinal muscular atrophy (progressive, AR)

519. Four disorders with absent deep tendon reflexes (DTRs)?

519. Friedreich's
SMA
CMT (no lower DTRs)
Riley-Day

520. A disorder of muscle with deep tendon reflexes present?

520. Muscular dystrophy

521. Three disorders with elevated CPK?

521. Muscular dystrophy
Limb girdle dystrophy
Polymyositis/dermatomyositis

522. A disorder with normal CPK?

522. Fascioscapulohumeral dystrophy

■ Cerebral Palsy

523. Is cerebral palsy (CP) an upper motor neuron (UMN) or lower motor neuron (LMN) disorder?

523. UMN

524. What does magnetic resonance imaging (MRI) of the brain show?

524. Periventricular leukomalacia

525. What are the three general types?

525. Spastic
Athetotic
Ataxic

Spastic

526. What is the relative frequency of spastic CP?

526. Most common type

527. What is the defining characteristic?

527. Slow restricted movements

528. Are surgical outcomes generally good or bad?

528. Good

Athetotic

529. What is the defining characteristic?

529. Slow involuntary movements

530. Are surgical outcomes generally good or poor?

530. Poor

531. With what condition is athetotic CP associated?

531. Erythroblastosis fetalis

Ataxic

532. What is the defining characteristic?

532. Inability to control movements

533. Are surgical outcomes generally good or poor?

533. Poor

534. What are the three components of an alternate classification of CP?

534. Hemiplegic
Diplegic
Quadriplegic

535. What two infantile reflexes are negative prognostically for ambulation if they persist?

535. Moro startle reflex
Parachute reflex

536. By which system is ambulatory function classified? What do higher numbers mean?

536. Gross motor function classification system (GMFCS)
Higher numbers mean poorer ambulatory function (4,5 = nonambulators)

537. What is the ambulatory prognosis for hemiplegic CP?

537. Very good

538. What is the ambulatory prognosis for diplegic?

538. Good

539. What is the ambulatory prognosis for quadriplegic?

539. Poor

540. What are two general predictors of good operative outcomes?

540. Voluntary motor control
Over 3 years old

541. How long does the effect of Botox generally last?

541. 6 months

542. What is Botox's mechanism of action?

542. Blocks release of ACh

543. Is there a downside to repeated Botox injections?

543. Effects decrease with more than three injections

Cerebral Palsy and Scoliosis

544. The highest scoliosis risk occurs in which CP patients?

544. Spastic quadriplegics

545. What are the two indications for operative intervention?

545. Over 50-degree curve
Worsening pelvic obliquity

546. If a severe pelvic obliquity is present, what generally needs to be done?

546. Combined anterior/posterior fusion from T-spine to pelvis

Cerebral Palsy and Hips

547. What are the two criteria for a hip at risk of subluxation?

547. Abduction <45 degrees
Partial head uncoverage

548. How can the extent of uncoverage be quantified?

548. Reimer's index (percentage outside acetabulum)

549. What is the treatment?

549. Adductor and psoas release

550. In what two areas are acetabuli of subluxed hips deficient?

550. Lateral
Posterior

551. In what area are acetabuli of dysplastic hips deficient?

551. Anterior

552. What are the three treatment options for a dislocated spastic hip?

552. Open reduction
Varus derotational osteotomy (VDRO) with or without shortening
Dega or Chiari osteotomy

553. What if dislocation is discovered late?

553. Leave dislocated

Cerebral Palsy and Knee Flexion Contracture

554. With flexion contracture, what tendon should be released?

554. Medial hamstring

555. What tendon should be preserved?

555. Lateral hamstring

556. What tendon should be transferred and where?

556. Rectus posteriorly

Cerebral Palsy and Feet

557. What is the benefit of a solid ankle-foot orthosis (AFO) in a CP patient?

557. Improved ankle kinetics

558. What is the benefit of a floor reaction AFO?

558. Correct crouch gait secondary to weak plantar flexors

559. How high should the AFOs extend?

559. To just below the knee

560. What are the two components of the operative treatment of equinovalgus foot?

560. Peroneus brevis lengthening
Calcaneal osteotomy

561. With an equinovarus foot, what must be checked?

561. Function of anterior and posterior tibialis to identify location of pathology

562. What are the two components of the operative treatment for equinovarus foot?

562. Split tendon transfer (complete transfer not recommended in CP)
Tendo-Achilles lengthening (TAL)

563. Overlengthening of the Achilles leads to what complication?

563. Crouch gait

Cerebral Palsy and the Upper Extremity

564. What four procedures are used to improve upper extremity function?

564. Shoulder derotation osteotomy
Biceps lengthening
Wrist arthrodesis or flexor carpi ulnaris (FCU) transfer
Flexor digitorum superficialis (FDS) to flexor digitorum profundus (FDP) transfer; flexor pollicis longus (FPL) lengthening

565. The selective dorsal rhizotomy ideal candidate is of what CP type?

565. Spastic diplegic

566. The selective dorsal rhizotomy ideal candidate is in what age group?

566. 4 to 8 years

567. The selective dorsal rhizotomy ideal candidate is ambulatory or nonambulatory?

567. Ambulatory

568. What are the two contraindications to selective dorsal rhizotomy?

568. Athetotic CP
Absent quadriceps function

Baclofen

569. What is baclofen's mechanism of action?

569. γ-aminobutyric acid (GABA) agonist

570. What is the effect?

570. Central decrease in tone

571. For what is baclofen commonly used?

571. CP spasticity

572. Has it been proven effective?

572. Yes

■ Arthrogryposis

573. Is arthrogryposis progressive or nonprogressive?

573. Nonprogressive

574. It is characterized by loss of what cells? Why?

574. Anterior horn cells
Vascular insult

575. What is the key feature of the joints?

575. Multiple joint contractures

576. What is the key feature of the intelligence?

576. Normal

577. What is the key feature of the hips?

577. Teratologic dislocation

578. What are the two key features of the feet?

578. Resistant clubfoot
Vertical talus

579. What is the key feature of the spine?

579. Neuromuscular scoliosis

580. What lower extremity condition should be addressed first?

580. Knee flexion contracture

581. Arthrogrypotic feet may require what operative procedure?

581. Talectomy

582. At what age should an upper extremity osteotomy be performed to optimize independent eating?

582. 4 years

583. What surgical procedure may improve the position of the wrist?

583. FCU transfer to extensors

584. A similar surgical intervention is often undertaken for what disorder?

584. CP

Larsen's Syndrome

585. What is the key feature of the joints?

585. Multiple joint dislocations

586. What is the key feature of the intelligence?

586. Normal

587. What is the key feature of the cervical spine? What is the treatment, if necessary?

587. Kyphosis due to hypotonia
Posterior spinal fusion if symptomatic

■ Myelomeningocele

588. What are the four risk factors for myelomeningocele (MM)?

588. Maternal diabetes
Valproic acid
Folate deficiency
Maternal hyperthermia

Which of the following are functional for each level (quads, medial hamstring, gluts, gastrocnemius)?

589. Thoracic/high lumbar: What are the functional muscle groups? What is the ambulatory function?

589. Thoracic/high lumbar: none is functional
No ambulation

590. Low lumbar: What are the functional muscle groups? What is the ambulatory function?

590. Low lumbar: quads, medial hamstrings
Ambulation with crutches and AFOs

591. High sacral: What are the functional muscle groups? What is the ambulatory function?

591. Quads
Medial hamstrings
Gluts
Ambulation with AFOs only

592. Low sacral: What are the functional muscle groups? What is the ambulatory function?

592. Quads
Medial hamstrings
Gluts
Gastrocnemius
Ambulation essentially normal

Myelomeningocele and Scoliosis

593. Is bracing effective?

593. No

594. At what age is the risk of curve progression maximal?

594. <15 years

595. What is the general rate of progression for curves over 40 degrees?

595. 5 degrees/year

596. What are the two indications for scoliosis surgery in a patient with MM?

596. Curve >50 degrees
Progressive kyphosis

Myelomeningocele and Lower Extremity Disorders

597. What is the most common level of MM with associated hip dislocation?

597. L3/4 (have hip adduction but not hip abduction)

598. What is the indication for treatment of hip dislocation?

598. Functioning quadriceps

599. What is the goal for hip flexion contractures in ambulatory patients?

599. Maintain <20 degrees

600. What is the operative indication for knee flexion contracture?

600. Over 20 degrees

601. External tibial torsion leads to what clinical problem?

601. Increased valgus stress at knee

602. Therefore, what is the indication for surgery?

602. Thigh-foot angle greater than 20 degrees

603. What is the treatment of mild ankle valgus?

603. Screw hemi-epiphysiodesis

604. What is the treatment of rigid clubfoot?

604. Open release

605. Is triple arthrodesis an option?

605. No; it is indicated only for severe hindfoot deformity in sensate feet

606. What is an alternative to triple arthrodesis?

606. Talectomy may be necessary if insensate

607. When designing a brace for MM, how many points of pressure are necessary if one joint is spanned? If two joints?

607. One joint: three-point pressure
Two joints: four-point pressure

Intrauterine Repair for Myelomeningocele: Recent Literature

608. What is the reported effect of intrauterine repair on the risk of hindbrain herniation?

608. Decreased

609. What is the reported effect of intrauterine repair on shunt dependence?

609. Decreased

610. What is the reported effect of intrauterine repair on functional outcome?

610. No functional difference

■ Neurofibromatosis

611. What is the inheritance?

611. AD

612. What is the mutation?

612. Neurofibromin on chromosome 17

613. What cells does the mutation affect?

613. Neural crest cells

614. What percentage of cases arise from new mutations?

614. 50%

615. What anatomic site is most commonly affected?

615. Spine

616. What are the five radiographic features of the spine with neurofibromatosis (NF)?

616. Vertebral scalloping
Enlarged neuroforamina
Penciling of transverse processes
Short, tight curves
Atlantoaxial instability

617. Penciling of transverse processes is a marker of what?

617. Impending curve progression

618. What are the two basic types of spine deformities with NF?

618. Dystrophic (kyphoscoliotic)
Nondystrophic (same as AIS, adolescent idiopathic scoliosis)

619. What is the threshold for treatment of dystrophic curves?

619. ASF/PSF (anterior/posterior spinal fusion) if over 20 degrees

620. This is the same threshold as what disorder?

620. Muscular dystrophy

621. What surgical complication is especially common in the neurofibromatosis patient?

621. Increased risk of pseudarthrosis

622. Therefore, one might consider what intervention?

622. Augmentation of fusion at 6 months

623. What test must be ordered preoperatively? Why?

623. MRI
To exclude neurofibromas and ectasia

■ Hematologic Disorders

Leukemia

624. What type is most common in children?

624. Acute lymphoblastic leukemia (ALL)

625. What is the age of ALL presentation?

625. Approximately 4 years

626. What are two common presenting symptoms?

626. Joint swelling
Night pain

627. What is the characteristic radiographic feature?

627. Metaphyseal leukemia lines

628. How is leukemia diagnosed?

628. Increased blasts on bone marrow biopsy

629. What are the two components of treatment?

629. Chemotherapy
Steroids

Sickle Cell Anemia

630. What is the inheritance?

630. AR

631. What are the two key features of the joints?

631. Septic arthritis
Osteonecrosis

632. What is the key feature of the spine?

632. Biconcave vertebrae

633. What is dactylitis?

633. Acute swelling of the hands and feet

634. What population is especially at risk for dactylitis?

634. Age <6 years

635. What causes sickle cell crises?

635. Hypoxemia and release of substance P

636. What two tests can help differentiate crisis from osteomyelitis?

636. Bone scan
Bone aspirate and culture

637. Is ESR valuable diagnostically?

637. No

638. Osteomyelitis classically affects what part of bone in children with sickle cell?

638. Diaphysis

639. What are the two most common causative organisms of osteomyelitis in patients with sickle cell?

639. *Staphylococcus aureus*
Salmonella

640. Quick review: what two complications are associated with THA (total hip arthroplasty) in sickle cell patients?

640. Infection
Loosening

Thalassemia

641. What are the two classic orthopaedic manifestations?

641. Bone pain
Leg ulcers

Hemophilia

642. What is the inheritance?

642. XLR

643. What factor is affected?

643. VIII

644. What is the definition of moderate disease?

644. Factor VIII concentration is 1 to 5% of normal level

645. What is the definition of severe disease?

645. Factor VIII concentration is less than 1% of normal level

646. What is the clinical problem with severe hemophilia?

646. Spontaneous bleeding

647. What are the two most common sites of bleeding?

647. Joints (e.g., knee)
Intramuscular bleeding (e.g., iliacus)

648. Why is hemarthrosis problematic?

648. Iron is an inflammatory stimulus
Results in hypertrophy of villi

649. What are the three classic radiographic findings in the knee?

649. Square patella
Square condyles
Very wide intercondylar notch

650. How is mild to moderate hemophilia generally treated?

650 Desmopressin

651. What are two basic treatment protocols for severe hemophilia?

651. Prophylactic factor administration
Demand treatment only

652. On demand treatment days 1 to 3, what level of factor VIII should be present?

652. Day 1: 80% of normal
Day 2: 40% of normal
Day 3: 40% of normal

653. What are the two indications for synovectomy?

653. Persistent synovitis or bleeding after 3 months of prophylaxis
Recurrent bleeding episodes within 1 year

654. What levels of factor VIII must be maintained preoperatively and postoperatively?

654. Preop: 100%
Postop: >50% for 10 days

655. What is the significance of the presence of immunoglobulin G (IgG) antibodies?

655. Contraindication to operative synovectomy

656. If IgG antibodies are present, what are the two treatment options?

656. Factor VII concentrate
Radiation

von Willebrand's Disease (vWD)

657. What is the inheritance?

657. AD

658. What are the two functions of von Willebrand's factor?

658. Stabilize factor VIII
Maintain normal platelet function

659. What is the usual treatment of vWD?

659. Desmopressin

660. If ineffective, then what?

660. Cryoprecipitate

■ Infections

Acute Hematogenous Osteomyelitis

661. What is the radiographic appearance of early osteomyelitis?

661. Soft tissue swelling

662. What is the radiographic appearance at 10 to 14 days?

662. Bone demineralization

663. What is the later radiographic appearance?

663. Sequestra (dead bone with surrounding tissue)
Involucrum (periosteal new bone formation)

664. What is the key diagnostic test for osteomyelitis?

664. Aspiration and culture

665. Until the culture results are available, what should treatment consist of?

665. Empiric antibiotic therapy based on age and history

666. In neonates, what is the most common causative organism?

666. Group B β-hemolytic streptococcus (GBBS)

667. What is the key physical exam finding?

667. Local warmth

668. What are the two antibiotic options?

668. Nafcillin
Cephalosporin

669. What is the most likely causative organism in all other children?

669. *Staphylococcus aureus*

670. What is the usual antibiotic treatment?

670. Nafcillin

671. For how long should intravenous antibiotics be continued?

671. 4 to 6 weeks (until laboratory tests normalize)

672. What is the best laboratory marker for monitoring response to treatment?

672. C-reactive protein (CRP)

673. What are the two indications for surgical treatment?

673. Abscess present
No response to conservative treatment

674. What is a Brodie's abscess?

674. Chronic subperiosteal pus surrounded by thick periosteum, fibrous tissue, bone

Septic Arthritis

675. What are the four diagnostic criteria for septic arthritis of the hip?

675. White blood count (WBC) >12,000
ESR >40
Inability to ambulate
Fever >101.5°F

676. What is the typical ESR with transient synovitis?

676. Generally <20

677. If three of four criteria are met, what is the likelihood of septic arthritis?

677. 93%

678. If four of four criteria are met?

678. 100%

679. What four joints have intraarticular metaphyses?

679. Hip
Elbow
Shoulder
Ankle

680. What are the four poor prognostic factors for children with septic arthritis?

680. <6 months old
Delayed diagnosis >4 days
Associated femoral osteomyelitis
S. aureus infection

681. What is the preferred operative approach for septic hip?

681. Anterior approach

682. If *Haemophilus influenzae* is the causative organism, what additional study should be performed?

682. Check CSF to rule out meningitis

683. What if *Neisseria gonorrhoeae* is the causative organism?

683. Operative intervention often unnecessary (penicillin alone is often effective)

■ Pediatric Lower Extremity

Intoeing: Differential Diagnosis and Management

Excess Femoral Anteversion

684. Excess femoral anteversion manifests clinically at what age?

684. 3 to 6 years

685. Spontaneous correction is usually seen by what age?

695. 10 years

686. What is the indication for surgery?

686. Less than 10 degrees external rotation by 10 years of age

687. What is the procedure of choice?

687. Intertrochanteric osteotomy

Tibial Torsion

688. How often is tibial torsion the cause of intoeing?

688. The No. 1 cause

689. At what age does it manifest?

689. 2 years

690. What is the usual outcome?

690. Spontaneously corrects

691. If necessary, what is the procedure of choice?

691. Supramalleolar osteotomy

Metatarsus Adductus

692. The deformity occurs at what location within the foot?

692. Tarsometatarsal (TMT) joint

693. What is the resultant gait pattern?

693. Intoeing gait

694. Where does the heel bisector normally fall?

694. Between the second and third web space

695. With what other musculoskeletal deformity is metatarsus adductus associated?

695. Developmental dysplasia of the hip (DDH) (15%)

696. What percentage spontaneously resolves?

696. 85%

697. What is the treatment if the foot actively corrects to neutral or passively beyond neutral?

697. None

698. What is the treatment if the foot passively corrects to neutral?

698. Stretching exercises

699. What is the treatment if the foot cannot passively correct to neutral?

699. Serial casting

700. When applying the cast, where should the pressure point be?

700. Calcaneocuboid joint

701. Where is the pressure point for clubfoot casting?

701. Lateral talus

702. At what age should surgery be performed if there is no response to conservative treatment?

702. After 5 years

703. Surgery involves what two procedures?

703. Cuneiform osteotomy
Medial release

704. What two structures must be released?

704. Abductor hallucis longus
Medial capsule

Developmental Dysplasia of the Hip

705. What are the four risk factors for developmental dysplasia of the hip (DDH)?

705. Breech
Female
Family history
First-born

706. What collagen abnormality is associated with DDH?

706. Increased type III collagen

707. A similar collagen abnormality is also seen in what condition?

707. Dupuytren

708. Which hip is most commonly affected?

708. Left

709. What are two extraarticular obstructions to concentric reduction?

709. Tight iliopsoas
Redundant capsule

710. What are four intraarticular obstructions to concentric reduction?

711. What is the definition of teratologic hip dislocation?

712. If teratologic, what is the appropriate treatment?

713. DDH is associated with what other packaging disorders?

714. Diagnosis on physical exam: what are the two key tests for children 6 months of age or older?

715. What is the key test for children 6 months of age or older?

716. If suspicious for DDH, radiographs should be obtained after what age?

717. What imaging study can be performed in younger children?

718. What is the normal acetabular index value?

719. What is the normal α angle?

720. What is the relationship between α angle and acetabular index?

721. What is the normal center-edge angle? What does it measure?

722. What is the normal β angle? What does it measure?

723. What is the role of arthrography?

724. What is the normal size of the medial dye pool?

725. What is the normal labrum appearance on arthrography?

726. If the labrum is infolded, what is it referred to as?

727. What is the treatment algorithm based on age at diagnosis?

728. When should reduction or osteotomy be considered in children over 8 years of age?

710. Inverted labrum (neolimbus)
Ligamentum teres
Transverse acetabular ligament
Pulvinar (fatty tissue)

711. Pseudoacetabulum present at birth

712. Early surgical intervention

713. Metatarsus adductus
Rotary atlantoaxial subluxation

714. Barlow
Ortolani

715. Decreased abduction

716. 3 months

717. Ultrasound of femoral head and acetabulum

718. <25 degrees (>30 degrees is abnormal)

719. >60 degrees

720. Complementary (add up to 90 degrees)

721. >25 degrees
Measures subluxation

722. <55 degrees
Measures lateral contour

723. To check concentricity after closed reduction

724. <7 mm

725. "Rose thorn"

726. Neolimbus

727. <6 months: Pavlik harness
6 to 18 months: closed reduction
>18 months to 3 years: open femoral derotation osteotomy
>3 years to 8 years: femoral derotation osteotomy and acetabular osteotomy
>8 years: if bilateral, leave alone until THA as adult

728. Unilateral dislocation

Pavlik Harness

729. Can the Pavlik harness be used in teratologic hip dislocations?

729. No

730. Why?

730. Requires normal muscle function

731. What are the two components of the desired position of the hip in the Pavlik harness?

731. 100 degrees flexion
Mild abduction (45 degrees)

732. What do the anterior straps control?

732. Hip flexion

733. What do the posterior straps control?

733. Hip abduction

734. If 45 degrees of abduction cannot be easily obtained, what procedure should be considered?

734. Adductor tenotomy

735. What is a possible consequence of placing the hips into excessive flexion?

735. Femoral nerve palsy

736. What vessel is associated with avascular necrosis (AVN) after Pavlik harness wear?

736. Medial femoral circumflex (posterosuperior retinacular artery)

737. How long after initiation of treatment should the hip be reimaged in Pavlik harness?

737. 2 weeks

738. What two steps should be taken if the reduction is unsatisfactory at that time?

738. Discontinue Pavlik treatment
Closed or open reduction when child is old enough

Open Reduction

739. What is the usual surgical approach for open reduction?

739. Anterior

740. Why?

740. Decreased risk to medial femoral circumflex artery

741. What is the other major advantage of the anterior approach?

741. All structures accessible

742. In patients of what age is the medial approach preferred?

742. Under 2 years

743. Through what approach can a femoral shortening be performed?

743. A separate lateral approach

744. What is the major risk of open or closed reduction?

744. AVN

745. What two structures are not accessible medially?

745. Acetabular roof (including labrum)
Superior hip capsule

746. What two procedures cannot be performed through a medial approach?

746. Capsular plication
Secondary bone procedures

747. What is the treatment if an inverted labrum is encountered when performing open reduction through the anterior approach?

747. Make radial cuts
Do not excise labrum

748. What is the end result of lateral growth arrest due to AVN?

748. Coxa valga

Acetabular Osteotomies

749. What are the two prerequisites for acetabular osteotomy?

749. Congruent reduction
Reasonable femoral sphericity

750. What study may be predictive of outcome?

750. Functional x-rays (abduction/internal rotation)

751. What three osteotomies are appropriate if the tri-radiate cartilage is open?

751. Salter
Pemberton
Dega

752. What two osteotomies are appropriate in the older child?

752. Steel (triple)
Ganz

753. What two osteotomies are appropriate as salvage procedures?

753. Shelf
Chiari

754. A Salter osteotomy enhances coverage where?

754. Superior and lateral

755. Does it medialize or lateralize the acetabulum?

755. Lateralize

756. What effect does it have on joint reaction force?

756. Increased

757. What is the age limit for Salter osteotomy?

757. Less than 8 years of age to rotate through symphysis

758. How is extremity length affected?

758. May lengthen 1 cm

759. On what structure does a Pemberton osteotomy bend?

759. Triradiate cartilage

760. What is the resultant effect?

760. Reduces acetabular volume

761. In what two situations is a Dega osteotomy appropriate?

761. Paralytic dislocation
Posterior deficiency

762. What is a Steel osteotomy?

762. Salter plus osteotomies of rami
Also known as triple

763. For whom is a Steel osteotomy indicated?

763. Older children who cannot rotate through symphysis

764. What is a Ganz osteotomy?

764. Periacetabular osteotomy
Leaves posterior column intact
Allows more rapid weightbearing

765. What osteotomy has greatest potential for increased coverage?

765. Ganz

766. Salvage procedures rely on what change taking place?

766. Tissue metaplasia

767. What is the disadvantage of a Chiari procedure?

767. Shortens leg by medializing hip

768. What osteotomy is an option for adults?

768. Ganz

769. What osteotomy leaves medial wall in place and redirects acetabulum?

769. Dial

770. How does it compare with others?

770. Others rotate teardrop also

Residuum of Hip Dysplasia in Adults

771. With what system is residual hip dysplasia classified?

771. Crowe

772. What is the Crowe system based on?

772. Degree of uncoverage

773. Where is the dysplastic acetabulum deficient?

773. Anteriorly

774. What is its size?

774. Small

775. A characteristic of the dysplastic femur is coxa ___?

775. Valga

776. What is the characteristic anteversion?

776. Excess

777. What is the characteristic canal size?

777. Small

778. What type of femoral arthroplasty component is generally required?

778. Modular

779. How much lengthening is tolerated before risk of developing CPN (common peroneal nerve) palsy increases significantly?

779. 2 cm

780. Sciatic nerve palsy generally occurs at what degree of lengthening?

780. 5 cm

781. If lengthening >2 cm, what procedure should be considered?

781. Femoral shortening

Coxa Vara

782. What is the basic defect that leads to coxa vara?

782. Triangular ossification defect in inferomedial femoral neck

783. What is the characteristic growth plate appearance?

783. Inverted Y

784. If developmental (i.e., not congenital), is the varus static or progressive?

784. Progressive

785. What is the inheritance?

785. AD

786. What is the key physical exam finding of coxa vara?

786. Decreased abduction

787. What is the classic gait pattern?

787. Trendelenburg

788. What is the significance of the Hilgenreiner epiphyseal angle? What is the prognosis if <45 degrees? 45 to 60 degrees? >60 degrees?

788. <45 degrees: spontaneously corrects
45 to 60 degrees: observe
>60 degrees: operative treatment

789. What is the neck shaft angle threshold for surgical intervention?

789. 110 degrees

790. What is the operative procedure of choice?

790. Pauwel osteotomy (valgus with or without DRO [derotation osteotomy])

791. What is the common complication of treatment?

791. Premature proximal femoral physeal closure

792. Therefore, what is recommended postoperatively?

792. Must follow for possible development of leg length discrepancy

Legg-Calvé-Perthes Disease

793. In general, what is the cause of Legg-Calvé-Perthes disease (LCPD)?

793. Vascular insult

794. What is the resultant effect?

794. Proximal femoral epiphyseal AVN

795. LCPD has been associated with what clinical conditions?

795. Hypercoagulable states

796. What are the two characteristics of the population at greatest risk?

796. Boys 4 to 8
2-year delay in skeletal maturity

797. What are the two classic signs and symptoms?

797. Hip pain and effusion
Decreased hip abduction and internal rotation

798. What is the usual gait pattern?

798. Trendelenburg

799. How frequently is involvement bilateral?

799. 15%

800. If bilateral disease is present, is it generally symmetric?

800. No: classically asymmetric

801. What are the four stages of disease?

801. Initial
Fragmentation
Reossification
Healed

802. Prognosis depends on what two factors?

802. Bone age
Lateral pillar classification

803. What classification system is based on initial stage of disease?

803. Salter-Thompson crescent

804. What classification system is based on fragmentation stage of disease?

804. Lateral pillar classification

805. The lateral pillar classification is assessed on what film?

805. AP

806. What are the three classification categories?

806. A: normal height
B: ≥50% height maintained
C: <50% height maintained

807. The worst clinical prognosis is associated with what two criteria?

807. Bone age >6 years old
B, C lateral pillar classification

808. What are five other poorly prognostic radiographic findings?

808. Lateral calcification
Gage's sign (defect in lateral physis)
Lateral subluxation
Metaphyseal cysts (not in MED)
Horizontalized growth plate

809. Long-term prognosis correlates with what MRI finding?

809. Percentage of physeal involvement

810. What are the two goals of LCPD treatment?

810. Maintain sphericity of femoral head
Contain the hip

811. What treatment is no longer commonly employed?

811. Bracing

812. Operative treatment is generally beneficial only in what stage of disease?

812. Fragmentation

813. Patients in what age group are most likely to benefit from surgery?

813. >8 years

814. Patients with what disease stage are most likely to benefit from surgery?

814. B

815. What is the general goal of surgery?

815. Improve containment

816. What is an example procedure?

816. Shelf osteotomy

817. What is the preferred treatment for a late osteochondritis dissecans (OCD) lesion in person with history of LCPD?

817. Nonoperative management

Slipped Capital Femoral Epiphysis

818. What patient population is at greatest risk for slipped capital femoral epiphysis (SCFE)?

818. African-American boys
Age 10 to 16

819. What are the two primary risk factors?

819. Family history
Obesity

820. How often is involvement bilateral?

820. 25%

821. What two other disorders are associated with SCFE development?

821. Hypothyroidism
Renal disease

822. What are two other iatrogenic associations?

822. Growth hormone therapy
Radiation treatment

823. What two effects does growth hormone have on the growth plate?

823. Stimulates proliferation
Inhibits maturation (keeps growth plate open)

824. What are two thyroid hormone effects?

824. Stimulates proliferation
Stimulates maturation (closure of the growth plate)

825. What four SCFE patient groups ought to have an endocrine evaluation?

825. <10 years old
>16 years old
<10th percentile for weight
Bilateral involvement

826. What does a biopsy of zone of provisional calcification show?

826. Granulation tissue between columns

827. In which two directions does the femoral neck slip?

827. Anterior
Superior

828. In which two directions does the epiphysis slip?

828. Posterior
Inferior

829. What are the three grades of slip?

829. I: $<\frac{1}{3}$
II: $\frac{1}{3}$ to $\frac{1}{2}$
III: $>\frac{1}{2}$

830. What key physical exam finding is suggestive of SCFE?

830. Obligate external rotation with flexion

831. Compare the rate of osteonecrosis with stable and unstable SCFE?

831. Stable: 0% develop AVN
Unstable: 50% develop AVN

832. When performing surgery on a patient <10 years old, what procedure should be considered?

832. Pinning of contralateral side also

833. Compare postoperative weight-bearing status with stable and unstable SCFE.

833. Stable: weight-bearing as tolerated (WBAT)
Unstable: non–weight-bearing (NWB)

Leg Length Discrepancies and Management

834. What is the best method for measurement of leg length discrepancy (LLD)?

834. Place blocks under shorter limb until pelvis level

835. General treatment guidelines: What is the treatment for a LLD <2 cm at maturity?

835. Shoe lift

836. … for an LLD of 2 to 5 cm?

836. Epiphysiodesis of long side

837. … for an LLD >5 cm?

837. Lengthening procedure

838. Generally speaking, what is the age of growth cessation in boys?

838. 16 years

839. … in girls?

839. 14 years

840. What is the annual growth rate of the proximal femur?

840. 1/8"

841. … of the distal femur?

841. 3/8" (10 mm)

842. … of the proximal tibia?

842. 2/8" (6 mm)

Proximal Femoral Focal Deficiency

843. Proximal femoral focal deficiency (PFFD) is associated with what three musculoskeletal disorders?

843. Coxa vara
Fibular hemimelia (50%)
Knee flexion contracture

844. PFFD is associated with what gene defect?

844. Sonic hedgehog

845. In what position do PFFD patients hold their hips?

845. Flexed, abducted, externally rotated

846. Trauma review: this is the same position as is seen with what fracture?

846. Subtrochanteric fracture

847. With the Aiken classification, what are the key features of classes A and B?

847. Femoral head present
So, can lengthen and reconstruct
Must have stable hip and knee to lengthen

848. … classes C and D?

848. Femoral head absent
So, amputation or femoral-pelvic fusion are options

849. What factor remains constant throughout growth?

849. Percentage of shortening

Disorders of Knee Alignment and Other Conditions of the Knee

Typical Knee Alignment

850. What is the expected alignment of the knees in a child less than 18 months of age?

850. Genu varum

851. ... 18 to 36 months of age?

851. Genu valgum

852. ... over 36 months of age?

852. Physiologic valgus

Angular Deformities of the Knees: General Principles

853. In general, conditions that present early result in what direction of knee deformity?

853. Excess varus

854. Conditions that present later result in what direction of knee deformity?

854. Excess valgus

855. What condition is the exception to this rule?

855. Adolescent Blount's (late presenting, but varus)

856. What is the most common nondysplastic cause of genu varum?

856. Blount's disease

Infantile Blount's Disease

857. What age group is affected?

857. 0 to 4 years

858. What are the three typical characteristics of affected children?

858. Obese
Ambulate before 1 year of age
Internal tibial torsion

859. How is Drennan's angle measured?

859. Draw first line through metaphyseal beaks
Draw second line along longitudinal tibial axis
Measure angle between intersecting lines

860. What is the normal range for Drennan's angle?

860. <12 degrees

861. What values are considered abnormal?

861. >16 degrees

862. What classification system is used for infantile Blount's disease?

862. Langenskiold

863. Stages V and VI are characterized by the presence of what?

863. Metaphyseal-epiphyseal bridge

864. What is the treatment for early, unilateral involvement?

864. Bracing

865. What are the two indications for surgery?

865. No response to bracing
>3 years old

866. What does surgical treatment generally involve?

866. Valgus producing osteotomy

867. What is the surgical treatment for stages V and VI?

867. Epiphysiolysis

Adolescent Blount's Disease

868. How does the severity of adolescent Blount's compare with that of infantile Blount's?

869. What patient population is particularly at risk?

870. Is adolescent Blount's more often unilateral or bilateral?

871. What is the treatment if growth potential remains?

872. How many months of remaining growth are necessary to consider epiphysiodesis?

873. What is the treatment if no growth potential remains?

868. Less severe than infantile Blount's

869. Obese children

870. Unilateral

871. Lateral proximal tibia/fibula epiphysiodesis

872. 15 months

873. Valgus osteotomy with or without lengthening

Genu Valgum

874. What measure of genu valgum is acceptable in children aged 2 to 6?

875. What is the most common cause of bilateral pathologic genu valgum?

876. What is the treatment if growth potential remains?

877. What are the two indications for surgery for genu valgum?

874. <15 degrees

875. Renal osteodystrophy

876. Medial physeal stapling

877. >10 years old
>10 cm between medial malleoli

Congenital Knee Dislocation

878. What are the two components of the nonoperative treatment for congenital knee dislocation?

879. What is the indication for surgery?

880. What two steps does surgical treatment include?

878. Serial casting
Reduction

879. <30 degrees of motion after 3 months of casting

880. V-Y lengthening
Collateral release

Baker's (Popliteal) Cyst in Children

881. What is the usual location of a Baker's cyst?

882. What is the general treatment?

883. How do pediatric Baker's cysts compare with those of adults?

881. Posteromedial (interval between medial gastrocnemius and semimembranosus)

882. Observation

883. In children not associated with intraarticular pathology (unlike adults)

General Algorithm for Osteochondritis Dissecans in Children

884. What is the key radiographic view for diagnosing knee OCD?

884. Tunnel view

885. What is the treatment for stable OCD lesions if relatively asymptomatic?

885. Activity restriction

886. What are the two components of the treatment for stable OCD lesions if symptoms are significant?

886. NWB
Immobilization

887. What is the treatment for stable OCD lesions if resolution with nonoperative treatment is incomplete?

887. Retrograde drilling

888. What are the two components of the treatment for unstable OCD lesions with subchondral bone attached to fragment?

888. Drill bed
Replace fragment

Bowing Deformities of the Tibia and Fibula: Significance

Apex Posteromedial

889. What is the most common cause of posteromedial bowing?

889. Physiologic

890. What structures are tight in this clinical situation?

890. Anterior structures

891. What is the position of the foot and ankle?

891. Calcaneovalgus

892. What is the preferred treatment?

892. Observe

893. What is the prognosis?

893. LLD of 3 to 4 cm

Apex Anterolateral

894. What is the most common cause of anterolateral bowing?

894. Congenital pseudarthrosis of tibia

895. What disease is associated?

895. 50% of time associated with neurofibromatosis

896. What cellular pathway is affected by this disease?

896. Ras pathway

897. What is the position of the foot and ankle?

897. Calcaneovalgus

898. What is the initial treatment?

898. Total contact brace

899. Despite bracing, what eventually occurs?

899. Inevitably goes on to fracture

900. What are the two components of the surgical treatment if fracture does not heal?

900. Intramedullary nail
Autograft

901. If two or three surgeries fail, then what?

901. Syme's amputation

902. Should you osteotomize to correct deformity?

902. No!

903. What other surgical options exist for children >5 years of age?

903. Distraction osteogenesis

904. In what two ways can the foot deformity be corrected safely?

904. Hemiepiphysiodesis
Synostosis

Tibial Hemimelia

905. What is the inheritance?

905. AD

906. What hand abnormality is associated with tibial hemimelia?

906. Lobster-claw

907. With hemimelia, where is the apex of the tibial bow?

907. Anterolateral

908. What is the position of the foot and ankle?

908. Equinovarus

909. What is the treatment if the tibia is entirely absent?

909. Knee disarticulation

910. What are two prerequisites for fibular transposition?

910. Presence of proximal tibia
Intact quadriceps function

911. What is the clinical problem?

911. Progressive knee flexion contracture

Apex Anteromedial

912. What is the most common cause of anteromedial bowing?

912. Fibular hemimelia

913. Fibular hemimelia is associated with instability of what joint?

913. Ankle

914. What is the position of the foot and ankle?

914. Equinovarus

915. What is the key feature of the rays of the foot?

915. Lateral rays are missing

916. What is the key feature of the tarsal bones?

916. Coalesced

917. What is the key feature of the femur?

917. Shortened

918. What is the treatment for severely short, nonfunctional foot?

918. Symes amputation

919. If the foot is functional, what is the treatment of choice?

919. Surgical reconstruction

Review of Foot/Ankle Positions

920. What position is associated with posteromedial and anterolateral "bowings"?

920. Calcaneovalgus

921. What position is associated with tibial hemimelia?

921. Equinovarus

922. What position is associated with fibular hemimelia?

922. Equinovalgus

Disorders of the Foot

Normal Radiographic Findings

923.	What is the range of normal values for the talocalcaneal angle on lateral film?	**923.** 35 to 50 degrees
924.	What is the range of normal values for the talocalcaneal angle on AP (Kite's angle) film?	**924.** 20 to 40 degrees

Clubfoot (Talipes Equinovarus)

925.	What gender is most commonly affected?	**925.** Male
926.	How often does bilateral involvement occur?	**926.** 50%
927.	What is Streeter's dysplasia?	**927.** Clubfoot with associated hand anomalies
928.	If a clubfoot is seen on prenatal ultrasound, what is the next step?	**928.** Amniocentesis to evaluate for other abnormalities
929.	What are the two key features of the forefoot position?	**929.** Adducted / Supinated
930.	What are the two key features of the hindfoot position?	**930.** Equinus / Varus
931.	What is the key classic radiographic feature?	**931.** Talocalcaneal parallelism
932.	What is the talocalcaneal angle on dorsiflexion lateral film?	**932.** <35 degrees
933.	What is the talocalcaneal angle on AP film?	**933.** <20 degrees
934.	Nonoperative treatment: What is the acronym for order of the four steps in deformity correction?	**934.** Acronym CAVE: Cavus / Adductus / Varus / Equinus
935.	How long should a Ponsetti cast be?	**935.** A long leg cast
936.	At which anatomic location should corrective pressure be applied?	**936.** Lateral talar head
937.	After casting has been completed, how can the correction be maintained?	**937.** Dennis-Browne bars
938.	80% of clubfoot patients ultimately require what adjunctive procedure?	**938.** Achilles lengthening
939.	25% of those patients also require what procedure?	**939.** Lateral transfer of tibialis anterior
940.	How long should cast treatment be attempted before operating on a resistant clubfoot?	**940.** 6 to 9 months

941. What artery is most commonly insufficient with clubfoot?

942. If a child presents late (8 to 10 years old) with clubfoot, what is the preferred surgical option?

943. A triple arthrodesis is contraindicated in what situation?

944. What is a better option for insensate patients?

Serpentine (Z) Foot (Skewfoot)

945. What systemic disorder is associated with bilateral skewfeet?

946. What is the key feature of the position of the TMT joint?

947. What is the key feature of the talonavicular position?

948. What is the key feature of the hindfoot position?

949. How is skewfoot treated?

Vertical Talus

950. What is the hindfoot position in vertical talus?

951. What is the forefoot position?

952. Bottom line: A foot with a vertical talus is essentially what?

953. What are the key radiographic features on a plantar flexion lateral film?

954. What is the key radiographic feature on an AP film?

955. How can vertical talus and oblique talus be distinguished?

956. What is the first step in the treatment of vertical talus?

957. At what age is surgery undertaken?

958. Surgical intervention must include what?

959. If vertical talus recurs, what procedure has been historically favored as the next step?

960. What if the foot is insensate?

961. More recently, what have the two first-line procedures been?

941. Dorsalis pedis

942. Triple arthrodesis

943. Insensate feet

944. Talectomy

945. Diastrophic dysplasia

946. Adduction

947. Lateral subluxation

948. Valgus

949. Operative intervention

950. Equinus

951. Abducted

952. Rigid flatfoot

953. Tarsometatarsal angle >20 degrees
Talocalcaneal angle >50 degrees

954. Talocalcaneal angle >40 degrees

955. Oblique talus corrects with plantar flexion

956. Casting for the first 3 months

957. 6 to 12 months of age

958. Extensive soft tissue release

959. Subtalar arthrodesis

960. Talectomy

961. Dorsal talonavicular approach (talonavicular fusion)
Tendo-Achilles lengthening

962. If vertical talus recurs, what procedure is currently favored as the next step?

962. Naviculectomy

963. How is oblique talus treated?

963. UCBL (University of California Biomechanics Laboratory) orthosis

Summary: Review of Foot Abnormalities

964. With clubfoot, what is the hindfoot position?

964. Varus

965. ... the talonavicular joint position?

965. Medial dislocation

966. ... the forefoot position?

966. Adducted

967. With metatarsus adductus, what is the hindfoot position?

967. Neutral

968. ... the talonavicular joint position?

968. Neutral

969. ... the forefoot position?

969. Adducted

970. With vertical talus, what is the hindfoot position?

970. Valgus

971. ... the talonavicular joint position?

971. Dorsal dislocation

972. ... the forefoot position?

972. Abducted

973. With skewfoot, what is the hindfoot position?

973. Valgus

974. ... the talonavicular joint position?

974. Lateral dislocation

975. ... the forefoot position?

975. Adducted

Tarsal Coalition: Another Cause of Rigid Flatfoot

976. What is the inheritance?

976. AD

977. Tarsal coalition is also referred to as what?

977. Peroneal spastic flatfoot

978. What are the two most common sites of coalition?

978. Calcaneonavicular
Subtalar

979. What site is more common in children who present between ages 10 and 12?

979. Calcaneonavicular

980. What site more common in ages 12 to 14?

980. Subtalar

981. What is the best imaging modality for diagnosis of a coalition?

981. Computed tomography (CT)

982. What is the initial treatment for all coalitions?

982. Casting, orthotics

983. What is the treatment for a resistant calcaneonavicular coalition?

983. Resection alone is usually adequate

984. What is the preferred surgical approach?

984. Lateral

985. With subtalar coalition: the coalition is in the ____ facet, but must also check the _____ facet.

985. Coalition in the middle facet
Must also check the posterior facet

986. What three factors are poorly prognostic in patients with subtalar coalition?

986. Coalition involves >50% of middle facet
Heel valgus >21 degrees
Posterior facet narrowing

987. Surgical treatment: what is the general rule of thumb?

987. <50% middle facet involved: resect
≥50% middle facet involved: fuse

988. What is the preferred surgical approach?

988. Medial

989. If this fails, what is the next procedure?

989. Triple arthrodesis

990. Bottom line: What is the treatment for hindfoot abnormalities identified late, with arthritis, or after failed initial surgery?

990. Triple arthrodesis

991. Triple arthrodesis is contraindicated in what patients?

991. Those with insensate feet

Flexible Flatfeet in Children (Pes Planovalgus)

992. What is pes planovalgus due to?

992. Ligamentous laxity

993. In comparison, what is the usual etiology of flatfeet in adults?

993. Posterior tibial tendon dysfunction

994. What is the hindfoot position?

994. Valgus

995. What is the forefoot position?

995. Supinated

996. What is the symptomatic association between flexible flatfeet and tight Achilles tendons?

996. Patients with tight Achilles are especially likely to develop symptoms

997. Radiographic features: what is Meary's line?

997. Talus–first metatarsal angle = plantar sag (talus "points" plantarly)

998. Is surgery necessary?

998. Very rarely

999. Surgical treatment includes what two procedures?

999. Calcaneal osteotomy
Posterior tibial tendon advancement

1000. What procedure is *not* included for flexible flatfoot treatment?

1000. Subtalar arthrodesis

Calcaneovalgus Foot

1001. What population is particularly at risk for calcaneovalgus feet?

1001. First-born children

1002. What is the foot deformity due to?

1002. Intrauterine position

1003. What is the preferred treatment?

1003. Passive stretching

1004. What other condition must be excluded in patients with calcaneovalgus feet?

1004. L5 myelomeningocele

1005. What is the associated direction of tibial bow?

1005. Posteromedial (physiologic)

Miscellaneous Pediatric Foot/Ankle Questions

1006. What is a "ball-and-socket" ankle?

1006. Talus shaped like a ball
Tibia and fibula are shaped like a socket

1007. With what three conditions is a ball-and-socket ankle associated?

1007. Fibular hemimelia/absent lateral rays (50%)
Tarsal coalition (50%)
Proximal femoral focal deficiency

1008. With overlapping toes, which toes are affected?

1008. Fifth toe overlaps the fourth

1009. What is the preferred treatment of overlapping toes?

1009. Stretching

1010. With curly (underlapping) toes, which toes are affected?

1010. Lateral three toes

1011. What is the preferred treatment?

1011. Flexor tenotomy

1012. Is there a conservative treatment option for a retained foreign body in the foot?

1012. Three weeks in short leg cast

1013. What organism is associated with a nail puncture through a sneaker?

1013. *Pseudomonas aeruginosa*

1014. What are the two components of the treatment of a penetrating injury through a shoe?

1014. Open debridement
Intravenous antibiotics (ceftazidime/Cipro)

1015. The accessory navicular is found in what tendon?

1015. Posterior tibial tendon

■ Pediatric Upper Extremity Malformations and Disorders

1016. Upper extremity malformations are associated with what parental risk factor?

1016. Advanced maternal age

1017. Hand formation (limb bud) occurs between which gestational days?

1017. Gestational days 26 to 56

1018. What is the most common congenital hand anomaly?

1018. Syndactyly

1019. What is the inheritance?

1019. AD

1020. What is acrosyndactyly?

1020. Digits are only fused distally

1021. What two digits are most commonly involved with syndactyly?

1021. Long
Ring

1022. What is the general rule of thumb for rates of involvement for each digit?

1022. 5–15–50–30
5% thumb–index
15% index–long
50% long–ring
30% ring–small

1023. At what age should syndactyly release generally be performed?

1023. 1 year

1024. With syndactyly surgery, what should never be done?

1024. Never release both sides of a digit at the same time

1025. For coverage, which type of graft should be used?

1025. Full-thickness skin graft (FTSG)

Camptodactyly

1026. What two entities is camptodactyly generally due to?

1026. Abnormal lumbrical insertion
Abnormal FDS

1027. What is the most common location for camptodactyly?

1027. Proximal interphalangeal (PIP) joint of the small finger

1028. What is the preferred treatment?

1028. Nonoperative (stretching, etc.)

1029. What is the operative treatment?

1029. Transfer to the radial lateral band

1030. What is the indication for surgery?

1030. PIP contracture greater than 60 degrees

1031. What is the definition of Kirner's deformity?

1031. Kirner's is a volar curve of the distal phalanx

Clinodactyly

1032. What is the preferred treatment if an associated delta phalanx is an extra bone?

1032. Early excision

1033. … is *not* an extra bone?

1033. Opening wedge osteotomy

1034. What are the four clinical features of Poland's syndrome?

1034. Unilaterally short fingers
Simple (soft tissue) complete syndactyly
Hand hypoplasia
Absent sternocostal head of pectoralis major (chest anomalies)

1035. What is the specific deformity that makes the fingers short in Poland's syndrome?

1035. Middle phalanx is short

1036. What are the six clinical features of Apert's syndrome?

1036. Bilateral complex (bony) syndactyly
Common nail
Acrocephaly
Hypertelorism
Craniosynostosis
Retardation

Radial Club Hand

1037. What bone is absent with radial club hand?

1037. Radius

1038. With what four disorders is radial club hand associated?

1038. Holt-Oram (cardiac)
Fanconi's
TAR (thrombocytopenia with absent radii)
VATER (vertebral defects, imperforate anus, tracheoesophageal fistula, radial and renal dysplasia)

1039. What does treatment usually consist of?

1039. Surgical

1040. What other option exists for mild cases of radial club hand?

1040. Cast

1041. The ulna should not be centralized if what contraindication to operative treatment exists?

1041. No elbow motion

1042. What is the key feature of the radius in TAR syndrome?

1042. No radii bilaterally

1043. What is the key feature of the thumbs in TAR syndrome?

1043. Normal thumbs

1044. What muscular procedure is required for improved outcomes?

1044. Excise brachiocarpalis muscle

Ulnar Club Hand

1045. What bone is absent with ulnar club hand?

1045. Ulna

1046. What is the most common clinical complaint of patients with ulnar club hand?

1046. Elbow stiffness

1047. What is the general rule for treatment?

1047. Conservative treatment

1048. Radioulnar synostosis is associated with what group of disorders?

1048. Sex chromosome developmental disorders

Symphalangism

1049. What joint is absent with symphalangism?

1049. Interphalangeal (IP) joint

1050. What is the clinical appearance of an affected digit?

1050. No skin crease

1051. What is the treatment of choice?

1051. No treatment is generally required

Preaxial Polydactyly

1052. Is preaxial polydactyly sporadic or inherited?

1052. Sporadic

1053. What is the most common type?

1053. Wassell IV (duplicate proximal phalanx)

1054. With treatment, which thumb is generally retained? Why?

1054. Retain ulnar thumb
To keep the ulnar collateral ligament (UCL) intact

1055. In what situation is the ulnar thumb not retained?

1055. Triphalangeal ulnar thumb

Macrodactyly

1056. What is the preferred treatment if one digit is severely affected?

1056. Amputation

Thumb Hypoplasia

1057. What is the treatment of thumb hypoplasia with an absent carpometacarpal (CMC) joint?

1057. Thumb amputation and index pollicization

1058. Why?

1058. Stable reconstruction cannot be achieved without functional CMC

Madelung's Deformity

1059. What is Madelung's deformity?

1059. Disruption of radial volar ulnar epiphysis

1060. What two clinical abnormalities may result?

1060. Excess radial inclination
Excess volar tilt

1061. What two things happen to the distal ulna?

1061. Subluxes
Enlarges

1062. What happens to the carpus?

1062. Becomes wedged

1063. What happens to the volar ligaments?

1063. Hypertrophy

1064. What happens to pronation/supination?

1064. Supination becomes very limited

1065. What is the treatment of painless Madelung's deformity?

1065. None generally required

1066. What are the two components of the treatment of painful Madelung's?

1066. Osteotomy of the radius
Distal ulna resection
May need to be corrected in more than one stage

1067. Constriction rings are seen with what syndrome?

1067. Streeter's dysplasia

1068. Why are constriction rings thought to develop?

1068. Amniotic fluid rupture

1069. How do the feet of affected children classically appear?

1069. Clubfeet

Congenital Radial Head Dislocation

1070. What radial head morphology is associated with congenital dislocation?

1070. Dome-shaped head

1071. What are the two treatment options if congenital dislocation is incidentally discovered? What is not a treatment option?

1071. Leave alone
Excise
Reduction is not an option

1072. What is the consequence of chronic congenital radial head dislocation?

1072. Limited flexion and rotation

■ Pediatric Trauma

General Principles

1073. What is the general treatment of nondisplaced Salter I and II fractures?

1073. Cast

1074. What is the general treatment of displaced Salter I, II fractures?

1074. Closed reduction and smooth pin fixation

1075. What is the general treatment of Salter III, IV fractures?

1075. Open reduction with internal fixation (ORIF)

1076. Fractures generally occur through what epiphyseal zone?

1076. Zone of provisional calcification

1077. What are the two most common anatomic sites of physeal injury?

1077. Distal radius
Distal tibia

1078. What physis must one be especially careful of?

1078. Distal femur: undulating growth plate

1079. Compare a fall onto an outstretched arm in children with greater versus lesser ligamentous laxity.

1079. Greater laxity: increased risk for supracondylar fractures
Lesser laxity: increased risk for distal radius fractures

Upper Extremity Trauma

Posteriorly Displaced Medial Clavicular Physis Fracture

1080. What is the treatment for a physeal fracture <10 days old?

1080. Closed reduction

1081. What is the treatment if irreducible?

1081. Leave alone

Proximal Humerus Fracture

1082. How much deformity is acceptable in patients over 12 years of age?

1082. <40 degrees

1083. What is the radiographic appearance of nursemaid's elbow?

1083. Normal

Pediatric Elbow: Supracondylar Distal Humerus Fractures

1084. What nerve is at risk with an extension type supracondylar fracture?

1084. AIN (anterior interosseus nerve)

1085. What nerve is at risk with an extension type and posteromedial displacement?

1085. Radial nerve

1086. What two nerves are at risk with an extension type and posterolateral displacement?

1086. Median nerve
Brachial artery

1087. What nerve is at risk with flexion type?

1087. Ulnar nerve

1088. What two complications are associated with casting the elbow in hyperflexion?

1088. Compartment syndrome
Volkmann's contracture

1089. In what compartment are the highest pressures present (same as in adult)?

1089. Deep volar compartment

1090. Compare resistance to varus and valgus stress: lateral pins only versus medial and lateral pins?

1090. Equivalent

1091. What construct provides better resistance to axial load?

1091. Medial and lateral pins better

1092. How can the strength of lateral-only fixation be improved?

1092. Cast also

1093. What are the three long-term complications of varus malunion?

1093. Poor cosmesis
Ulnar neuropathy
Posterolateral rotatory instability

Lateral Condylar Fractures

1094. What is the usual age of injury?

1094. 6 years

1095. How much displacement is acceptable?

1095. 2 mm

1096. What is the treatment if less than 2 mm displacement?

1096. Cast

1097. What is critical about nonoperative lateral condylar fracture treatment?

1097. Must follow very closely

1098. Like a supracondylar fracture, what is fracture stability dependent on?

1098. Integrity of cartilaginous hinge

1099. What is the treatment for lateral condylar fracture with 2 to 5 mm of displacement?

1099. Closed reduction and percutaneous pinning

1100. How long after surgery should the pins be removed?

1100. 4 weeks

1101. At what time point is radiographic evidence of healing first seen?

1101. 6 weeks

1102. What is the treatment for lateral condylar fracture with over 5-mm displacement?

1102. ORIF

1103. What is a key caveat?

1103. Avoid posterior dissection to preserve blood supply

1104. How is a nonunion with <1 cm displacement best treated?

1104. Leave alone

1105. What is the preferred treatment for a nonunion with ≥1 cm displacement?

1105. ORIF

1106. What are the two key caveats?

1106. No soft tissue stripping
Anatomic reduction unnecessary

Medial Epicondylar Fracture

1107. What is the usual age of medial epicondylar fracture?

1107. 9 to 14 years

1108. How much displacement is considered acceptable?

1108. 10 mm

1109. How is late-presenting Monteggia fracture with chronic radial head dislocation treated?

1109. ORIF
May require ulnar osteotomy

Radial Head Fractures

1110. How are radial head fractures with 0 to <40 degrees of angulation treated?

1110. Nonoperative

1111. How are radial head fractures with 40 to 60 degrees of angulation?

1111. Closed reduction and percutaneous pinning

1112. How are radial head fractures with over 60 degrees of angulation?

1112. ORIF

1113. What should be tried before ORIF?

1113. Closed reduction (with Kirschner [K] wire hinge, for example) to improve angulation

Wrist and Forearm Fractures

1114. What are the three recently reported risk factors for wrist and forearm fractures in children?

1114. Decreased bone density
Poor balance
Increased body mass index

1115. What two steps are proven to protect against wrist and forearm fractures in sports?

1115. Wrist guards
Decreased ball size

1116. How much rotation is acceptable in both-bone forearm (BBF) fractures in patients <10 years of age?

1116. 45 degrees

1117. What bone is at greater risk of developing growth disturbance: radius or ulna?

1117. Ulna

1118. What is the likely diagnosis for a child with healed BBF and inability to extend the fourth and fifth distal interphalangeals (DIPs)?

1118. Tethering of the fourth and fifth FDP tendons within the fracture callus

1119. What is the advantage to pinning a pediatric distal radius fracture?

1119. Decreased rate of loss of reduction

1120. How do outcomes of pinning and nonoperative treatment compare?

1120. Equivalent

1121. If median nerve symptoms are present, how does this affect treatment?

1121. Should be pinned

Phalangeal Neck Fractures After Crush or Extraction Injury

1122. What are the two treatment options for phalangeal neck fracture?

1122. Closed reduction percutaneous pinning
ORIF

1123. What structures must be identified and protected in surgery?

1123. Preserve collateral ligaments

Distal Phalanx Fractures

1124. What is Seymour's fracture?

1124. Distal phalanx fracture with associated nail-bed laceration
Incarceration of germinal matrix in physis

1125. How is it treated?

1125. Requires exploration, nail-bed repair, fracture reduction

Lower Extremity Trauma

Pediatric Hip Fractures

1126. What are the four components of pediatric hip fracture classification?

1126. Transepiphyseal (with or without dislocation)
Transcervical
Cervicotrochanteric
Intertrochanteric

1127. What is the rate of AVN with transepiphyseal fractures? How are they treated?

1127. Nearly 100% develop AVN
ORIF is the preferred treatment

1128. What is the rate of AVN with transcervical and cervicotrochanteric fractures? In what two ways are they treated?

1128. 25% AVN
ORIF
Closed reduction and percutaneous pinning with postoperative spica

1129. How are pediatric intertrochanteric fractures most commonly treated?

1129. Spica cast

1130. An acetabular fracture ORIF in a patient under 10 years of age may result in what complication?

1130. Premature closure of triradiate cartilage

1131. What is the consequence of early triradiate cartilage closure?

1131. Shallow acetabulum

Femoral Shaft Fractures

1132. How are femoral shaft fractures generally treated in patients <6 years of age?

1132. Spica cast

1133. … in patients 6 to 13 years of age

1133. Flexible intramedullary nails

1134. in patients over the age of 13 years?

1134. Rigid intramedullary (IM) nail

1135. How much shortening is acceptable?

1135. 2.5 cm

1136. What is the biggest disadvantage of using external fixation for treatment?

1136. Increased risk of refracture

1137. What are two possible complications of pediatric femoral shaft fracture?

1137. Patients under 10 years: femoral overgrowth
Tibial tubercle growth arrest with resulting recurvatum deformity

Pediatric Distal Femur Fracture

1138. Pediatric distal femur fractures tend to fall into what direction?

1138. Varus

1139. These fractures are usually a Salter-Harris __?

1139. II

1140. What key complication must one closely observe for?

1140. Physeal growth arrest

1141. Physeal bridges: consider resection in patients with what two characteristics?

1141. >2 cm remaining growth
<50% physeal involvement

1142. If >50% physis involved, what are the two surgical procedures?

1142. Ipsilateral completion
Contralateral epiphysiodesis

1143. What two populations are especially at risk for pediatric knee dislocation?

1143. Down syndrome
Arthrogryposis

1144. What two structures may be trapped and block reduction of a tibial eminence fracture?

1144. Anterior horn of meniscus
Transverse meniscal ligament

Proximal Tibial Physis Fracture ("Physis Torn Off")

1145. What two injuries are potentially associated with these high-energy fractures?

1145. Popliteal artery injury
Compartment syndrome

1146. Proximal tibial physis fractures are analogous to what problem in adults?

1146. Knee dislocation

1147. If the physeal fracture goes into malalignment, in what direction does it usually fall?

1147. Varus

1148. In what direction does a proximal tibial metaphyseal fracture usually fall?

1148. Valgus

1149. How can malalignment be prevented?

1149. Long leg cast in extension

1150. What is the prognosis if malalignment does occur?

1150. Usually remodels

1151. With a pediatric tibial shaft fracture, is reaming acceptable?

1151. Not if physes are open

Distal Tibial Physis Fractures

1152. In which order do the three distal tibial physes close?

1152. Central
Medial
Lateral

1153. What fracture tends to affect a younger age group: triplane or Tillaux?

1153. Triplane occurs earlier

1154. What is the radiographic appearance of a triplane fracture on AP film?

1154. Looks like Salter-Harris III

1155. What is the radiographic appearance of a triplane fracture on lateral view?

1155. Looks like a Salter-Harris II

1156. But it is actually which Salter-Harris classification?

1156. Salter-Harris IV

1157. How are distal tibial physeal fractures treated?

1157. ORIF

1158. What part of physis has already closed with a Tillaux fracture?

1158. Medial

1159. What part of physis is injured?

1159. Lateral

1160. What is the Salter-Harris stage of a Tillaux fracture?

1160. III

1161. How are Tillaux fractures treated?

1161. ORIF

1162. What is the surgical approach?

1162. Anteriorly

Overuse Injuries

1163. Young gymnasts are at risk for stress fractures at what four sites outside of the spine?

1163. Scaphoid
Distal radius
Elbow
Clavicle

1164. What of these is most common?

1164. Distal radius

1165. What is the most sensitive physical examination test for stress fracture at this site?

1165. Tenderness to palpation

1166. What are the two potential long-term complications of stress fracture?

1166. Premature physeal closure
Ulnar overgrowth

1167. Young throwers and racquet handlers develop stress fractures at what site?

1167. Proximal humerus (Little Leaguer's shoulder)

Child Abuse

1168. What six fracture locations are most suspicious for child abuse?

1168. Metaphyseal corner fractures
Rib fractures
Scapula
Spinous process
Sternum
Hangman's fracture

1169. What three bones are actually most commonly involved in child abuse?

1169. Humerus
Tibia
Femur

1170. Overall, are diaphyseal or metaphyseal abuse injuries more common?

1170. Diaphyseal

1171. What is the single most common fracture pattern of abuse?

1171. Transverse fracture, long bone

■ High-Yield Pediatric Review

List the disorders for each of the following descriptions:

1172. Four disorders with sporadic inheritance?

1172. Wassell IV polydactyly
Ollier
Mafucci
McCune-Albright

1173. Three disorders with café-au-lait spots?

1173. McCune-Albright
Neurofibromatosis
Jaffe-Campanacci

1174. Clubfoot surgery requires what artery to be patent?

1174. Posterior tibial artery

1175. What artery is often deficient in clubfoot?

1175. Dorsalis pedis

1176. What other procedure relies on a patent posterior tibial artery?

1176. Syme's amputation

1177. Increased paternal age is associated with what disorder?

1177. Achondroplasia

1178. How about increased maternal age?

1178. Limb deformities

1179. Polyphasic potentials are seen with what two disorders or physiologic processes?

1179. Friedreich's ataxia
Reinnervation

1180. Cubita valga is seen with what three conditions?

1180. Lateral condylar fracture
Turner syndrome
Ellis–van Creveld

1181. Five disorders with preceding febrile or viral illnesses?

1181. Guillain-Barré
Grisel's syndrome
Caffey
Polymyositis/dermatomyositis
Transient synovitis

1182. Three autosomal dominant inherited lower extremity disorders?

1182. Coxa vara
Tibial hemimelia
Tarsal coalition

1183. Four demyelinating disorders?

1183. Charcot Marie Tooth
Multiple sclerosis
Guillain-Barré syndrome
POEMS (myeloma)

1184. Four leg-length discrepancy–producing conditions in children?

1184. Femoral fracture
Posteromedial tibial bowing
Juvenile rheumatoid arthritis
Coxa vara after correction (proximal physeal deficiency)

1185. Three chromosome 15 disorders?

1185. Prader-Willi (imprinting paternal)
Angelman (imprinting maternal)
Marfan

1186. Two conditions associated with short metacarpals?

1186. Mucopolysaccharidoses (bullet metacarpals)
Albright syndrome

1187. A condition associated with a short middle phalanx?

1187. Poland syndrome

1188. Three disorders associated with protrusio?

1188. Marfan syndrome
Rheumatoid arthritis
Inflammatory arthropathies (ankylosing spondylitis, etc.)

10

Basic Science

■ Bone

Osteoblasts, Osteoclasts, and Osteocytes

Osteoblasts

1. From which cells do osteoblasts arise?

1. Undifferentiated mesenchymal stem cells (MSCs)

2. What seven growth factors influence osteoblast differentiation?

2. Interleukins (ILs)
Insulin-like growth factor (IGF-I)
Platelet-derived growth factor (PDGF)
Bone morphogenic proteins (BMPs)
Transforming growth factor-β (TGF-β)
Osterix
Runx 2 (formerly Cbfa 1)

3. What is the function of IGF?

3. Osteosynthesis

4. Through what intracellular signaling pathway does it work?

4. Tyrosine kinase

5. What is the function of PDGF?

5. Chemotaxis

6. Through what intracellular signaling pathway does it work?

6. Tyrosine kinase

7. What is the function of BMP?

7. Stimulates mesenchymal cell differentiation

8. Through what intracellular signaling pathway does it work?

8. Serine/threonine kinase through SMAD proteins

9. Is BMP osteoinductive or osteoconductive?

9. Osteoinductive

10. TGF-β stimulates mesenchymal cells to produce what two substances?

10. Type II collagen
Proteoglycans

11. TGF-β also indirectly stimulates osteoblasts to produce what?

11. Type I collagen

12. Through what intracellular signaling pathway does it work?

12. Serine/threonine kinase

13. What four substances do osteoblasts produce?

13. Alkaline phosphate
Type I collagen

Osteocalcin
RANK ligand

14. Osteoblasts respond directly to what five factors?

14. Parathyroid hormone (PTH)
Glucocorticoids
Prostaglandins
1,25–vitamin D
Estrogen

15. Which two of these favor osteogenesis?

15. 1,25–vitamin D
Estrogen

16. Which three favor resorption?

16. PTH (resorption releases calcium)
Glucocorticoids
Prostaglandins

17. What two factors upregulate adenylate cyclase at the cellular level?

17. PTH
Prostaglandins

18. What factor downregulates adenylate cyclase?

18. Estrogen

19. What factor also decreases calcium absorption at the level of the gut?

19. Glucocorticoids

Osteoclasts

20. From what cells do osteoclasts arise?

20. Monocyte progenitors

21. How do osteoclasts bind to the surface of bone?

21. With integrins (vibronectin)

22. Where does resorption occur?

22. Howship's lacunae

23. What are the two products of osteoclasts?

23. Hydrogen ions (through carbonic anhydrase)
Tartrate resistant acid phosphatase

24. What do osteoclasts respond directly to?

24. Calcitonin

25. What is the effect of calcitonin on the osteoclast?

25. Inhibits osteoclast function

26. What is the effect of IL-1?

26. Stimulates osteoclast function

27. What is the effect of IL-10?

27. Inhibits osteoclast function

28. What is the effect of IL-11?

28. Increases production of RANK ligand

29. What is the function of RANK ligand?

29. Links osteoblast and osteoclast function

30. What cell contains RANK ligand?

30. Osteoblast

31. How does RANK ligand work?

31. Binds to and stimulates osteoclasts

32. What cofactor is required?

32. Macrophage colony-stimulating factor (M-CSF)

33. What inhibits the RANK stimulation of osteoclasts?

33. Osteoprotegerin

34. How?

34. Blocks RANK binding to the osteoclast, competitive inhibition

Hormonal Effects on Bone Metabolism

35. If considering estrogen replacement therapy, when should it be started for maximal benefit?

35. Within 5 to 10 years of menopause

36. Generally speaking, how does estrogen work?

36. Decreases both bony resorption and formation
    But resorption is decreased much more than formation

37. What are two pharmacologic alternatives to estrogen therapy?

37. Alendronate
    Raloxifene

Osteocytes

38. What are osteocytes stimulated by?

38. Calcitonin

39. What are osteocytes inhibited by?

39. PTH

40. How does mechanical stimulation work?

40. Increases prostaglandin E_2 production (stimulus)

41. How are osteons connected to one another?

41. By haversian canals

42. What are the extensive networks of osteonal processes that allow communication?

42. Canaliculi

43. What is the outer osteonal border called?

43. Cement line

44. What lies in between osteons?

44. Interstitial lamellae

Composition of Bone

45. What is the principal organic component of bone?

45. Type I collagen

46. What is the composition of a collagen fibril?

46. Two α_1 chains
    Two α_2 chains

47. How is collagen secreted?

47. Secreted as procollagen

48. Then what happens?

48. Cross-linked after secretion

49. What is the difference between a hole and a pore?

49. Holes are the spaces between the ends of collagen molecules
    Pores are the spaces between the sides of the collagen molecules

50. What are the three noncollagenous matrix proteins of bone?

50. Osteocalcin
    Osteonectin
    Osteopontin

51. What stimulates osteocalcin production?

51. 1,25–vitamin D

52. What inhibits osteocalcin production?

52. PTH

53. Osteocalcin attracts what cell type?

53. Osteoclasts

54. What are osteocalcin levels a marker of?

54. Bone metabolism

55. Bone mineralization consists of what two processes? What are the key features of each?

55. Initiation (sialoproteins, pores, high-energy requirement)
    Growth (osteocalcin, coalescing areas of mineralization)

56. What are the three laboratory markers of bone resorption?

56. Urinary hydroxyproline
    Urinary pyridoline
    N-telopeptide

57. What are the laboratory markers of bone formation?

57. Alkaline phosphate

Properties of Mature Bone

58. Normal mature bone is of what type?

58. Lamellar

59. What is the defining characteristic of lamellar bone?

59. Remodeled along lines of stress

60. What are the two subtypes of lamellar bone?

60. Cortical
    Cancellous

61. In contrast, immature or pathologic bone is of what type?

61. Woven

62. Bone is strongest in what direction? Weakest in what direction?

62. Strongest in compression
    Weakest in shear

63. When bone is under torsion, where is the greatest load experienced?

63. Maximum load experienced at 45 degrees to the long axis of the bone

64. What is the basic premise of Wolff's law?

64. Increased stress leads to increased bone formation

65. Piezoelectric charges: is compression electropositive or negative?

65. Compression results in a negative charge

66. The negative charge then leads to what process?

66. Bone formation

67. Is tension electropositive or negative?

67. Positive charge

68. What does the positive charge lead to?

68. Bone resorption

69. What is the Heuter-Volkmann law? Give an example of where this law applies.

69. Compression inhibits growth
    Tension stimulates growth
    Example: scoliosis

70. At what age is peak bone mass achieved?

70. End of the third decade of life (the 20s)

71. What is the annual rate of bone loss after peak?

71. 0.3 to 0.5% per year

72. What is the annual rate of bone loss after menopause, without treatment?

72. 2 to 3% per year for 6 to 10 years after menopause

73. Is the observed postmenopausal decline simply estrogen related?

73. Not just estrogen, but changes in calcium metabolism also
    Decreased intestinal calcium absorption
    Increased calcium losses

Blood Supply of Mature Bone

74. Is the nutrient system high or low pressure?

74. High pressure

75. What does it supply?

75. Inner two thirds of bone

76. Is the periosteal system high or low pressure?

76. Low pressure

77. What does it supply?

77. Outer one third of bone

78. In what direction does blood flow in the adult?

78. Nutrient to periosteal

79. In what direction does blood flow in immature bone?

79. Opposite direction of flow

Fracture Healing

80. What is the principal determinant of fracture healing?

80. Blood supply

81. What are the three components of the sequence of changes in blood supply after fracture?

81. Immediate decrease in blood supply
Increased vascularity (maximal at 2 weeks)
Return to normal by 3 to 5 months

82. What is the effect of reaming?

82. Destroys endosteal blood supply

83. What are the three effects of nicotine on fracture healing?

83. Increased time to fracture healing
Increased risk of nonunion
Decreased fracture callus strength

84. Nicotine use is associated with increased risk of fractures at which locations?

84. Increases risk of wrist and hip fractures

85. How does smoking affect lumbar fusion rates?

85. Increases the pseudarthrosis rate of lumbar fusion by 500%

86. What is the two-step sequence of callus types formed after fracture?

86. Bridging (soft) callus within 2 weeks
Replaced by woven bone (hard callus)

87. Callus is ultimately remodeled over what period?

87. Remodeled to lamellar bone within 7 years

88. What two types of bone formation are seen with cast treatment of fracture?

88. Periosteal bridging callus
Enchondral ossification

89. Is there any difference with intramedullary (IM) nail treatment?

89. IM nail treatment also results in medullary callus formation late

90. Under what two conditions can intramembranous bone formation (no cartilage precursor) be seen after fracture?

90. Low strain
High oxygen tension

91. What type of chondrocytes are present in the first 10 days after fracture?

91. Proliferative chondrocytes

92. What collagen type do they produce?

92. Type II

93. What other collagen type is present in the chondroid phase?

93. Type IX: cross-linking function

94. After 14 days, what chondrocyte type is present?

94. Hypertrophic chondrocytes

95. What type of collagen do they produce?

95. Type X

96. What are the next three steps?

96. Calcification
Osteoclasts resorb matrix
Osteoblasts lay down new bone

97. How do hypertrophic nonunions heal?

97. Mineralization of fibrocartilage

98. What other treatment modality has a similar mechanism?

98. Pulsed electromagnetic field treatment (bone stimulator)

99. Rate the four tissue types from highest to lowest strain tolerances?

99. Granulation tissue (100% strain tolerance)
Fibrous tissue
Cartilage
Bone

Additional Fracture Treatment Modalities

100. At what phase of fracture healing does direct current exert an effect?

100. Inflammatory-response phase

101. At what phase of fracture healing does alternating current exert an effect?

101. Repair phase (callus)

102. What is the effect of pulsed electromagnetic fields?

102. Initiates fibrocartilage calcification

103. What is the classic application of this technology?

103. Nonhealing pseudo-Jones fracture

104. What are the two benefits of pulsed low-intensity ultrasound?

104. Accelerated fracture healing
Increased callus strength

105. What are the two detrimental effects of radiation?

105. Decreased cellularity
Decreased callus strength

Distraction Osteogenesis

106. How long should the latency phase last?

106. 5 to 7 days

107. What is the desired rate of distraction during distraction phase?

107. 1 mm/day

108. What is the duration of the consolidation phase?

108. Twice as long as the distraction phase

109. What is the weight-bearing status throughout treatment?

109. Weight-bearing as tolerated (WBAT)

110. What changes are seen in blood vessels?

110. Proliferation of vasa vasorum

111. What is the oxygen tension with distraction osteogenesis?

111. High oxygen tension

112. So what type of bone formation is seen under these low-strain, high oxygen tension conditions?

112. Intramembranous bone formation (no cartilage precursor)

Calcium and Phosphate Metabolism: Key Concepts

Calcium

113. What is the daily calcium intake recommendation for healthy children and adults?

113. 750 mg

114. What is the daily calcium intake recommendation for teenagers, pregnant women, and individuals with healing fractures?

114. 1500 mg

115. What is the daily calcium intake recommendation for lactating mothers?

115. 2000 mg

116. What is the mechanism of calcium absorption in the duodenum?

116. Active transport

117. What is the mechanism of calcium absorption in the jejunum?

117. Passive diffusion

118. What is the mechanism of calcium absorption in the kidney?

118. Proximal tubular resorption

119. What percentage of total body calcium is within plasma?

119. 1%

120. What are the relative proportions of bound vs. unbound plasma calcium?

120. Bound = unbound

121. What are the two principal regulators of plasma calcium concentration?

121. PTH
1,25–vitamin D

Phosphate

122. What are the relative proportions of bound vs. unbound plasma phosphate?

122. Unbound predominates

123. What is the principal site of phosphate resorption within the kidney?

123. Proximal tubule

Parathyroid Hormone

124. What type of molecule is parathyroid hormone (PTH)?

124. Peptide

125. Where is PTH produced?

125. Chief cells of the parathyroid gland

126. What is the stimulus for release of PTH?

126. Low plasma calcium concentration

127. What receptor detects calcium concentration?

127. Calcium sensing receptor (CaSR)

128. In what organ and gland can this receptor be found?

128. Kidney
Parathyroid gland

129. What type of receptor is CaSR?

129. G-protein–coupled receptor

130. What are the three effects of CaSR activation within the parathyroid gland?

130. PTH secretion
PTH gene expression
Cellular proliferation

131. In what organ and in what cells can PTH receptors be found?

131. Kidney
Osteoblasts

132. What are PTH's two actions on the kidney?

132. Increase 1,25–vitamin D production
Decrease resorption of renal phosphate

133. What are PTH's three actions on the bone?

133. Stimulate osteoblasts
Osteoblasts produce RANK ligand
RANK ligand stimulates osteoclasts

134. What is the net effect of PTH on plasma calcium and phosphate concentrations?

134. Increased plasma calcium
Decreased plasma phosphate

1,25–Vitamin D

135. What type of molecule is 1,25–vitamin D?

135. Steroid

136. As vitamin D is activated to 1,25–vitamin D, what are the two sites of hydroxylation?

136. First: liver
Second: kidney

137. What are the three stimuli for release of 1,25–vitamin D?

137. Low serum calcium concentration
Low serum phosphate concentration
Elevated PTH levels

138. What are the two effects of 1,25–vitamin D?

138. Increased intestinal absorption of calcium and phosphate
Increased osteoclast activity

139. What is the net effect of 1,25–vitamin D on plasma calcium and phosphate concentrations?

139. Increased plasma calcium
Increased plasma phosphate

Calcitonin

140. What type of molecule is calcitonin?

140. Peptide

141. Where is calcitonin produced?

141. Clear cells (parafollicular cells) of the thyroid gland

142. What is the stimulus for release of calcitonin?

142. Elevated serum calcium

143. What is the effect of calcitonin?

143. Inhibits osteoclast activity

Calcium and Phosphate Metabolism: Pathologic States

Primary Hyperparathyroidism

144. What is a common cause of primary hyperparathyroidism?

144. Adenoma of one parathyroid gland

145. If four glands are affected, what diagnosis must be considered?

145. Multiple endocrine neoplasia (MEN) syndrome

146. What is the effect of primary hyperparathyroidism on 1,25–vitamin D levels?

146. Increased 1,25–vitamin D

147. What is the effect of primary hyperparathyroidism on serum calcium concentration?

147. Increased serum calcium

148. What is the effect of primary hyperparathyroidism on serum phosphate concentration?

148. Decreased serum phosphate

149. What is the hydration status of hypercalcemic patients?

149. Generally dehydrated as hypercalcemia leads to polyuria

150. What is osteitis fibrosa cystica?

150. Resorption of bone due to PTH overactivity and replacement with fibrous tissue

151. What are the two characteristic histologic features of brown tumors?

151. Giant cells
Hemosiderin

152. What are the other systemic effects of hypercalcemia?

152. Renal stones
Psychiatric disorders
Abdominal pain

153. What are the four available hypercalcemia treatment methods?

153. Saline hydration
Loop diuretics
Dialysis
Mobilization

Hypoparathyroidism

154. What is the most common cause of hypoparathyroidism?

154. Iatrogenic

155. What is the effect on serum calcium concentration?

155. Decreased serum calcium

156. What is the effect on serum phosphate concentration?

156. Increased serum phosphate (because low PTH levels)

157. What is the effect on 1,25–vitamin D levels?

157. Decreased 1,25–vitamin D

158. What is the characteristic radiographic finding on skull films?

158. Calcification of the basal ganglia

Pseudohypoparathyroidism

159. What is the cause of pseudohypoparathyroidism?

159. No PTH effect at target cells

160. Inheritance?

160. X-linked dominant (XLD)

161. Quick review: what other disorder has a similar inheritance pattern?

161. Hypophosphatemic rickets

162. What gene is involved?

162. *GNAS1*

163. Mutation?

163. Gα subunit

164. Quick review: in what two other clinical situations do G-proteins play a vital role?

164. Fibrous dysplasia
CaSR function

165. What is the PTH level in pseudohypoparathyroidism?

165. Normal or high

166. What is the serum calcium concentration?

166. Low serum calcium

167. What is the serum phosphate concentration?

167. Elevated serum phosphate (again, no PTH effect)

168. What is the effect on 1,25–vitamin D levels?

168. Low 1,25–vitamin D

169. Give an example of a disorder associated with pseudohypoparathyroidism?

169. Albright syndrome

170. What are the four characteristic features of pseudohypoparathyroidism?

170. Short metacarpals
Bony exostoses
Obesity
Mental retardation

171. Quick review: what is another disorder that is associated with obesity and mental retardation?

171. Prader-Willi

Pseudopseudohypoparathyroidism

172. Pseudopseudohypoparathyroidism is phenotypically similar to what?

172. Pseudohypoparathyroidism

173. What is the serum calcium concentration?

173. Normal

174. What is the target cell response to PTH?

174. Normal

Renal Failure Osteodystrophy

175. What are the two general types of renal failure osteodystrophy?

175. High turnover
Low turnover (excess aluminum leads to decreased metabolic activity)

176. With the high turnover type, what is the serum phosphate level?

176. Elevated due to renal failure/inability to dump phosphate

177. … the serum calcium level?

177. Low because with elevated phosphate, calcium precipitates out of solution

178. … the PTH level?

178. Elevated, because high phosphate levels lead to secondary hyperparathyroidism

179. What are the two components of the treatment for high turnover renal osteodystrophy?

179. Phosphate binders (antacids)
Activated oral vitamin D

180. With the low turnover type, what is the serum calcium level?

180. Normal

181. … the serum phosphate level?

181. Normal

182. … the PTH level?

182. Low

183. … the 1,25–vitamin D level?

183. Low because of impaired renal hydroxylase

184. With renal osteodystrophy, what is the clinical appearance of the spine?

184. Rugger jersey spine

185. What other disorder also exhibits a rugger jersey spine?

185. Osteopetrosis

186. What other generalized bony changes are present?

186. Osteitis fibrosa cystica due to secondary hypoparathyroidism

187. Chronic dialysis treatment also leads to what disorder?

187. Amyloidosis

Renal Tubular Acidosis

188. With renal tubular acidosis, what two ions are lost in the urine?

188. Sodium
Calcium

189. What is the key lab value for diagnosis?

189. Urine calcium > serum calcium

190. What is the treatment of renal tubular acidosis?

190. Alkalinize the urine

191. Renal tubular acidosis is phenotypically similar to what disorder?

191. Rickets

192. Quick review: What are three other situations in which calcium losses can exceed intake?

192. Postmenopausal woman (increased urine calcium, decreased absorption)

Elevated glucocorticoids (increased urine calcium)

Osteogenic rickets (fibroblast growth factor-23 [FGF-23])

Rickets

Nutritional Rickets: Vitamin D Deficiency

193. What is the suggested daily intake of vitamin D for healthy adults?

193. 200 international units (IU)

194. What is the suggested daily intake of vitamin D for children, pregnant women, and lactating mothers?

194. 400 IU

195. What is the only natural dietary source of vitamin D?

195. Oily fish

196. What is the serum calcium level with vitamin D deficiency?

196. Decreased (due to decreased absorption)

197. What is the resulting effect on PTH?

197 Increased (in response to low calcium)

198. What two clinical features of nutritional rickets are most sensitive and specific?

198. Wrist enlargement
Costochondral enlargement

199. What is the serum phosphate level?

199. Decreased (due to high PTH)

200. What does treatment of vitamin D deficiency rickets consist of?

200. 5000 IU per day of vitamin D

Nutritional Rickets: Calcium Deficiency

201. Deficient calcium intake has what effect on PTH levels?

201. PTH levels become elevated

202. What effect does this have on vitamin D levels?

202. Increases vitamin D levels (attempt to absorb greater amounts of calcium, phosphate)

203. What are serum phosphate levels?

203. May actually be low (due to elevated PTH)

204. What is the treatment of calcium deficiency rickets?

204. 750 mg/day of calcium

Nutritional Rickets: Phosphate Deficiency

205. Deficient phosphate intake has what effect on PTH levels?

205. None (PTH responds only to high phosphate)

206. What effect does low serum phosphate have on vitamin D levels?

206. Increases vitamin D levels (attempt to absorb greater amounts of phosphate)

207. What is the treatment of phosphate deficiency rickets?

207. Oral phosphate supplementation

Vitamin D–Dependent Rickets Type I

208. Inheritance?

208. Autosomal recessive (AR)

209. Mutation?

209. Defect in renal 1,25-hydroxylase

210. What is the effect of defective hydroxylase?

210. No conversion of inactive vitamin D to active form

211. What is the characteristic clinical feature?

211. Rachitic rosary responsive to vitamin D

212. What is the resulting serum calcium level?

212. Decreased

213. What is the resulting serum phosphate level?

213. Decreased (due to decreased absorption)

214. What is the resulting serum PTH level?

214. Elevated (in response to low calcium)

215. What is the treatment of vitamin D–dependent rickets (VDDR) type I?

215. Oral activated vitamin D

Vitamin D–Dependent Rickets Type II

216. Defect?

216. No receptor for 1,25–vitamin D at target cells

217. What is the serum level of 1,25–vitamin D?

217. Very high

218. What is the serum level of active vitamin D in type I?

218. Very low in type I

219. What are the two characteristic clinical features?

219. Alopecia
Rachitic rosary unresponsive to vitamin D therapy

220. What is the treatment of VDDR type II?

220. Vitamin D analogue

221. What is the relative severity of both types of vitamin D dependent rickets vs. nutritional rickets?

221. Vitamin D dependent rickets I and II are more severe

Hypophosphatemic Rickets

222. What is the relative frequency of hypophosphatemic rickets as a cause of rickets?

222. Most common cause in the United States

223. What is the inheritance?

223. XLD

224. What is the mutation?

224. Impaired renal tubular absorption of phosphate

225. What is the gene?

225. *PHEX*

226. This disorder is also known as what?

226. Vitamin D resistant rickets

227. What is the serum phosphate level?

227. Low, because a lot of phosphate is lost in the urine

228. What is the resulting PTH level?

228. Normal (no PTH response to low serum phosphate)

229. What is the serum calcium level?

229. Normal

230. What is the classic triad of clinical features?

231. What are the two components of treatment of hypophosphatemic rickets?

Hypophosphatasia

232. What is the inheritance?
233. What is the defect?

234. Clinical features are similar to what group of disorders?
235. How is hypophosphatasia diagnosed?

236. What is the treatment of hypophosphatasia?

Review of Key Points of Confusion

237. High-turnover renal osteodystrophy displays clinical features similar to what other disorder?
238. The renal osteodystrophy spine has what appearance?
239. This spine appearance is also associated with what other disorder?
240. Hypophosphatasia displays clinical features similar to what other disorder?
241. The spine has what appearance in hypophosphatasia?

Paget's Disease

242. What are three proposed viral etiologies for Paget's disease?

243. What is the typical clinical presentation of Paget's?
244. Within a given bone, how does Paget's progress?
245. What is the radiographic appearance of progression?
246. Laboratory findings include increased levels of what four substances?

---

230. Short child
Lower limb deformities
Low serum phosphate

231. High-dose phosphate replacement
High-dose vitamin D (to facilitate phosphate absorption)

232. AR
233. Enzymatic deficiency leads to low levels of alkaline phosphate
234. Nutritional rickets

235. Elevated urinary phosphoethanolamine
236. No good options exist

237. Primary hyperparathyroidism (for example, osteitis fibrosa cystica)

238. Rugger jersey spine

239. Osteopetrosis

240. Nutritional rickets

241. Rachitic rosary (like rickets)

242. Respiratory syncytial virus (RSV)
Paramyxovirus
Canine distemper virus

243. Bone pain

244. Starts at one end and progresses to the other
245. Leading "lytic flame"

246. Alkaline phosphate
Urinary hydroxyproline
Osteocalcin
N-telopeptide

247. What are the three key histologic features?

247. Osteoclasts with viral inclusion bodies (paramyxovirus)

Cement lines

Relative osteoblastic or osteoclastic appearance depends on phase of disease

248. What is the treatment of Paget's disease?

248. Bisphosphonates

249. What other clinical conditions occur secondary to Paget's disease in the spine?

249. Spinal stenosis

250. What other clinical conditions occur secondary to Paget's disease in the heart?

250. High output cardiac failure

251. What other clinical conditions occur secondary to Paget's disease in the auditory system?

251. Deafness

252. What does the new onset of severe pain and swelling in a patient with known Paget's suggest?

252. Malignant osteosarcoma

253. How often does this occur?

253. In 10% of patients

Osteoporosis

Aging and Bone Metabolism

254. What effect does aging have on stomach acidity?

254. Decreased acidity

255. What effect does the change in acidity have on calcium absorption?

255. Decreased calcium absorption

256. What effect does aging have on vitamin D requirements?

256. Increased vitamin D requirements with age

Osteoporosis

257. Is osteoporosis a quantitative or qualitative deficiency of bone?

257. Quantitative (not enough bone)

Compare to rickets (qualitative; poor quality bone)

258. What are the common laboratory findings in patients with osteoporosis?

258. Generally normal

259. What is the definition of osteoporosis in terms of T-score?

259. T-score of –2.5 or less

260. What are the two indications for treatment of osteoporosis?

260. T score of –2.5

History of any osteoporotic fracture

261. Compare the definitions of T-score and Z-score?

261. T-score is the number of standard deviations away from mean peak bone mass (comparison to 25-year-old population)

Z-score is the number of standard deviations away from mean bone mass in age-matched population (comparison to population of the same age as the patient)

262. What two imaging modalities are most commonly used to arrive at a T-score?

262. Dual-energy x-ray absorptiometry (DEXA) scan
Quantitative computed tomography (CT) scan

263. How much bone must be lost before a change in plain x-ray appearance is evident?

263. 30%

264. Does a DEXA scan evaluate cancellous and cortical bone individually?

264. No, together

265. Does a quantitative CT scan evaluate cancellous and cortical bone individually?

265. Yes, can separate

266. What is the downside of quantitative CT?

266. Increased radiation

267. What test is the most accurate for determining bone density?

267. Quantitative CT

268. What test is the most reliable for predicting fracture risk?

268. DEXA scan

269. What are the two general types of osteoporosis?

269. Type I: postmenopausal
Type II: age related (>75 years old)

270. With type I osteoporosis, what type of bone is principally affected?

270. Trabecular bone (cancellous)

271. Give two examples of typical type I fractures?

271. Vertebral body fractures
Distal radius fractures

272. With type II osteoporosis, what type of bone is principally affected?

272. Trabecular and cortical bone

273. Give two examples of typical type II fractures?

273. Hip fracture
Pelvic fracture

274. How do bisphosphonates affect osteoclast microstructure?

274. Disrupt microtubules within the ruffled border

275. How do they disrupt macrostructure?

275. Disrupt protein prenylation

276. What disadvantageous effect do high-dose bisphosphonates have?

276. Disrupt calcium deposition also, not just resorption

Osteoporosis in the Spinal Cord Injured Patient

277. Over what period of time does the peak bone loss occur?

277. First 16 months after injury

278. After that period of time, how much bone mass remains?

278. Two thirds of the preinjury bone mass

279. What anatomic region is most affected by bone loss?

279. Knee

280. What anatomic region is most spared by bone loss?

280. Skull

Bone Grafts and Bone Alternatives

281. What are the two products of stem cell division?

281. Another stem cell
Progenitor cell

282. Why is it desirable to select out stem cells from other cells within grafts?

282. Because the greater the total number of cells, the greater the metabolic needs
Greater metabolic needs lead to a lower cell survival depth

Allografts

283. What is the main advantage of fresh allograft?

283. Contains osteoinductive BMPs

284. What is the main disadvantage?

284. Immunogenic

285. Is fresh allograft osteoconductive or inductive?

285. Both

286. What are the two advantages of fresh frozen allograft?

286. Still contains osteoinductive BMPs
Less immunogenic

287. Is fresh frozen allograft osteoconductive or inductive?

287. Both

288. What is the main advantage of freeze-dried allograft?

288. Lowest immunogenicity

289. What are the two main disadvantages?

289. Does not contain BMPs
Structural properties may be compromised with freeze drying

290. How does freeze-dried stiffness and compactability compare to fresh allograft?

290. Same maximal stiffness
More compactable

291. Based on recent literature, what type of allograft results in superior stem fixation?

291. Freeze-dried has superior stem fixation

292. What does the recent literature on use of freeze-dried allograft in adolescent idiopathic scoliosis surgery indicate?

292. Significantly lowers fusion rates

293. What is demineralized bone matrix?

293. Digested allograft and BMP

294. Is it osteoconductive or inductive?

294. Both

295. What are the three key points to know about BMP mechanism of osteoinductivity?

295. Serine/threonine kinase intracellular signaling pathway
Acts via cytokines
Facilitated by SMAD proteins

296. What is the main disadvantage of osteochondral allografts?

296. Cartilage is immunogenic

297. How does cryogenic preservation affect chondrocyte number?

297. Very few remain

298. After implantation of osteochondral allograft, what happens to host chondrocytes?

298. Not preserved

299. How long is transplanted cartilage preserved?

299. 2 to 3 years

300. What is the histological appearance thereafter?

300. Transplanted cartilage covered by fibrocartilage

301. Bottom line: How does the strength of cortical and cancellous grafts change over time?

301. Cortical grafts are strongest day 1; then resorbed and remodeled
Cancellous grafts get progressively stronger through process of creeping substitution

Ceramics

302. What is the two-step sequence of chemical conversion of tricalcium phosphate (TCP)?

302. TCP rapidly broken down
But slowly converted to hyaluronic acid (HA)

303. Is TCP osteoconductive or inductive?

303. Osteoconductive only

304. Is TCP immunogenic?

304. No

305. What is the ideal ceramic pore size?

305. 150 µm

Anti-Allograft Antigenicity

306. What two factors determine the extent of allograft incorporation?

306. Cellularity
Major histocompatability complex (MHC) compatibility

307. What cells mediate the immune response?

307. T cells

308. What surface structure on transplanted cells is recognized by host immune cells?

308. Surface glycoprotein

309. Mechanical properties of allograft change at what dose of radiation?

309. 3 Mrad

■ Articular Cartilage

Chondrocytes

Growth Factors

310. What four growth factors act on chondrocytes?

310. IGF-I
TGF-β
Fibroblast growth factor (FGF)
PDGF

311. What is the effect of IGF-I on the chondrocyte?

311. Stimulates matrix production

312. TGF-β has what three effects on the chondrocyte?

312. Stimulates production of proteoglycans
Suppresses production of type II collagen
Turns on the expression of SMAD3—chondroprotective

313. Quick review: what other commonly tested role do Smads have?

313. Facilitate signaling and activity of BMPs

314. What are the two other key points about BMP?

314. Intracellular signaling through serine/threonine kinase pathway
Contains cytokines

315. What is the net effect of FGF on chondrocytes?

315. Synthetic

316. PDGF is particularly important in what clinical situation?

316. Osteoarthritis

Composition of Cartilage

Collagens

317. What is the predominant collagen type in articular cartilage?

317. Type II

318. What is the principal function of type II collagen?

318. Provides tensile strength

319. What three other collagen types may also be present in articular cartilage?

319. Type VI
Type X
Type XI

320. Are type VI collagen levels higher with normal aging or with osteoarthritis?

320. Osteoarthritis

321. In what situation are type X collagen levels particularly elevated?

321. During enchondral ossification

322. Type X collagen is produced by what cells?

322. Hypertrophic chondrocytes

323. When does this occur?

323. >14 days after fracture

324. Type X collagen is generally associated with what process?

324. Calcification of cartilage

325. Type X collagen is deficient in what inherited syndrome?

325. Schmid metaphyseal chondrodysplasia

326. What is the principal function of type XI collagen?

326. Acts as an adhesive holding collagen together

Proteoglycans

327. What is the principal function of proteoglycans?

327. Provide compressive strength

328. How do they achieve this function?

328. By maintaining water within the matrix

329. What limits the total water content of normal cartilage?

329. The ordered structure of proteoglycan and collagen

330. What are proteoglycan subunits called?

330. Glycosaminoglycans (GAGs)

331. What are three commonly tested GAGs?

331. Chondroitin 4 sulfate
Chondroitin 6 sulfate
Keratan sulfate

332. What GAG increases most significantly in concentration with normal aging?

332. Keratan sulfate

333. What GAG increases most significantly with osteoarthritis development?

333. Chondroitin 4 sulfate

334. What GAG concentration remains relatively constant despite aging or osteoarthritis?

334. Chondroitin 6 sulfate

335. How are GAGs bound to the protein core?

335. Sugar bonds

336. GAGs and the protein core form what molecules?

336. Aggrecan

337. What is the role of link proteins?

337. Stabilize aggrecan molecules to hyaluronic acid (HA)

338. Several aggrecan molecules stabilized to HA form what?

338. Proteoglycan aggregate

339. What is the half-life of a proteoglycan aggregate?

339. 3 months

Mature Cartilage

340. How can mature cartilage be differentiated from immature cartilage?

340. Mature cartilage has no stem cell population

Cartilage Zones

341. What are the five zones of articular cartilage?

341. Gliding zone (superficial)
Transitional zone (middle)
Radial zone (deep)
Tidemark
Calcified zone

342. In general, where is water content the highest?

342. At the surface

343. In general, where is proteoglycan concentration the highest?

343. In the deep layers

344. Within the gliding zone, what is the fiber orientation?

344. Tangential

345. What is the function of this zone?

345. Resists shear

346. What is the level of metabolic activity?

346. Low

347. Within the transitional zone, what is the fiber orientation?

347. Oblique

348. What is the function of this zone?

348. Resists compression

349. What is the level of metabolic activity?

349. High

350. Within the radial zone, what is the fiber orientation?

350. Vertical

351. What is the function of this zone?

351. Resists compression

352. What is the collagen size?

352. Large

353. Within the tidemark, what is the fiber orientation?

353. Tangential

354. What are the two functions of this zone?

354. Resists shear
Acts as a barrier

355. Is the tidemark seen best in adults or children?

355. Adults

356. Is the tidemark present in cartilaginous exostoses?

356. No, joints only (articular cartilage)

357. In the calcified zone, what is the key component?

357. Hydroxyapatite crystals

358. What is the function?

358. Acts as an anchor

359. How do these zones make cartilage biphasic?

359. Fluid layers shield solid matrix from stress

Synovium and Cartilage Lubrication

360. What two cell types are present within synovium?

360. Type A: responsible for phagocytosis
Type B: produces synovial fluid

361. Does synovium have a basement membrane?

361. No; facilitates fluid transport

362. What three components of plasma are absent in synovial fluid?

362. Red blood cells
Hemoglobin
Clotting factors

363. Compare complement levels in synovial fluid with rheumatoid arthritis and ankylosing spondylitis.

363. Rheumatoid arthritis: decreased levels of complement
Ankylosing spondylitis: normal levels of complement

364. How does the viscosity of synovial fluid change with shear? What does that say about synovial fluid?

364. Viscosity increases as shear decreases
So synovial fluid is non-newtonian

365. Under conditions of high strain, what two things happen to the hyaluronan within synovial fluid?

365. Becomes entangled and forms a relatively solid cushion
Relative proteoglycan concentration increases

366. Under conditions of instability, what happens to the hyaluronan within synovial fluid?

366. Hyaluronan content and efficacy decrease

367. Under conditions of disuse, what happens to the hyaluronan within synovial fluid?

367. No change

368. What are the two key lubricating components of synovial fluid?

368. Lubricin: a glycoprotein
Superficial zone protein (SZP)

369. What is hydrodynamic lubrication?

369. A thin film completely separates two articulating surfaces

370. What is elastic lubrication?

370. Articular surfaces deform slightly when loaded to create pockets of fluid

371. What is the primary method by which normal articular cartilage is lubricated?

371. Elastohydrodynamic: a combination of elastic and hydrodynamic lubrication

372. Comparison/review: What is the primary lubrication method for hard-on-soft articular bearings?

372. Boundary method
Some points of contact between surfaces but separation adequate to minimize wear

373. Comparison/review: What is the primary lubrication method for hard-on-hard articular bearings?

373 Mixed: hydrodynamic and boundary methods

374. What does "weeping" refer to?

374. Under conditions of loading, fluid shifts to loaded areas of articular cartilage

Aging Cartilage

375. What is the half-life of articular cartilage?

375. 117 years

376. Because cartilage has such a long half-life, what is the rate of cartilage synthesis in adulthood?

376. Markedly diminished relative to earlier in life

377. What is the basic mechanism by which normal cartilage ages?

377. Passive glycation

378. What is the net effect of this process?

378. Increased cartilage stiffness (modulus of elasticity)

Other Changes Observed with Normal Cartilage Aging

379. With aging, what changes are seen in chondrocyte number?

379. Decreases

380. What changes are seen in chondrocyte size?

380. Increases

381. What changes are seen in collagen variability?

381. Increases

382. What changes are seen in total proteoglycan concentration?

382. Decreases

383. What is the corresponding change in water content?

383. Decreases

384. In normal aging, what happens to chondroitin 4 concentration as a percentage of total chondroitin?

384. Decreases

385. What happens to keratan sulfate concentration?

385. Increases

386. Again, what is the net effect on modulus of elasticity?

386. Increased (increased cartilage stiffness)

Cartilage Injury and Healing

387. Do superficial cartilage lacerations heal?

387. No, because cartilage is avascular

388. Do lacerations deep to the tidemark heal?

388. Yes, blood supply is available

389. What cell type is involved in healing?

389. Mesenchymal cells produce fibrocartilage

Relevant Literature

390. Is motion beneficial or detrimental to the healing of deep lacerations?

390. Beneficial

391. After BMP-7 application, what effect is seen at 4 weeks? At 8 months?

391. 4 weeks: accelerated healing observed
8 months: same as control

392. Is there an observed difference in outcomes between microfracture and autologous chondrocyte implantation?

392. No demonstrated difference

393. What sequence of three steps is involved in autologous chondrocyte implantation?

393. Harvest cartilage
Expand population of chondrocytes
Reimplant at site of injury

394. What is the maximum defect area for which this technology is applicable?

394. 8 cm

395. What are the two potential benefits of hyaluronic acid injection?

395. Stimulation of fibroblasts
Facilitates meniscal healing

396. Have any chondroprotective effects been proven?

396. No

397. What location is the most reliable for successful injection into the knee?

397. Superolaterally

Osteoarthritis

Microscopic Features

398. What two families of enzymes are involved with the development of osteoarthritis?

398. Metalloproteinases
Cathepsins

399. What are three examples of metalloproteinases? What is a common factor among them?

399. Collagenase
Gelatinase
Stromelysin
Zinc is a common factor for all three

400. What are the roles of tumor necrosis factor-α (TNF-α) and interleukin-1 (IL-1)?

400. Catabolic
Upregulate metalloproteinase production

401. What is more detrimental to articular cartilage: shear or compression?

401. Shear (e.g., instability)

Other Changes Observed in Articular Cartilage with Osteoarthritis Development

402. With osteoarthritis development, what changes are seen in collagen order and relative concentration?

402. Increasingly disordered
Relative increase in concentration as proteoglycan concentration decreases

403. What changes are seen in DNA within the chondrocytes?

403. No change; remains essentially normal

404. What changes are seen in rate of proteoglycan degradation?

404. Markedly increased

405. What changes are seen in proteoglycan concentration?

405. Decreases

406. What changes are seen in water content?

406. Increases

407. So, if a proteoglycan concentration determines water content, why does the water content increase in osteoarthritis when proteoglycan concentration decreases?

407. Because the ordered structure of proteoglycan and cartilage in normal cartilage limits total water content

In osteoarthritis, although total proteoglycan concentration decreases, structure falls apart

As a result, the water content increases in osteoarthritic cartilage

408. In osteoarthritis, what happens to chondroitin 4 concentration as a percentage of total chondroitin?

408. Increases

409. What happens to keratan sulfate concentration?

409. Decreases

410. What happens to modulus of elasticity?

410. Decreases (decreased stiffness)

Macroscopic Features

411. What joint is most commonly affected by osteoarthritis?

411. Knee

412. What are two subchondral changes?

412. Sclerosis
Subchondral cyst development

413. How do gross changes in cartilage appear?

413. As microfractures

414. What is the four-part Outerbridge classification of cartilage injury?

414. I: cartilage softening
II: fragmentation, fissuring
III: crabmeat appearance
IV: exposed bone

Rheumatoid Arthritis

Microscopic Features

415. With rheumatoid arthritis, what are the two key associated enzymes?

415. IL-1
TNF-α

416. What are the two key human leukocyte antigen (HLA) associations?

416. DR4
DW4

417. What virus may possibly be associated with rheumatoid arthritis development?

417. Epstein-Barr virus

418. What cell type is responsible for inciting inflammatory response?

418. T-cell

419. What cell type is responsible for the associated destruction?

419. Monocyte

Macroscopic Features

420. What are the two key elements of the history and exam?

420. Morning stiffness
Swelling and nodules

421. What four laboratory findings may be present in rheumatoid arthritis?

421. Elevated erythrocyte sedimentation rate (ESR)
Elevated C-reactive protein (CRP)
Positive rheumatoid factor
Low levels of complement

422. What is rheumatoid factor?

422. An immunoglobulin M (IgM) antibody against IgG

423. What are the two classic radiographic findings of rheumatoid arthritis?

423. Periarticular erosions
Osteopenia

Treatment Alternatives

424. What are the four classic disease-modifying antirheumatologic agents (DMARDs)?

424. Methotrexate
Gold
Sulfasalazine
Cyclosporine

425. What drug is anti IL-1?

425. Anakinra

426. What three drugs are anti–TNF-α?

426. Etanercept: may be associated with demyelination as side effect
Infliximab: may be associated with congestive heart failure (CHF)
Adalimumab

427. What drug is anti–B-cell?

427. Rituximab

Syndromes Associated with Rheumatoid Arthritis

428. What are the three characteristics of Felty's syndrome?

428. Rheumatoid arthritis
Splenomegaly
Leucopenia

429. What are the three characteristics of Still's disease?

429. Acute fever
Rash
Arthritis

Juvenile Rheumatoid Arthritis

430. By definition, symptoms must last for how long to be considered juvenile rheumatoid arthritis (JRA)?

430. At least 6 weeks

431. What is the age criterion for JRA diagnosis?

431. 16 years old or less

432. What joint is most commonly affected?

432. Knee

433. Are most JRA patients rheumatoid factor positive or negative?

433. Negative

434. What is the significance of rheumatoid factor positive JRA?

434. Increased likelihood of developing adult form of rheumatoid arthritis

435. How many joints must be affected for JRA to be considered polyarticular?

435. Five

436. What gender is most affected by early-onset pauciarticular JRA?

436. Female

437. What is the usual age at onset?

437. 2 to 3 years old

438. What are two associated conditions to watch for?

438. Iridocyclitis
Leg length discrepancy development

439. What gender is most affected by late-onset pauciarticular JRA?

439. Male

440. What is the usual age at onset?

440. Teenage years

441. What is the classic treatment for JRA?

441. High-dose aspirin

Ankylosing Spondylitis

Macroscopic Features

442. Ankylosing spondylitis (AS) patients generally feel stiffest at what time of day?

442. Morning

443. What joint is most often the first affected?

443. Sacroiliac joint

444. What physical exam finding is most specific for AS?

444. Decreased chest wall expansion

445. What are the two classic ocular findings?

445. Iritis
Anterior uveitis

446. What two associated conditions may also severely complicate AS?

446. Pulmonary fibrosis
Aortic regurgitation and other cardiac valvular and conduction abnormalities

447. What two tests can be used to evaluate bone density in ankylosing spondylitis patients?

447. DEXA scan of the hip
Quantitative CT scan

Spine Manifestations

448. What are the three classic spine findings of AS?

448. Bamboo spine
Marginal syndesmophytes
Square vertebrae

449. What is the two-part treatment for low-energy neck trauma in AS patients? Why?

449. Strict immobilization
Thorough evaluation for fracture
Occult fracture or instability may not be immediately apparent on radiographic studies

450. What additional test may be beneficial in excluding an occult fracture?

450. Bone scan

451. Cervical spine fractures in AS patients may be associated with what complication? How can this be evaluated?

451. Epidural hemorrhage
Evaluate with magnetic resonance imaging (MRI)

452. What are two treatment options for cervical fractures in ankylosing spondylitis?

452. Halo vest
Surgery

453. In general, surgical intervention on the spine of AS patients requires what approach?

453. Combined anterior and posterior approaches

454. What is the preferred osteotomy for treatment of AS-related kyphosis?

454. Pedicle subtraction osteotomy

455. What is the general rule for the amount of correction this osteotomy can give you?

455. 30 degrees per level

456. At which level should cervical kyphosis generally be corrected?

456. C7-T1

457. At which levels should umbar kyphosis generally be corrected?

457. L2 or below

458. Quick review of syndesmophytes: What are the two key characteristics of the syndesmophytes associated with AS and inflammatory bowel diseases?

458. Marginal
Thin, symmetric

459. What are the two key characteristics of the syndesmophytes associated with Reiter syndrome and psoriasis syndesmophytes?

459. Nonmarginal
Thick, asymmetric

460. What are the two aspects of the classic radiographic appearance of disseminated idiopathic skeletal hyperostosis (DISH)?

460. Nonmarginal syndesmophytes
Intervertebral disk is spared

Gout

461. What is the composition of the crystals associated with gout?

461. Monosodium urate

462. What are the two aspects of the appearance of crystals under plane-polarized light?

462. Yellow
Negatively birefringent

463. Where do articular erosions generally appear in patients with gout?

463. Generally away from the joint surface itself

Treatment Strategies

464. What is the drug of choice to inhibit associated inflammatory mediators?

464. Colchicine

465. What two drugs act to inhibit phagocytosis?

465. Phenylbutazone
Indomethacin

466. What is the mechanism of action of allopurinol? When it is indicated?

466. Xanthine oxidase inhibition
For chronic gout suppression

467. What is the relationship between myeloproliferative syndrome (MPS) and gout?

467. Chemotherapy for MPS may precipitate an attack of gout

Chondrocalcinosis

468. What are five potential causes of chondrocalcinosis?

468. Calcium pyrophosphate deposition disease (CPPD, positively birefringent crystals)
Ochronosis
Hyperparathyroidism
Hypothyroidism
Hemochromatosis (primarily affects small joints)

Other Conditions Associated with Arthritis or Spondylitis

Systemic Lupus Erythematosus

469. What is the primary site of arthritic involvement with systemic lupus erythematosus (SLE)?

469. Hands and wrists

470. What is the classic clinical feature of SLE?

470. Malar (butterfly) rash

471. What are the two key lab values?

471. Generally ANA+
Occasionally RF+ also

472. How is SLE treated?

472. Generally the same as rheumatoid arthritis

473. Mortality from SLE is generally due to what?

473. Renal disease

474. Quick review: In general, when given a patient with avascular necrosis (AVN), what should always be in the differential diagnosis?

474. AVN secondary to chronic steroid therapy

475. What are two commonly tested disorders that may present this way?

475. Systemic lupus erythematosus
Rheumatoid arthritis

Ochronosis (Alkaptonuria)

476. What is the associated mutation?

476. Homogentisic acid oxidase deficiency

477. This deficiency results in the accumulation of what substance?

477. Homogentisic acid, which is then deposited within joints

478. In what two ways is alkaptonuria diagnosed?

478. Urine is black
Can check urine homogentisic acid concentration

479. What are two characteristics of the associated spondylitis?

479. Disk space narrowing
Calcification of the disk

Relapsing Polychondritis

480. What is the classic clinical presentation of relapsing polychondritis?

480. Episodic attacks of arthritic pain

481. What patient population is most commonly affected?

481. Elderly

482. Other clinical manifestations include what two organs?

482. Ears
Eyes

Acute Rheumatic Fever

483. What organism is responsible for acute rheumatic fever?

483. Group A streptococcus

484. What are the two relevant diagnostic tests?

484. Antistreptolysin O (ASO) titer
Elevated ESR

485. What is the key point about the resultant arthritis?

485. Migratory

486. Acute rheumatic fever preferentially involves joints of what size?

486. Large

487. Other systemic manifestations include what process in the heart?

487. Carditis

488. ... in the skin?

488. Erythema marginatum

489. ... in the neurologic system?

489. Chorea (movement disorder)

Reiter Syndrome

490. What is the classic triad of Reiter's syndrome?

490. Arthritis
Uveitis
Urethritis

491. What is the key clinical feature of the hand and wrist?

491. Tenosynovitis of the dorsal hand and wrist (especially if gonorrhea)

492. What is the key clinical feature of the skin?

492. Pustular lesions on palms and soles

493. What is the key clinical feature of the mucosal surfaces?

493. Oral ulcers

494. How frequently are the sacroiliac joints involved?

494. In 60% of patients

495. How often are Reiter syndrome patients HLA-B27 positive?

495. 80 to 90%

Tuberculous Arthritis

496. What are the characteristic synovial fluid findings of tuberculosis?

496. Rice bodies (fibrin globules)

■ Muscle

Composition of Muscle

Microstructure

497. What is the smallest functional unit of muscle?

497. The sarcomere

498. What is the function of tropomyosin?

498. Prevents actin cross-bridge binding

499. What is the function of troponin?

499. Modifies tropomyosin to allow cross-bridge binding

500. Troponin function is sensitive to what?

500. Changes in calcium level

501. A collection of sarcomeres forms what larger unit?

501. Myofibril

502. How are the myofibrils supplied with calcium?

502. Via the T-tubules

503. And a collection of myofibrils forms what larger unit?

503. The individual muscle fiber

Macrostructure

504. What structure surrounds individual muscle fibers?

504. Endomysium

505. What structure surrounds each fascicle?

505. Perimysium

506. What structure surrounds each muscle bundle?

506. Epimysium

Energy Generation and Utilization

First 20 Seconds of Intense Activity

507. What energy generation system predominates in this time period?

507. Adenosine triphosphate (ATP)-creatine phosphate system

508. What is the mechanism of action?

508. Stored carbohydrates in muscle are converted into ATP

509. Is this process aerobic or anaerobic?

509. Anaerobic

510. Is lactate generated in this process?

510. No

511. When is carbohydrate loading most beneficial?

511. 48 to 72 hours prior to event

21 to 120 Seconds of Intense Activity

512. What energy generation system predominates in this time period?

512. Lactic anaerobic system

513. What is the mechanism of action?

513. Glucose is converted into lactate plus 2 ATP molecules

514. Is this process aerobic or anaerobic?

514. Anaerobic

515. Is lactate generated in this process?

515. Yes

Over 120 Seconds of Intense Activity

516. What two energy sources are recruited?

516. Glucose
Fatty acids

517. How many ATP molecules are generated in the process?

517. 34

518. Is this process aerobic or anaerobic?

518. Aerobic

Muscle Physiology and Training

519. The cross-sectional area of muscle determines what?

519. Muscle force

520. The volume and mass of muscle determine what?

520. Muscle work

Strength Training

521. Is strength training a static or dynamic form of exercise?

521. Static

522. Strength training involves ____ force and ____ number of repetitions.

522. high
low

523. Does training alter the ratio of type I/type II fibers?

523 No
Training may alter ratio of type IIA/IIB, however

524. In general, what muscle fiber changes do occur with strength training?

524. Hypertrophy of type II fibers

525. What changes are seen in muscle innervation with strength training?

525. Increased simultaneous firing percentage

526. What is the best form of exercise for rapidly increasing strength?

526. Isokinetic exercise

527. What form of exercise is more efficient for increasing strength: concentric or eccentric?

527. Eccentric

Endurance Training

528. Is endurance training a static or dynamic form of exercise?

528. Dynamic

529. How does endurance training increase cardiac output?

529. By increasing stroke volume

530. Endurance training involves _____ force and ___ number of repetitions?

530. low
high

531. What effect does endurance training have upon muscle itself?

531. Improved metabolism

532. What effect is seen on vascularity? What benefit does this have?

532. Increased capillary density
Decreased fatigability

533. What systemic effect has endurance training been shown to provide?

533. Improved lipid profile

Other Key Exercise and Training Questions

534. What is the best form of exercise for increasing power?

534. Plyometric exercise

535. What does that form of exercise entail?

535. Rapid shortening (eccentric)

536. What muscle changes are seen with isometric exercise?

536. Muscle hypertrophy

537. What is delayed-onset muscle soreness?

537. Muscle soreness 24 to 72 hours after exercise

538. At the level of the sarcomere, where are changes seen?

538. At the I-band

539. What two modalities have been proven beneficial for delayed-onset muscle soreness?

539. Nonsteroidal antiinflammatory drugs (NSAIDs)
Massage

540. What is the best way to replace fluid losses during exercise?

540. Weight for weight replacement (replace to maintain constant weight)

541. What is the ideal fluid osmolality for replacement?

541. <10%

542. When fluid and food are restricted for weight reduction, what effect is seen on cardiac output?

542. Decreased

543. … on heart rate?

543. Increased

544. … on stroke volume?

544. Decreased

545. … on oxygen consumption?

545. Decreased

Other Conditions Associated with Athletes and Athletics

Commonly Asked Questions

546. What are the two most common causes of sudden death in young athletes?

546. Hypertrophic obstructive cardiomyopathy (HOCM)
Anomalous coronary arterial supply

547. What is the most common reason for disqualification of an athlete on a preparticipation physical?

547. A condition of the musculoskeletal system

548. What is the classic injury suffered by rowers?

548. Stress fracture of a rib

549. What is the classic injury suffered by surfers?

549. Saphenous nerve injury

Hypertrophic Obstructive Cardiomyopathy

550. What is the inheritance?

550. Autosomal dominant

551. What are the two key clinical exam findings?

551. II/IV systolic ejection murmur
Increased murmur with Valsalva, standing

552. What is the best means of screening for HOCM?

552. History and physical exam

553. What is the best confirmatory test?

553. Echocardiogram

Eye Injuries

554. Children under 14 years of age are most likely to sustain an eye injury in what sport?

554. Baseball

555. Children 14 years old and over are most likely to sustain an eye injury in what sport?

555. Basketball

Heat Exhaustion and Heat Stroke

556. What are the core temperature criteria for differentiating heat exhaustion and heat stroke?

556. <104°F: heat exhaustion
≥104°F: heat stroke

557. What is the most important factor in determining the amount of core temperature increase?

557. Water deficit

558. What is the exam criterion for differentiating the two conditions?

558. Patients with heat stroke exhibit central nervous system changes

559. To prevent these conditions, vigorous training should be avoided if?

559. Wet-bulb temperature exceeds 82°F degrees

Muscle Injury and Healing

General Principles of Soft Tissue Healing

560. What are the four soft tissue healing phases?

560. Hemostasis
Inflammation
Organogenesis
Remodeling

561. How is hemostasis achieved within the first 5 minutes?

561. Primary platelet plug

562. What changes occur within 10 to 15 minutes of soft tissue injury?

562. Secondary clot formation via coagulation cascade and fibrin

563. What is the mechanism of aspirin activity?

563. Directly inhibits cyclooxygenase

564. What is the mechanism of acetaminophen activity?

564. Inhibits prostaglandin E production via IL-1β

565. When in the time course of soft tissue healing has ultrasound been shown to provide benefit?

565. Early (within the first 12 days)

566. What is the difference between iontophoresis and phonophoresis?

566. Iontophoresis uses direct current to deliver topical medication
Phonophoresis uses ultrasound to deliver topical medication

Muscle Injury

567. What cell is the first to appear after muscle injury?

567. Neutrophil arrives to begin phagocytosis

568. What is the ideal position for immobilization of an injured muscle?

568. Lengthened position

569. What is the adverse effect of prolonged immobilization?

569. Immobilization leads to increased muscle fatigability

570. This change predisposes to what type of injury?

570. Strain injury risk increased

571. What is the ultimate outcome of surgical repair for muscle belly tear?

571. Regain approximately half the original muscle strength

572. What is the general sequence of five steps through which muscle rehabilitation progresses?

572. Passive range of motion (ROM) exercises
Closed-chain exercises
Axially loaded active ROM
Open-chain exercises
Plyometrics and sport-specific exercises

573. In the first 10 days of rehabilitation, strength gains are due to what?

573. Improved neural coordination

574. Subsequent strength gains are due to what?

574. Muscle and ROM improvements

575. What is the definition of a closed-chain exercise?

575. Agonist and antagonist muscles co-contract

576. What is the advantage of a closed-chain exercise program upon the muscle?

576. Decreased shear forces

577. How do anabolic steroids compare to corticosteroids for treatment of muscle contusion?

577. Anabolic steroids superior

Muscle Changes with Aging

578. What changes are observed in the fiber composition of muscle with normal aging?

578. Decrease seen particularly in type II (fast) muscle fibers

579. How does the collagen content of muscle change with age?

579. Increased collagen content

580. What effect does this have on muscle stiffness?

580. Increased muscle stiffness with age

581. Decreased strength in what particular muscle group tends to increase risk of falls with age?

581. Quadriceps

Metabolism: Pathologic and Pharmacologic

Supplements

582. What effect do anabolic steroids have on protein synthesis?

582. Increased

583. Do anabolic steroids provide any aerobic benefit?

583. No

584. What effect do they have on the physes of skeletally mature individuals?

584. Premature closure

585. What effect does growth hormone have on muscle?

585. Selective hypertrophy of type I muscle fibers

586. What effect does growth hormone have on the physis?

586. Proliferation without maturation (no premature closure)

587. What effect does creatine have on work (force × distance)?

587. Increased work during the first few anaerobic trials

588. What effect does creatine have on peak force generated?

588. None

Paralytic Agents

589. What are two nondepolarizing drugs?

589. Curare
Pancuronium

590. How do nondepolarizing drugs work?

590. Through competitive inhibition of acetylcholine receptors

591. What is the clinical effect of nondepolarizing drugs?

591. Relatively long duration of muscle paralysis

592. What is an example of a depolarizing drug?

592. Succinylcholine

593. How do depolarizing drugs work?

593. Temporary binding to the acetylcholine receptor site

594. What is the clinical effect of depolarizing drugs?

594. Shorter duration muscle paralysis

595. What class of drugs can be used for reversal of these agents?

595. Anticholinesterases

596. What are two examples of anticholinesterases?

596. Neostigmine
Edrophonium

597. Because they block the consumption of acetylcholine, what do their side effects include?

597. Parasympathetic activation (acetylcholine hangs around longer)

■ Tendons and Ligaments

Tendons

598. Tendons connect what two structures?

598. Muscle
Bone

599. What is the four-part sequence of transitional tissue as tendon attaches to bone?

599. Tendon
Fibrocartilage
Mineralized fibrocartilage (Sharpey's fibers)
Bone

600. Describe the toe region of the tendon stress-strain curve? Why?

600. Small toe region ("tendons have tiny toes")
Because of high collagen content within tendons (85% collagen)

Tendon Injury, Healing, and Repair

601. Paratenon covered tendons vs. sheathed tendons: which heal more readily and why?

601. Paratenon covered tendons heal better
Because they have a rich capillary system that provides excellent vascularity

602. When reinserting tendon to bone, is there a proven benefit to creating a bony trough?

602. No demonstrated benefit

603. What is the advantage of early active motion after tendon injury?

603. Improved ROM relative to immobilization

604. What is the disadvantage of early active motion?

604. Stresses repair and healing tissue

605. What is the preferred form of motion after tendon repair?

605. Controlled passive motion

606. What three microscopic changes are seen in tendon composition after prolonged immobilization?

606. Decreased collagen diameter
Increased collagen disorder
Decreased cellularity

607. What effect do these changes have on tendon strength?

607. Reduced

Ligaments

608. How does the collagen content of ligaments compare to that of tendons?

608. Decreased: ligaments have 70% collagen content vs. 85% (tendons)

609. What effect does this have on the stress-strain curve of ligaments?

609. Ligaments have a larger toe region

610. What else is significant about the composition of ligaments relative to tendons?

610. Ligaments have greater elastin content

611. How are ligaments supplied with blood?

611. Vascular supply from ligament insertion
Distributed throughout ligament through uniform microvascularity

612. Are ligaments innervated?

612. Yes; nerve endings provide proprioceptive feedback and contribute to joint stability

613. What two types of bony insertions are seen with ligaments?

613. Indirect
Direct

614. What type is more common?

614. Indirect

615. Indirect ligament insertions: describe the superficial and deep fibers.

615. Superficial fibers attach at an acute angle to the periosteum
Deep fibers attach to Sharpey's fibers (mineralized fibrocartilage)

616. Direct ligament insertions: in what two ways are the fibers different?

616. Have superficial fibers also
But deep fibers attach perpendicular to the bone and go through four transitional tissue phases (like tendons)

Ligament Injury, Healing, and Repair

617. Is a ligament capable of plastic deformation?

617. No

618. What is the most common mechanism by which a ligament fails?

618. Sequential rupture of collagen bundles

619. Where does the failure occur most commonly: compare children vs. adults.

619. Children: avulsion at the junction of unmineralized and mineralized fibrocartilage zones
Adults: midsubstance injury

620. What type of collagen predominates in the early healing phase?

620. Type III collagen

621. What type of collagen predominates in the late healing phase?

621. Type I

622. What is the effect of prolonged immobilization on ligament repair strength?

622. Reduced (similar to tendons)

■ The Immune System and Infection

Cells

623. Where do B lymphocytes mature?

623. Within the lymph nodes and spleen

624. What do they become?

624. Plasma cells

625. What do they produce?

625. Immunoglobulins

626. What immunoglobulin is the most prevalent in humans?

626. IgG

627. What type of immunoglobulin is produced first by the fetus?

627. IgM

628. What immunoglobulin is the mediator of type I hypersensitivity?

628. IgE

629. What cells produce cytokines in response to foreign antigen?

629. T cells

630. The HLA gene is found on which chromosome?

630. Chromosome 6

631. Is HLA associated with T-cell or B-cell immunity?

631. B cell

Antibiotics

632. What is the mechanism of action for each of the following groups of antibiotics: β-lactams (e.g., penicillin, cephalosporins) and vancomycin?

632. Inhibit peptidoglycan synthesis; acts against the cell wall

633. Quinolones?

633. Inhibit DNA gyrase

634. Metronidazole?

634. Creates free oxygen radicals

635. Polymyxin/nystatin?

635. Increase cellular permeability

636. Most others (aminoglycosides, linezolid, clindamycin, etc.)?

636. Inhibit protein synthesis (e.g., through ribosomal activity, etc.)

637. What is the definition of inherent antibiotic resistance? Example?

637. Cell features that prevent antibiotic activity
Example: absence of a metabolic pathway

638. What is the definition of acquired antibiotic resistance? Example?

638. Resistance acquired through new cellular elements
Example: plasmids or transposons

639. How does staphylococcus develop resistance to penicillin? What gene is involved?

639. Penicillin-binding protein 2a (PBP2a)
mecA

640. What is the spectrum of organisms generally susceptible to bacitracin?

640. Gram positive only

641. What two antibiotics can be added to bacitracin to broaden its spectrum?

641. Polymyxin
Neomycin

642. By what route is bacitracin administered?

642. Topically

643. What antibiotic achieves the highest concentration in bone?

643. Clindamycin

644. When antibiotics are added to cement, how long does the maximal effect last?

644. Approximately 2 weeks

645. After how long has all of the effectiveness generally been exhausted?

645. 8 weeks

Osteomyelitis and Septic Arthritis in the Adult

Osteomyelitis in Adults

646. What is the x-ray appearance of osteomyelitis: initially? At 7 to 10 days?

646. Initially: soft tissue swelling only
After 7 to 10 days: bone demineralization (e.g., lucencies) or disk space narrowing

647. When does subperiosteal elevation show up on x-ray?

647. At approximately 14 days

648. What is the radiographic appearance at 6 months?

648. Reactive bone

649. What is the MRI appearance of osteomyelitis: T1? T1 with gadolinium? T2?

649. T1: low intensity
T1 with gadolinium: high intensity
T2: high intensity

650. What is the key treatment sequence of six steps for osteomyelitis in adults?

650. Identify organism
Surgical resection
Begin appropriate systemic or local antibiotics
Stabilization (e.g., external fixator)
Delayed closure (e.g., soft tissue coverage)
Bone graft as necessary

651. What are the two best means to identify the etiologic organism?

651. Aspiration of multiple deep sites
Culture

652. Is a gram stain sufficient?

652. No, gram stain is not sufficiently sensitive

653. Should empiric antibiotic therapy be used for osteomyelitis in adults?

653. No; treatment should be organism-specific

654. What may inadequate or inappropriate antibiotic treatment lead to?

654. Chronic osteomyelitis

Subacute Osteomyelitis

655. Subacute osteomyelitis is essentially what?

655. Slowly developing osteomyelitis

656. With subacute osteomyelitis, are white blood count (WBC) and blood cultures generally valuable?

656. No, these studies are often normal

657. What three diagnostic tests are preferred?

657. CRP/ESR
Radiographs
Bone aspiration and culture

Diskitis/Vertebral Osteomyelitis in Adults

658. What are the two key imaging studies to visualize diskitis and vertebral osteomyelitis?

658. MRI
Technetium and gallium bone scan

659. Is a biopsy generally necessary to identify the etiologic organism?

659. Yes, must biopsy as in other cases of adult osteomyelitis

660. What is the initial preferred treatment?

660. Antibiotics if no epidural abscess or neurologic compromise

661. What is the indication for surgical intervention?

661. Failure of antibiotic therapy

Epidural Abscess

662. What are the two key imaging studies to visualize epidural abscesses?

662. MRI
Contrast CT scan

663. Is a biopsy generally necessary?

663. No, immediate operative intervention if neurologic deficit; antibiotic therapy

Pediatric Infections

664. In what two ways is the neonatal physis unique?

664. Blood vessels course across the physis until 18 months of age
Infection can therefore cross into the epiphysis

Chronic Recurrent Multifocal Osteomyelitis

665. Does chronic recurrent multifocal osteomyelitis generally result in unilateral or bilateral involvement?

665. Bilateral, symmetric bony involvement

666. What sites are generally involved?

666. Clavicle
Other metaphyseal sites

667. What organism is most commonly identified?

667. None

668. What is the treatment of choice?

668. NSAIDs

Chronic Sclerosing Osteomyelitis

669. What age group is most commonly affected?

669. Adolescents

670. What is the classic radiographic feature of chronic sclerosing osteomyelitis?

670. Intense periosteal proliferation

671. What organisms are most commonly identified?

671. Anaerobes

672. What is the treatment of choice?

672. Appropriate antibiotic therapy

Diskitis in Children

673. Is a biopsy generally necessary to identify the organism?

673. No; in general, biopsy is only necessary if patient fails antibiotic therapy Generally assume *Staphylococcus aureus* is the etiologic organism and treat empirically

674. In vertebral osteomyelitis in adults, is a biopsy generally necessary?

674. Yes, a biopsy must be performed as with other cases of osteomyelitis in adults

Postoperative Infection

675. Is the WBC a reliable marker for the diagnosis of postoperative infection?

675. No, not sufficiently reliable

676. How long after surgery do CRP values begin to rise?

676. 6 hours

677. When do postoperative CRP values peak?

677. 3 days

678. How long after surgery have CRP values generally returned to normal?

678. 1 week

679. How long after surgery do ESR values begin to rise?

679. 2 days

680. When do postoperative ESR values peak?

680. 5 days

681. How long after surgery have ESR values generally returned to normal?

681. 3 weeks

Other Specific Infectious Conditions

Tetanus

682. What are the characteristic features of tetanus-prone wounds: Age? Depth? Contamination?

682. Age >6 hours
Depth >1 cm
Gross contamination with devitalized tissue

683. If a wound does not meet these criteria, what are the two indications for a tetanus booster?

683. Unknown history of tetanus vaccination
History of fewer than three tetanus shots

684. If a wound is tetanus prone, what is the prophylactic treatment if the patient has had a tetanus booster within the past 5 years?

684. No booster necessary

685. What is the prophylactic treatment if the patient has not had a tetanus booster within the past 5 years?

685. Administer tetanus vaccine

686. What is the two-part prophylactic treatment if the history of vaccination is unknown?

686. Administer tetanus vaccine
Administer immunoglobulin antibody

687. What is the two-part treatment for established tetanus?

687. Diazepam to decrease spasm
Penicillin

Necrotizing Fasciitis

688. What are the key organisms responsible for necrotizing fasciitis?

688. Group A streptococcus is more commonly isolated than other organisms
But polymicrobial infection is more common than group A streptococcus alone

689. What is the treatment of choice?

689. Emergent operative debridement

690. What are the two preferred antibiotics?

690. Penicillin
Meropenem

Gas Gangrene

691. What is the key organism responsible for gas gangrene?

691. *Clostridium* species

692. What is the treatment of choice?

692. Emergent operative debridement

693. What are the two preferred antibiotics?

693. Penicillin
Clindamycin

Toxic Shock Syndrome

694. What are the two key organisms responsible for toxic shock syndrome?

694. *S. aureus*
Group A streptococcus

695. What is the preferred antibiotic?

695. Nafcillin

Wound Contamination by Water Exposed to Shellfish

696. What is the key organism?

696. *Vibrio vulnificus*

697. What is the preferred antibiotic?

697. Ceftazidime

Rabies

698. What is the appropriate treatment for a patient bitten by a healthy dog or cat?

698. Observe for 10 days

699. What are the two components of the appropriate treatment for a patient bitten by a symptomatic animal?

700. What is the appropriate treatment for a patient bitten by a skunk, raccoon, bat, or fox?

699. Immunoglobulin
Rabies vaccination

700. Assume the animal is rabid
Treat immediately as if animal was symptomatic

Cat-Scratch Fever

701. What is the key organism responsible for cat scratch fever?

702. Is incision and drainage usually necessary?

703. What is the preferred antibiotic?

701. *Bartonella henselae*

702. No, generally not

703. Azithromycin

Pseudomonas Aeruginosa

704. What is the classically tested means by which a pseudomonas infection occurs in the foot?

705. What are the two components of the appropriate antibiotic treatment?

704. Puncture wound through a tennis shoe

705. Ceftazidime
Ciprofloxacin

Lyme Disease

706. What species of tick is associated with Lyme disease?

707. What organism is responsible?

708. Lyme disease is classically associated with what two skin findings?

709. What joint is most commonly affected?

710. What are the three stages of disease progression?

711. How is Lyme disease definitively diagnosed?

712. What two antibiotics are commonly used to treat Lyme disease?

706. *Ixodes* tick

707. *Borrelia burgdorferi*

708. Erythema migrans
"Bull's-eye" lesion

709. Knee joint

710. Rash
Neurologic findings
Arthritis

711. Enzyme-linked immunosorbent assay (ELISA)

712. Amoxicillin
Doxycycline

Review of Stains and Culture Media

713. What is the special stain and medium for mycobacterium?

714. What is the special stain for herpes?

715. What is the medium for *Neisseria gonorrhoeae*?

713. Ziehl-Nielson stain
Lowenstein-Jensen medium

714. Tzanck prep

715. Thayer-Martin medium (chocolate agar)

716. What organism has been potentially associated with malignancy?

716. *Clostridium septicum*

717. What is the two-part preferred laboratory sequence for diagnosing hepatitis C virus?

717. ELISA
Immunoblot assay

718. What is the most sensitive test for early detection of hepatitis C infection?

718. Polymerase chain reaction (PCR)

■ Coagulation, Thrombosis, and Blood Products

719. What are the final two enzymatic conversions of the clotting cascade?

719. Prothrombin to thrombin
Fibrinogen to fibrin

720. What is the first reaction in clot dissolution?

720. Conversion of plasminogen to plasmin
Plasmin then dissolves fibrin clot

721. Heparin binds to what substance?

721. Antithrombin III

722. Once bound, heparin inhibits what two factors?

722. Activated factor II (IIa)
Activated factor X (Xa)

723. What is the general threshold for platelet transfusion?

723. Transfuse if platelets <5000

724. Duplex ultrasound is 90% sensitive for what type of clot?

724. Deep venous thrombosis (DVT) proximal to the trifurcation

725. What type of ultrasound has the highest sensitivity?

725. Color

726. What is the risk of a fatal pulmonary embolism (PE) after arthroplasty if no prophylaxis is administered?

726. 0.1 to 0.5% after total hip or total knee arthroplasty

727. How does the risk of a fatal postoperative PE change with prophylaxis?

727. Reduced by one half

728. Is prophylaxis against DVT necessary after spine surgery?

728. Generally not; only SCDs (sequential compression devices) are used

729. Other than direct venous compression, by what mechanism are SCDs thought to also work?

729. Enhance endogenous fibrinolytic activity

730. What type of spine surgery is associated with an increased risk of DVT?

730. Combined anterior/posterior fusions

731. What treatment should be considered with a PE in a patient acutely after spine surgery?

731. IVC (inferior vena cava) filter
Anticoagulation may lead to epidural hematoma development

732. What is the threshold hemoglobin value below which there is an increased risk of needing a postoperative transfusion?

732. Hemoglobin <13

733. What is the association between transfusion and the postoperative infection rate?

733. Transfusions increase the risk of postoperative infection

734. What nontranfusion technique achieves transfusion rates equivalent to those with autologous donation?

734. Normovolemic dilution

735. For which viral infection is blood not routinely screened?

735. Cytomegalovirus (CMV)

736. What blood product should be administered for a low intraoperative fibrin value?

736. Cryoprecipitate

737. Following tourniquet use, electromyograph (EMG) abnormalities can be detected in what percentage of postoperative patients?

737. 70%

738. After 90 minutes of tourniquet use, how long should the tourniquet be deflated to achieve equilibrium?

738. 5 minutes

739. How about after 3 hours of tourniquet use?

739. Deflate for 15 minutes before reinflating

Pain

740. What is transduction?

740. The process by which pain receptors (nociceptors) convey pain through the dorsal column and spinothalamic tracts

741. What is modulation?

741. The interpretation of the transduced pain signals by the brain

742. Which of these processes is the target of prostaglandin inhibitors?

742. Transduction

743. What is the target of opioids?

743. Modulation

744. How do local anesthetics achieve their effect?

744. Block nerve conduction

745. In what two ways does capsaicin work?

745. Blocks substance P
Results in an increased pain threshold

746. What is the normal value for nerve latency on EMG?

746. <3.5 msec

747. What is the normal conduction velocity on EMG?

747. >50 meters/second

■ Imaging Modalities: Key Facts

Bone Scan

748. With a bone scan, onto what substance is technetium absorbed?

748. Hydroxyapatite crystals

749. To diagnose osteomyelitis, a technetium bone scan should be combined with what two elements?

749. Gallium
Indium

750. In general, a technetium bone scan is good for what three diagnoses?

750. Infection
Trauma
Malignancy

751. In general, a gallium bone scan is good for what two diagnoses?

751. Infection; improved specificity when combined with WBC tagged scan
Malignancy

752. In general, an indium bone scan is good for what diagnosis? Except in what situation?

752. Infection
Except in the spine, where indium is not helpful for diagnosing an infection

Magnetic Resonance Imaging

753. What does the magic angle refer to?

753. A bright artifact on the MRI that may appear to be real pathology

754. What is the typical value of the magic angle?

754. 55 degrees

755. What MRI sequence does the magic angle affect?

755. T1

756. What is the repeat time for T1-weighted images?

756. <1000 msec

757. What is the repeat time for T2-weighted images?

757. ≥1000 msec

758. What MRI study is preferred for diagnosing a recurrent disk herniation? Why?

758. MRI with gadolinium
Gadolinium highlights scar tissue on T1-weighted images

759. What two MRI sequences best demonstrate marrow edema?

759. Short tau inversion recovery (STIR)
Fat-suppressed T2

760. Why does osteonecrosis appear black on T1-weighted images?

760. Because fatty marrow cells have been destroyed

761. How does acute or rapid flowing blood appear on T1? T2?

761. Dark on T1
Dark on T2

762. What is the MRI appearance of chronic or slow flowing blood on T1? T2?

762. Bright on T1
Bright on T2

763. What two advantages does multidetector CT provide over MRI?

763. Improved resolution along longitudinal axis
Decreased metal artifact

■ Orthopaedic Biomechanics and Materials

Key Biomechanical Concepts

764. Where is the center of gravity located at the level of the pelvis in the sagittal plane?

764. Anterior to the body of S2

765. What is the principal determinant of the magnitude of the JRF (joint reaction force)?

765. Muscle activity around the joint

766. Define stress and strain.

766. Stress = force/area (measure of internal strain)
Strain = change in length/original length (measure of deformability)

767. How is strain energy represented on the stress-strain diagram?

767. Area under the curve

768. Strain energy is a measure of what material property?

768. Toughness

769. What is the definition of toughness?

769. Ability of a material to absorb energy before it fails

770. What is the definition of stiffness?

770. Resistance of a material to deformation from an applied load

771. Compare the stress-strain curve appearances of brittle and ductile materials.

771. Brittle materials have linearly perfect stress-strain curves; no plastic deformation
Ductile materials allow for a large amount of plastic deformation

772. If cortical bone is the midline, working away from the midline in the direction of increasing elastic modulus are what four materials?

772. Titanium
Stainless steel
Cobalt chrome
Ceramic/alumina

773. Working away from the midline in the direction of decreasing elastic modulus are what three materials?

773. Polymethylmethacrylate
Polyethylene
Cancellous bone

774. What is the definition of fatigue failure?

774. Failure after many cycles of repetitive submaximal load

775. Fatigue failure will never occur if what condition is met?

775. Force is below the endurance limit of the material

Viscoelastic Materials

776. As the strain rate increases, viscoelastic materials become more what?

776. Stiff (higher elastic modulus)

777. What is the definition of hysteresis?

777. Hysteresis refers to energy dissipation such that unloading and loading does not follow the same path

778. Stress relaxation of a liquid is essentially the same as what?

778. Creep

779. What formula determines the bending rigidity of a rectangle?

779. Base * height^3

780. What formula determines the bending rigidity of a cylinder?

780. Radius^4

781. The area moment of inertia is a measure of what?

781. Resistance to bending

782. What is the mass moment of inertia?

782. Measures resistance to rotation

783. What is the polar moment of inertia?

783. Measures resistance to torsion

Corrosion

784. Pitting and crevice corrosion are most likely with what material?

784. 316L stainless steel is most likely to be associated with pitting and crevice corrosion

785. There is a classically increased risk of galvanic corrosion between what two metals?

785. 316L stainless steel
cobalt chrome

Principles of Fixation

Bone Screws

786. Inner (root) diameter determines what property?

786. Tensile strength

787. Outer diameter determines what property?

787. Pullout strength

788. What three screw dimensions maximize pullout strength?

788. Small inner diameter
Large outer diameter
Fine pitch

789. What is the most important factor determining pedicle screw pullout strength?

789. Bone density

790. A screw hole reduces the strength of bone by how much?

790. 50%

791. When does the strength return to baseline?

791. 9 to 12 months after the screw has been removed

792. Is an oval hole or a rectangular hole biomechanically superior?

792. Oval hole

Intramedullary Nails

793. What mechanical advantage does a closed nail have over a slotted nail?

793. Closed nails have greater torsional stiffness

794. What then is the advantage of a slotted nail?

794. Decreased hoop stress on insertion

External Fixators

795. What are the top two factors determining the stability of an external fixation construct?

795. Contact between the two ends of bone
Pin diameter

796. What is the most stable circular external fixation construct that can be achieved with two implants?

796. 1 olive wire and 1 half-pin at 90 degrees to each other

797. How does construct stability vary with ring diameter?

797. Stability increases with decreasing ring diameter

11

Orthopaedic Oncology

■ Tumor Growth and Metastasis

1. Tumor cells secrete what substance?

2. PTHrP then stimulates what cells?
3. What do the osteoblasts secrete when stimulated?
4. This ligand then binds to osteoclasts and stimulates the secretion of what two substances?

5. What is the net effect of these growth factors?

6. What cofactor is required to facilitate the RANK–RANK ligand interaction?
7. What is the cause of osteogenic rickets?
8. What is the resultant effect?
9. What is the sequence of five events leading to metastasis?

10. What are the five most common tumors that metastasize to bone?

11. What type of thyroid cancer is especially likely to metastasize to bone?

1. Parathyroid hormone–related peptide (PTHrP)

2. Osteoblasts
3. RANK ligand

4. Transforming growth factor-β (TGF-β) Insulin-derived growth factor (IGF)

5. Tumor growth
Release of more PTHrP (cycle repeats itself)

6. Macrophage colony-stimulating factor (M-CSF)
7. Secretion of fibroblast growth factor-23 (FGF-23)
8. Decreased renal reabsorption of calcium
9. Tumor growth and increased vascularity
Metalloproteinases degrade type IV collagen (present within the basement membrane)
Tumor cells enter the bloodstream
Tumor cells embolize
Tumor invades vessel wall to grow at a new location

10. Breast
Prostate
Lung
Kidney
Thyroid

11. Follicular

12. What is the No. 1 location to which bony metastases go?

12. Thoracic vertebral body

13. Besides lung cancer, what other cancer also metastasizes distally (e.g., to hands)?

13. Renal cell

14. What four sarcomas classically metastasize to lymph nodes?

14. Rhabdomyosarcoma
    Synovial sarcoma
    Epithelioid sarcoma
    Clear cell sarcoma

15. What is the usual function of P-glycoprotein?

15. Pumps out cellular toxins

16. What is the significance of P-glycoprotein and chemotherapy?

16. Pumps out chemotherapeutic agents and may contribute to chemotherapy resistance

---

■ Key Genetic and Immunohistochemical Concepts

DNA: Normal Physiology

17. Approximately how many genes are there in human DNA?

17. 30,000

18. What is the difference between an intron and an exon?

18. Intron: noncoding sequence within DNA
    Exon: directly codes for protein

19. What is an oncogene?

19. Tumor-inducing agent
    Arises from proto-oncogenes after mutation or increased expression

20. What is a proto-oncogene?

20. Normal gene
    Codes for proteins that regulate cell growth and differentiation

21. What is an anti-oncogene?

21. Tumor suppression gene
    Suppresses growth in damaged cells to inhibit tumors
    If function is lost, allows tumor growth

22. What is a gene promoter?

22. DNA sequence required for transcription

23. What is a gene enhancer?

23. Region of DNA that provides a binding site for transcription factors

24. What happens after a transcription factor binds to a region of DNA?

24. Recruits RNA polymerase
    Enables RNA synthesis from the coding region of the gene

25. What is a consensus sequence?

25. Shared sequence of nucleotides in different DNA and RNA sequences
    Plays the same role in different locations (e.g., binding site for regulatory proteins)

26. What transcription factor is critical for enchondral ossification?

26. SOX-9

27. A deficiency of this transcription factor results in which dysplasia?

27. Camptomelic dysplasia

28. What transcription factor is associated with intramedullary ossification?

28. CBFA -1 (core binding factor 1)

29. What dysplasia is associated with deficiency of this factor?

29. Cleidocranial dysostosis

Laboratory Techniques for Manipulating DNA

30. What is DNA ligation? What is an example of a clinical application?

30. Joining linear DNA fragments together with covalent bonds
Example: attachment of human genes to plasmids

31. Two fragments of DNA can be linked to form what?

31. Recombinant DNA

32. What is transformation? What is an example of an application where transformation is used?

32. The genetic alteration of a cell resulting from uptake and expression of foreign material
Example: Inserting a recombinant plasmid into a bacteria

33. What is the difference between therapeutic cloning, reproductive cloning, and embryo cloning?

33. Therapeutic: a specific organ or tissue is produced from a stem cell
Reproductive: an animal is produced that is genetically identical to the host
Embryo: several genetically identical animals are produced

34. How is a transgenic animal made?

34. A foreign gene is inserted into a one-cell embryo
Transgene is then represented in every cell of the animal

35. What is the difference between Southern, Northern, and Western hybridization?

35. Southern hybridization can identify a DNA sequence
Northern hybridization can identify an RNA sequence
Western hybridization can identify proteins expressed after translation

Genetics in Orthopaedic Oncology

36. What is gene translocation? What is the clinical significance?

36. Movement of a gene fragment from one chromosomal location to another
May alter or abolish gene expression

37. What are the two methods by which translocations are identified?

37. Polymerase chain reaction (PCR)
Fluorescence in situ

38. PCR is used for the amplification of what?

38. DNA

39. Real-time PCR is used for the amplification of what?

39. RNA

40. What translocation is associated with Ewing sarcoma?

40. 11:22

41. What translocation is associated with myxoid liposarcoma?

41. 12:16

42. What translocation is associated with clear cell sarcoma?

42. 12:22

43. What translocation is associated with synovial sarcoma?

43. X:18

44. What translocation is associated with rhabdomyosarcoma?

44. 2:13

45. What translocation is associated with myxoid chondrosarcoma?

45. 9:22

46. What gene is associated with osteosarcoma and retinoblastoma?

46. *Rb1*

47. With what syndrome is a p53 mutation associated?

47. Li-Fraumeni

48. What is the inheritance pattern of this genetic mutation?

48. Autosomal dominant (AD)

49. What four other classes of tumors have been associated with p53 mutations?

49. Adrenal tumors
Brain tumors
Soft tissue sarcomas
  (e.g., rhabdomyosarcoma)
Breast cancer

Key Immunohistochemistry Concepts

50. Lymphoma stains positive for what marker?

50. Leukocyte common antigen (LCA)

51. What other disorder also stains positive for this marker?

51. Leukemia

52. What three disorders are associated with a positive keratin stain?

52. Metastatic carcinoma
Synovial sarcoma
Adamantinoma

53. What disorder is associated with a positive vimentin stain? Example?

53. Mesothelial tumors
Example: sarcoma

54. What disorder is associated with positive desmin and actin stains? Example?

54. Tumors with myodifferentiation
  (stains for muscle components)
Example: rhabdomyosarcoma

55. What disorder is associated with a positive smooth muscle actin stain?

55. Leiomyosarcoma

56. What three disorders are associated with S-100 positivity?

56. Chondroid tumors and chordoma
Neural tumors (for example,
  neurofibromatosis)
Melanocytic tumors

57. What two disorders are associated with factor VIII antigen positivity?

57. Hemangioma
Hemangioendothelioma

58. What four disorders are associated with α-fetoprotein positivity?

58. Nephroblastoma (Wilms')
Testicular cancer
Ovarian cancer
Malignant teratoma

59. What four disorders are associated with high α-fetoprotein levels in pregnancy?

59. Spina bifida
Anencephaly
Chromosomal abnormalities
(e.g., trisomy 21 and trisomy 18)
Omphalocele

60. What disorder is associated with CD138?

60. Myeloma

61. What disorder is associated with a ring chromosome/giant marker?

61. Liposarcoma

62. What disorder is associated with CA-125?

62. Metastatic ovarian cancer

63. What disorder is associated with CK-7?

63. Metastatic brain/lung cancer

64. What disorder is associated with CK-20?

64. Metastatic colon cancer

■ Basic Orthopaedic Tumor Principles

Workup and Staging

65. What is the role of computed tomography (CT), magnetic resonance imaging (MRI), and technetium (Tc) bone scan in evaluating bony lesions?

65. CT: determines amount of bone destruction and soft tissue calcification
MRI: determines lesion extent, edema, and presence of soft tissue extension
Tc bone scan: determines total number of lesions

New Soft Tissue Mass Workup

66. What is the imaging study of choice for evaluation of a soft tissue mass?

66. MRI with contrast

67. What is the classic MRI appearance of a malignant tumor on T1? T2?

67. Low T1
High T2

68. Quick review: what is the typical MRI appearance of a hemangioma on T1? T2?

68. High T1
High T2

69. What does rim enhancement suggest?

69. Mass is likely a cyst

70. What if the entire mass enhances?

70. Mass is likely a tumor

71. If the mass is indeterminate in appearance (benign versus malignant), what is the next study?

71. Needle or open biopsy

72. What does a positron emission tomography (PET) scanner measure?

72. Fluorodeoxyglucose (FDG) accumulation

73. This is an indirect measure of what?

73. Glucose utilization rate

74. Why does a suspected hematoma require careful follow-up?

74. May be clinically difficult to differentiate hematoma and developing sarcoma
    Must follow patient regularly until mass has resolved

75. From what tissue line do sarcomas originate?

75. Mesenchyme

76. In general, what is the significance of sarcoma size?

76. >5 cm is more likely to metastasize

77. What is the significance of sarcoma location?

77. If sarcoma is below the deep fascia, the prognosis is poorer

78. In general, which study is ordered to evaluate for sarcomatous metastases?

78. CT chest

79. What studies are ordered to evaluate for liposarcoma metastases?

79. CT chest/abdomen/pelvis

Additional Evaluation of Bony Tumors

80. Complete staging of osteosarcoma requires what two imaging studies?

80. CT chest
    Bone scan

81. What additional test is routinely performed for Ewing sarcoma?

81. Bone marrow biopsy

82. What additional test is routinely performed for rhabdomyosarcoma? Why?

82. Local node biopsy
    One of four sarcomas that metastasizes to lymph nodes

Stage and Grade

83. What are the three stages of benign tumors?

83. Latent
    Active
    Aggressive

84. In the Enneking staging of malignant tumors, what do I and II refer to?

84. Whether the tumor is low grade (I) or high grade (II)

85. What is the significance of grade?

85. High-grade tumors are more likely to metastasize

86. What is the 5-year survival rate for high-grade sarcomas?

86. 50%

87. What do A, B, and C refer to?

87. Whether the tumor is intracompartmental (A), extracompartmental (B), or metastatic (C)

88. What other system is commonly employed to stage malignant tumors?

88. American Joint Committee on Cancer (AJCC) system

89. What is the major difference in this system?

89. Includes a classification for "skip" metastases

90. What are the four key prognostic factors for malignant tumors in descending order of importance?

90. Stage (includes grade and metastases)
Whether metastases are present
Grade
Size greater than or less than 8 cm

91. For what can flow cytometry be used?

91. To quantify the amount of abnormal DNA present

92. What are Mirel's four criteria?

92. Site
Pain
Lesion type
Size

93. What is the clinical application of Mirel's score?

93 To predict the likelihood that a metastatic bony lesion will go on to fracture

94. How are lesions scored based on site?

94. 1: upper limb
2: lower limb
3: trochanteric

95. How are lesions scored based on pain?

95. 1: mild
2: moderate
3: pain with activity

96. How are lesions scored based on type of lesion?

96. 1: blastic
2: mixed
3: lytic

97. How are lesions scored based on size?

97. 1: <⅓ diameter
2: ⅓ to ⅔ diameter
3: >⅔ diameter

98. What was the mean score for the population that went on to fracture?

98. 10

99. What was the mean score for the nonfracture population?

99. 7

Radiographic Examination Pearls

100. What are the five key differential diagnoses for destructive lesions of bone in young patients?

100. Osteosarcoma
Ewing sarcoma
Leukemia/lymphoma
Osteomyelitis
Eosinophilic granuloma

101. What are the five key differential diagnoses for destructive lesions of bone in older patients?

101. Metastases
Myeloma
Lymphoma
Chondrosarcoma
Malignant fibrous histiocytoma (MFH)

102. What are the five key differential diagnoses for processes that affect both sides of a joint?

102. Bone infarcts (x-ray: smoke signal; histology: empty lacunae)
Tuberculosis/coccidioidomycosis (histology: spores, Langerhans' cells)
Pigmented villonodular synovitis (PVNS; x-ray: lytic)
Gout (histology: tophaceous material)
Rheumatoid arthritis

103. What are the three key differential diagnoses for eccentric metaphyseal lesions?

103. Nonossifying fibroma (NOF): "bubbly" x-ray appearance
Chondromyxoid fibroma (CMF): "bubbly"
Aneurysmal bone cyst (ABC): not bubbly

104. What are the six key differential diagnoses for a calcified lesion on the surface of bone?

104. Osteochondroma
Periosteal osteosarcoma
Parosteal osteosarcoma
Myositis ossificans
Periosteal chondroma
Periosteal chondrosarcoma

105. If you see a multiple-lesion process, what are the three most likely etiologies in children <5 years of age?

105. Metastases from neuroblastoma
Metastases from nephroblastoma
Histiocytosis

106. What is the most likely etiology at ages 15 to 40?

106. Vascular tumor (e.g., hemangioendothelioma)

107. What are the three most likely etiologies at age >40?

107. Metastases
Multiple myeloma
Lymphoma

108. What two other multiple-lesion processes can affect patients at a variety of ages?

108. Fibrous dysplasia
Paget's disease

109. What three tumors often demonstrate predominantly cortical involvement or tunneling?

109. Ewing sarcoma (occasionally)
Osteomyelitis (cortical tunneling classically)
Osseofibrous dysplasia

110. What are the five key differential diagnoses for a lytic lesion within the sacrum?

110. Chordoma
Chondrosarcoma
Giant cell tumor
Metastasis
Myeloma

111. What is the key differential diagnosis for a centrally located lytic lesion in a pediatric humeral shaft without periosteal reaction?

111. Unicameral bone cyst

112. What are the three key differential diagnoses for a pagetoid-looking pelvis and unilateral femoral involvement?

112. Polyostotic fibrous dysplasia
Ollier disease
Paget's disease

113. A widened femoral metaphysis may suggest what disorder?

113. Multiple hereditary exostoses (MHE)

114. What six tumors classically involve the anterior vertebral body?

114. Eosinophilic granuloma
Giant cell tumor
Osteosarcoma
Hemangioma
Metastases
Myeloma

115. What three tumors classically involve the posterior spinal elements?

115. Aneurysmal bone cyst (ABC)
Osteoid osteoma/blastoma
Osteochondroma

116. What tumors classically involve the neuroforamina?

116. Neurofibromatosis (NF)

117. What are the five components of the differential diagnosis of an intramedullary destructive lesion of the hand or foot?

117. Enchondroma
Giant cell tumor (no bone on histology)
Giant cell reactive granuloma (bone present on histology)
Aneurysmal bone cyst (ABC)
Metastases

118. What are punched-out lytic lesions?

118. Lytic lesions that look as if they were created by a hole punch in bone

119. Among younger patients, what lesion classically has this appearance?

119. Eosinophilic granuloma

120. What lesion classically has this appearance among older patients?

120. Multiple myeloma

Histologic Examination Pearls

121. When interpreting the histology of a bony tumor, what does lamellar bone indicate?

121. A section that is not part of the tumor

122. How do you go about evaluating the histology of a bony tumor with woven bone present?

122. First, look for osteoblastic rimming
If osteoblastic rimming is present, then the bone is reactive
If no osteoblastic rimming is present, then the bone is neoplastic
Second, look at stroma to determine if the neoplasm is benign or malignant

123. What are the two features of malignant stroma?

123. High cellularity and necrosis
High mitotic rate and atypia

124. What are three examples of lesions with woven bone and osteoblastic rimming?

124. Osseofibrous dysplasia
Osteoblastoma
Paget's disease (also see coarse trabeculae on x-ray)

125. If the histology resembles osseofibrous dysplasia but no osteoblastic rimming is present, consider what lesion?

125. Fibrous dysplasia

126. Metastases often have what cells on histology? How do they generally appear?

126. Epithelial cells
Appear as clumps (stuck together) or as glands

127. What are the three aspects of the histologic appearance of normal cartilage?

127. Relatively sparse cells
One nucleus per cell
One cell per lacuna

128. Myxoid lesions are characterized by what two areas of distinct histologic appearance?

128. White (myxoid) area
Dense or cartilage looking area

129. When present in bone, such lesions often represent what?

129. CMF

130. When present in soft tissue, a myxoid lesion often represents what?

130. Schwannoma with Antoni A and Antoni B areas

131. What is the acronym and what are the five components of the differential diagnosis for a tumor that has small round cells on histology?

131. Acronym: La HEIM
Lymphoma
Histiocytosis
Ewing sarcoma
Infection
Metastases/myeloma

132. If you see a giant cell tumor with bone present, consider what lesion in what location?

132. Giant cell reactive granuloma
Hands

133. Nuclear inclusions on electron microscopy are suggestive of what two tumors?

133. Paget's disease
Eosinophilic granuloma

134. In eosinophilic granuloma, what are the nuclear inclusions called?

134. Birbeck granules

General Treatment Concepts: Resection, Reconstruction, Chemotherapy, and Radiation

135. What are the two major drawbacks to plate-and-screw fixation of allograft to native bone for reconstruction after tumor surgery?

135. High allograft fracture rate
10% deep infection rate

136. What anatomic location is particularly prone to complications with this method?

136. Proximal tibia

137. What is the relative advantage of this method of fixation?

137. Relatively high rates of union

138. What three tumors are the classic low-grade malignant tumors of bone?

138. Adamantinoma
Parosteal osteosarcoma
Chordoma

139. Because they are low grade, how are these tumors generally treated?

139. Wide resection only

140. Chemotherapy is generally helpful for what four tumors?

140. Acronym: MOLE
Metastases
Osteosarcoma
Lymphoma
Ewing sarcoma

141. Radiation therapy is generally helpful for what five tumors?

141. Acronym: ELMMS
Ewing sarcoma
Lymphoma
Multiple myeloma
Metastases
Soft tissue sarcoma

142. By what mechanism is radiation therapy thought to act?

142. Oxygenates intracellular water
Damages DNA of tumor cells

143. What are the two potential therapeutic uses of strontium in patients with neoplasms?

143. Control pain from bony metastases
Localizes selectively within bone and irradiates bony metastases from within

144. What complication is classically associated with doxorubicin?

144. Cardiac toxicity

■ Specific Neoplasms

Bony Tumors

Osteoid Osteoma

145. In what three anatomic locations is an osteoid osteoma most commonly found?

145. Hip
Tibia
Spine (approximately 10%)

146. What syndrome is associated with multiple osteomas?

146. Gardner's syndrome

147. What are two other characteristics of this syndrome?

147. Multiple colon polyps
Tumors outside the colon

148. What is the inheritance pattern of Gardner's syndrome?

148. AD

149. What is the general size threshold for osteoid osteoma?

149. <1.5 cm
Above that size, it is generally an osteoblastoma

150. Does osteoid osteoma light up on a bone scan?

150. Yes

151. When osteoid osteoma occurs within the spine, in what direction is the scoliosis?

151. Bends toward side of lesion
Lesion is on the concave side of the main curve

152. Scoliosis is more likely to improve postoperatively if the lesion is treated in what time frame?

152. Fewer than 15 months after onset

153. What is the target temperature range for radiofrequency ablation (RFA) treatment?

153. 50° to 100°C

154. How does RFA work? What is the effect?

154. Generates frictional heat through rapid ionic agitation
Causes coagulative necrosis and protein denaturation

Osteoblastoma

155. At what two locations does osteoblastoma most often occur?

155. Posterior elements of the spine
Metadiaphyseal regions of long bones

156. What is the general radiographic appearance of osteoblastoma?

156. Lytic with central ossification/calcification

157. This appearance helps differentiate osteoblastoma from what other disorder?

157. ABC

158. What is the treatment of choice for osteoblastoma?

158. Curettage

Classic Osteosarcoma

159. What population is most commonly affected by osteosarcoma?

159. Children and teenagers

160. What are the three most common anatomic locations?

160. Knee
Hip
Shoulder

161. What are the two histologic features of the tumor cells?

161. Tumor cells make osteoid
No osteoblastic rimming

162. What are the two histologic features of the stromal cells?

162. Stromal cells demonstrate malignant features
May contain spindle cells, giant cells, or small cells

163. What two imaging studies should be ordered to thoroughly evaluate the involved anatomic area?

163. Plain radiographs
MRI

164. What is the radiographic appearance of osteosarcoma?

164. Metaphyseal lesion with soft tissue extension and new bone formation
Periosteal reaction is common ("sunburst" or "hair-on-end" appearance)

165. What are the two staging studies?

165. CT chest
Bone scan

166. What percentage of patients have metastases at the time of diagnosis?

166. 20%

167. What is the worst prognostic indicator?

167. Skeletal metastases

168. What are the three components of the general treatment regimen for osteosarcoma?

168. Preoperative chemotherapy
Wide resection
Maintenance chemotherapy

169. What are the six factors that indicate a poor prognosis?

169. Expression of P-glycoprotein
High serum alkaline phosphatase
High lactic dehydrogenase (LDH) levels
Vascular invasion
No alteration of DNA ploidy after chemotherapy
Absence of antishock protein 90 antibodies after chemotherapy

170. For what other disorder are high LDH levels also poorly prognostic?

170. Ewing sarcoma

171. What is a good preoperative kill percentage for chemotherapy?

171. >99%

172. What preoperative kill percentage is negative prognostically?

172. <90%

173. What is the local recurrence rate?

173. 5 to 10%

174. Is there a difference in overall survival between limb salvage techniques and amputation?

174. No difference overall

175. What are the two relative advantages of amputation?

175. Decreased local recurrence rate
Potentially fewer complications

176. What is the mean 5-year survival with no metastases?

176. 60 to 70%

177. What is the mean 5-year survival with metastases?

177. 25%

Telangiectatic Osteosarcoma

178. How does telangiectatic osteosarcoma appear on plain radiographs?

178. Destructive and lytic with no bone production

179. This looks similar to what other lytic bony lesion?

179. ABC

Parosteal Osteosarcoma

180. What population (age, sex) is most commonly affected by parosteal osteosarcoma?

180. Middle age
Female

181. What anatomic location is most commonly affected?

181. Posterior knee

182. Is parosteal osteosarcoma a low-grade or high-grade tumor?

182. Low-grade

183. What is the usual treatment?

183. Wide resection only

Periosteal Osteosarcoma

184. What two anatomic locations are most commonly affected by periosteal osteosarcoma?

184. Tibial diaphysis
Femoral diaphysis

185. What is the radiographic appearance?

185. Extracortical sunburst on a "saucerized" cortical depression

186. What are the histologic features?

186. Lots of bone and cartilage formation

Ewing Sarcoma

187. What population is particularly at risk?

187. Children (over 5 years old) and young adults

188. What is the key translocation?

188. 11:22

189. What genetic marker may indicate a better prognosis?

189. *EWS fly1*

190. What are two classic symptoms on presentation?

190. Localized pain
Fevers

191. What are the two key laboratory value findings?

191. Elevated erythrocyte sedimentation rate (ESR)
Elevated white blood count (WBC)

192. What are four poorly prognostic factors?

192. Tumor in spine or pelvis
Tumor greater than 100 cm³
Poor response to chemotherapy (less than 90% necrosis)
Elevated LDH

193. What three anatomic locations are most commonly affected?

193. Hip
Knee
Shoulder

194. What are the two typical locations in bone of Ewing sarcoma?

194. Metaphysis
Diaphysis

195. What are two plain radiographic characteristics?

195. Onion-skin lifting of periosteum
Soft tissue mass

196. What is the key histologic feature?

196. Small blue cells

197. Differential diagnosis: what are two other conditions with small blue cells in patients <5 years old?

197. Leukemia
Metastatic neuroblastoma

198. What are three other conditions with small blue cells in patients >30 years old?

198. Metastases
Myeloma (plasma cells)
Lymphoma

199. How is neuroblastoma histologically different from Ewing sarcoma?

199. Pseudorosettes (round cells in circles around pink center)

200. What is the immunohistochemical marker for Ewing sarcoma?

200. CD99

201. Ewing sarcoma also stains positive for what?

201. Glycogen

202. What two components does the treatment of Ewing sarcoma generally include?

202. Chemotherapy
Resection

Cartilaginous Tumors

Chondroma

203. What four anatomic locations are most commonly affected by chordoma?

203. Hip
Knee
Shoulder
Hand

204. What is the typical location within bone?

204. Metaphysis of long bones

205. How does chordoma appear on plain radiographs?

205. Stippled area within bone

206. Is the bone scan positive or negative?

206. Positive

207. What is the histologic appearance?

207. Benign cartilage

208. What is the usual treatment?

208. None usually necessary (if asymptomatic)

209. Where are periosteal chondromas seen on bones?

209. On the surface of long bones

210. What is the plain radiographic appearance of periosteal chondroma?

210. Cortical defect with adjacent spicules

211. If treatment is required for symptomatic periosteal chondroma, what is it?

211. Marginal excision

212. What two syndromes are associated with multiple chondromas? What are their characteristics?

212. Ollier syndrome (multiple chondromas, 30% malignancy rate)
Mafucci syndrome (also soft tissue angiomas, 100% malignancy rate)

213. What is the inheritance pattern for these syndromes?

213. None; sporadic mutation

Osteochondroma (Exostosis)

214. What three anatomic locations are most commonly affected by osteochondroma?

214. Hip
Knee
Shoulder

215. What is key to note about the medullary cavity on radiographs? Cortex?

215. Bony medullary space continuous with that of the exostosis
Cortex of the lesion is confluent with that of the bone

216. What is the general rule about size of cartilage cap? What is an exception?

216. 2 to 3 mm thick cartilage cap
May be thicker in growing children

217. Osteochondroma is histologically similar in appearance to what?

217. Normal physis

218. How frequently does malignant degeneration occur?

218. Fewer than 1% of patients

219. What are two warning signs of malignant degeneration?

219. Pain without mechanical symptoms
Growth after puberty with large cartilage cap

220. If malignant degeneration does occur, what is the usual grade of the malignancy?

220. Low grade

221. What syndrome is associated with multiple exostoses?

221. Multiple hereditary exostoses (MHE)

222. What is the inheritance?

222. AD

223. What is the mutation?

223. *EXT 1, 2 genes*

224. What is the overall risk of malignancy with MHE?

224. 10%

225. If a malignancy does develop, what is it and where is it most common?

225. Secondary chondrosarcoma
Especially around shoulder

226. What are the two key clinical features of the characteristic wrist deformities?

226. Ulna short
Distal radius angular malalignment

Chondroblastoma

227. What population is most commonly affected by chondroblastoma?

228. What three anatomic locations are most commonly affected?

229. What is the typical location within bone?

230. Quick review: what other tumor is commonly found at the same location within bone?

231. What is the MRI appearance of chondroblastoma? Similar to what two nonneoplastic conditions?

232. What are the two key histologic features?

233. What are two key phrases on the histology description?

234. What are the two components of the usual treatment of chondroblastoma?

235. How frequently does chondroblastoma metastasize?

236. Metastatic pattern and frequency are similar to what other lesion?

237. How often does chondroblastoma recur?

227. Young adults

228. Hip
Knee
Shoulder

229. Epiphysis

230. Giant cell tumor

231. Lytic epiphyseal lesion with
surrounding edema
Similar to osteochondritis dissecans
(OCD) and osteomyelitis

232. Chondroblasts: polygonal cells
Giant cells scattered throughout

233. Cobblestone
Chicken wire

234. Curettage and graft
Consider treating with phenol also

235. Metastasizes to lungs in 2% of patients

236. Giant cell tumor

237. 10%

Chondromyxoid Fibroma

238. What gender is most commonly affected?

239. What bone is most commonly affected?

240. What is the typical clinical presentation of chondromyxoid fibroma?

241. What are the classic plain radiographic findings?

242. What are the classic histologic features?

243. What is the usual treatment of chondromyxoid fibroma?

238. Male

239. Tibia
May occur in other long bones as
well

240. Pain

241. Eccentric lytic metaphyseal lesion

242. Myxoid (white) with cartilage (blue);
see lobules of cartilage/fibrous
tissue/giant cells

243. Marginal resection

Chondrosarcoma

244. What are the two components of the plain radiographic appearance of chondrosarcoma?

244. Bone destruction (lytic)
Mineralization (if chronic)

245. What grade are most chondrosarcomas?

245. Low

246. How is chondrosarcoma treated?

246. Wide resection

247. How can a dedifferentiated chondrosarcoma be identified histologically?

247. Biphasic appearance with low- and high-grade areas

248. What are the two components of the treatment of dedifferentiated chondrosarcoma?

248. Wide resection
Chemotherapy

249. Quick review: what is the cortical involvement in enchondroma versus chondrosarcoma?

249. Enchondroma: partial cortical involvement, but remains within cortex
Chondrosarcoma: through cortex sometimes with a soft tissue mass

250. What are the x-ray changes over time in the adult in enchondroma versus chondrosarcoma?

250. Enchondroma: no radiographic progression with time
Chondrosarcoma: progresses with time

251. Is there pain in enchondroma and chondrosarcoma?

251. Enchondroma usually painless
Chondrosarcoma often painful (especially at night)

252. Clear cell chondrosarcoma occurs at what location within bone?

252. Epiphyseal

Chordoma

253. Can chordomas be found outside of the sacrum?

253. Yes; especially in vertebral bodies

254. What characteristic cells are seen on histology?

254. Physaliferous cells (large clear cells)

255. What are the two components of the treatment of chordoma?

255. Resection
Radiation

256. How often do metastases occur?

256. 50%

Fibrous Tumors

Nonossifying Fibroma (NOF) (Metaphyseal Fibrous Defect)

257. What population is most commonly affected?

257. Young (usually <20 years old)

258. What are the two most common anatomic locations?

258. Knee
Ankle

259. What is the usual location within bone of NOF?

259. Eccentric, metaphyseal

260. What is the plain radiographic appearance of NOF?

260. Eccentric lucent lesion with or without cortical erosion
Can be "bubbly" in appearance

261. What else may have a similar radiographic appearance?

261. CMF

262. What are two key histologic features?

262. Whorled fibroblasts
Hemosiderin

263. What is the treatment if the NOF occupies 50 to 75% of the bony diameter?

263. Curettage and graft

264. Otherwise, how should a symptomatic NOF be treated?

264. Cast immobilization

265. What syndrome is associated with multiple NOFs?

265. Jaffe-Campanacci

266. What are the three classic features of this syndrome?

266. Café-au-lait spots
Mental retardation
Multiple NOFs

Malignant Fibrous Histiocytoma (MFH) and Fibrosarcoma

267. What population is most commonly affected by these disorders?

267. 30 to 80 years of age
Male > female

268. Are they benign or malignant?

268. Malignant

269. What is the classic physical exam finding?

269. Mass with or without associated pain and swelling

270. What are four key histologic findings for MFH?

270. Storiform spindles
Short fascicles radiating around a common center
Indented nuclei
Giant cells

271. What are two key fibrosarcoma histologic features?

271. Herringbone spindles
Intersecting fascicles with perpendicular nuclei

272. What are the two components of the treatment for MFH and fibrosarcoma of soft tissue?

272. Wide resection
Radiation

273. What are the two components of the treatment for MFH and fibrosarcoma of bone?

273. Wide resection
Chemotherapy

Extraabdominal Desmoid Tumor

274. What population is most commonly affected?

274. Young adults

275. Is extraabdominal desmoid benign or malignant?

275. Benign

276. Is extraabdominal desmoid aggressive or latent?

276. Very aggressive

277. What is the key physical exam finding?

277. "Rock hard" mass on palpation

278. What are the two components of the usual treatment?

278. Wide resection
Radiation

Fatty Tumors

Lipoma

279. Is lipoma generally painful on presentation? Is there an exception?

279. Not generally painful
Angiolipoma is the exception, as it can be painful

280. What are the two components of the MRI appearance of a lipoma?

280. Well-demarcated mass
Same MRI signal as adjacent fat (bright T1 and T2, dark on fat-suppressed and shout tau inversion recovery [STIR])

281. How is a lipoma treated?

281. Marginal resection

Liposarcoma

282. What cells are classically associated with the histology of liposarcoma?

282. Signet ring cells (lipoblasts)

283. What is the size of the tumor at presentation? Why?

283. Large (5 to 15 cm)
Because it is a slow-growing deep asymptomatic mass

284. What factor predicts the likelihood of metastasis? How?

284. Grade
Low grade: <10% metastasize
High grade: >50% metastasize

285. What is the MRI appearance of a liposarcoma?

285. Dark on T1
Bright on T2, STIR, and fat-suppressed images

286. What is unique about liposarcoma staging as compared with staging for other sarcomas?

286. Liposarcoma: CT chest/abdomen/pelvis
Other sarcomas: CT chest

Neural Tissue Tumors

Neurilemmoma

287. Neurilemmoma is also known as what?

287. Benign schwannoma

288. What are the three most common locations?

288. Spinal nerve roots
Mediastinal nerves
Retroperitoneal nerves

289. What are the four components of the general histologic appearance?

289. Myxoid in soft tissue
Well encapsulated
Two organized structural areas
No mitotic figures

290. What are the two regions seen on histology called?

290. Antoni A: highly ordered compact spindle cells with twisted nuclei
Antoni B: less orderly with a myxoid matrix

291. What are the characteristic bodies seen with neurilemmoma? Appearance?

291. Verocay bodies
Palisading of nuclei around eosinophilic areas

292. What bodies are associated with Morton's neuroma?

292. Renaut bodies

293. What does neurilemmoma stain positive for?

293. S-100

294. How is neurilemmoma treated?

294. Surgical resection of mass, sparing the nerve

Neurofibroma

295. How many lesions are typically found in affected adults?

295. Usually a solitary mass in adults

296. How many lesions are typically found in patients with von Recklinghausen's disease?

296. Multiple nodules at different sites with different rates of growth

297. What is the inheritance pattern of von Recklinghausen's?

297. AD

298. What are two other key features of this syndrome?

298. Café-au-lait spots
Cystic bone lesions

299. What other neoplasm do the bony lesions generally resemble?

299. Nonossifying fibroma (NOF)

300. What are the three typical histologic features of neurofibroma?

300. No capsule (compare with neurilemmoma)
Spindle cells with rare mitoses
S-100 positive

301. How frequently does malignant degeneration occur with neurofibroma?

301. 5 to 30% of cases

302. What is the treatment of choice?

302. Marginal excision

Other Key Sarcomas

303. What four sarcomas classically metastasize to lymph nodes?

303. Rhabdomyosarcoma
Synovial sarcoma
Epithelioid sarcoma
Clear cell sarcoma

Rhabdomyosarcoma

304. What are the two components of the population most commonly affected?

304. Age <20 years old
Males > females

305. What is the relative frequency of rhabdomyosarcoma among sarcomas in this population?

305 Most common sarcoma in children and young adults

306. What subtype is most common?

306. Alveolar

307. What is the histologic appearance of rhabdomyosarcoma?

307. Racquet-shaped cells and spindles

308. What are the three components of the treatment?

308. Preoperative chemotherapy
Wide resection
Radiation

Synovial Sarcoma

309. Synovial sarcoma is the most common sarcoma in what location?

309. Foot

310. Where is the mass generally located in relation to the joint?

310. Proximal to the joint

311. Synovial sarcoma must be differentiated from what two conditions?

311. Synovial chondromatosis (nondestructive; no bony involvement)
Heterotopic ossification (25% of synovial sarcomas have calcification within lesion)

312. What is the histologic appearance of synovial sarcoma?

312. Biphasic (epithelial and spindle cell components)

313. What are the two components of treatment?

313. Wide resection
Radiation

Epithelioid Sarcoma

314. What population (age, sex) is most commonly affected? What is the overall frequency of this tumor?

314. Ages 10 to 35
Male
Rare tumor

315. Epithelioid sarcoma is the most common sarcoma in what location?

315. Most common upper extremity soft tissue sarcoma

316. What is the classic physical exam finding?

316. Subcutaneous nodule within the hand

317. What are the two histologic features of epithelioid sarcoma?

317. Nodules
Epithelioid cells with eosinophilic cytoplasm and necrotic center

318. Quick review: what two other conditions are also associated with hand nodules in young patients?

318. Calcified aponeurotic fibroma
Nodular fasciitis

319. Is calcifying aponeurotic fibroma benign or malignant?

319. Benign

320. Is calcifying aponeurotic fibroma painful or painless?

320. Painless

321. In what anatomic location does nodular fasciitis most commonly occur?

321. Volar surfaces of the upper extremity

322. Is nodular fasciitis painful or painless?

322. Painful

323. Is nodular fasciitis slowly or rapidly progressive?

323. Rapidly progressive

324. Quick review: what organism may cause an infection with hand nodules?

324. *Mycobacterium marinum*

Clear Cell Sarcoma

325. With what translocation is clear cell sarcoma associated?

325. 12:22

326. Clear cell sarcoma is histologically similar to what other neoplasm?

326. Melanoma (see pigmented melanin)

327. How can clear cell sarcoma be differentiated from liposarcoma on histology?

327. Clear cell sarcoma has fewer cells with clear cytoplasm

Vascular Tissue Tumors

Hemangioma

328. What is the classic plain radiographic appearance of vertebral body hemangioma?

328. Jail-house striations

329. How is the CT appearance classically described?

329. Polka dot vertebral body

330. Compare with the plain radiographic appearance of soft tissue hemangioma.

330. May reveal small phleboliths

331. What is the histologic appearance of hemangioma?

331. Endothelial-cell lined vascular channels

Hemangioendothelioma

332. What population is at risk of developing hemangioendothelioma?

332. All ages affected

333. Is it benign or malignant?

333. Malignant

334. What is the plain radiographic appearance?

334. Multiple small lytic ovals in one bone

335. What is the histologic appearance?

335. Tumor cells form vascular spaces

336. What is the treatment of low-grade hemangioendothelioma?

336. Radiation alone

Lymphoma and Myeloma

Lymphoma

337. What population is at risk for developing lymphoma?

337. All ages affected
Peak in 60s and 70s

338. Lymphoma may also occur at the end stage of what disease process?

338. HIV

339. What is the histologic appearance of lymphoma?

339. Sheets of small blue cells (B cells) without significant matrix

340. What are three immunohistochemistry markers?

340. LCA
CD45
CD20

341. What are the two components of the treatment of lymphoma?

341. Chemotherapy
Radiation

Myeloma

342. What age group is most commonly affected?

342. 50 to 80 years

343. Myeloma is similar in age distribution to what two other tumors?

343. Chondrosarcoma
Fibrosarcoma

344. In patients with myeloma, what is the typical laboratory value for hemoglobin?

344. Low

345. ... for calcium?

345. High

346. ... for creatinine?

346. High

347. ... for erythrocyte sedimentation rate (ESR)?

347. High

348. What is the plain radiographic appearance of myeloma?

348. Punched-out lytic lesions

349. What is the typical radiographic appearance of involved vertebral body?

349. Collapsed "fish-mouth" vertebra

350. What is the histologic appearance?

350. Sheets of plasma cells (clock face)

351. What two key growth factors do plasma cells secrete?

351. Interleukin-6 (IL-6)
MIP-1α (MIP = macrophage inflammatory protein)

352. What are four factors that indicate a poor prognosis for myeloma?

352. Translocations
Chromosome 13 deletion
Low albumin
High β_2-microglobulin

353. How is myeloma treated?

353. Chemotherapy

354. What is the overall survival with multiple myeloma?

354. Survival is related to stage of disease
With chemotherapy, survival times of >3 to 5 years are increasingly common

355. What are the two criteria for diagnosis of a solitary myeloma?

355. Single plasmacytoma
<10% plasmacytosis

356. What is the treatment for solitary myeloma?

356. Radiation alone

357. How does solitary myeloma survival compare with multiple myeloma?

357. Improved

358. What is osteosclerotic myeloma? Frequency?

358. Myeloma with a demyelinating polyneuropathy
Rare

359. What is the direction of demyelination? What is it similar to?

359. Distal to proximal
Similar to Guillain-Barré syndrome

360. What is the acronym and what are the five features of osteosclerotic myeloma?

360. Acronym: POEMS
Polyneuropathy
Organomegaly
Endocrinopathy
M protein
Skin changes

Fibrous Dysplasia and Related Conditions

Fibrous Dysplasia (FD)

361. Mutation?

361. Gsα activating subunit defect

362. Is fibrous dysplasia more commonly monostotic or polyostotic?

362. Monostotic (good prognosis)

363. Clinical features of fibrous dysplasia: what is the appearance of the femoral neck?

363. Progressive varus deformity ("shepherd's crook")

364. What is the classic radiographic appearance?

365. What is the histologic appearance?

366. In general, what is the treatment of fibrous dysplasia?

367. How is an impending pathologic fracture of the upper extremity treated in patients with FD?

368. What is the treatment of an impending pathologic fracture of lower extremity?

369. Is autograft or allograft preferable in patients with fibrous dysplasia?

370. Polyostotic fibrous dysplasia can be associated with what syndrome?

371. What are the two other features of this syndrome?

Osseofibrous Dysplasia

372. What age group is at risk for osseofibrous dysplasia (OFD)?

373. What anatomic location is most commonly involved?

374. What is the typical location in bone?

375. Osseofibrous dysplasia may be a precursor to what condition?

Adamantinoma

376. What age group is at risk?

377. What is the most common anatomic location?

378. Is adamantinoma benign or malignant?

379. Is it painful or painless?

380. How many lesions are usually present?

381. With the exception of multiple lesions, adamantinoma is otherwise similar to?

382. What are the two radiographic features of adamantinoma?

383. How can adamantinoma and OFD be differentiated on plain radiographs?

384. What are the two histologic features of adamantinoma?

---

364. Ground-glass lesion with distinct margins

365. Irregular woven bone
"Chinese letters" or "alphabet soup"

366. Observation
If large or symptomatic lesions, curette and bone graft

367. Do not use internal fixation

368. Open reduction and internal fixation (ORIF)

369. Do not use autograft
Use cortical allograft instead

370. McCune-Albright syndrome

371. Café-au-lait spots (irregular)
Precocious puberty

372. Age <10

373. Tibia

374. Cortices

375. Adamantinoma

376. Young adults (generally over 20 years old)

377. Tibia

378. Low-grade malignant lesion

379. Painful

380. Multiple lesions

381. CMF

382. Bubbly diaphyseal lesion
Permeative throughout tibial diaphysis

383. OFD: cortical
Adamantinoma: permeative throughout tibial diaphysis

384. Epithelioid "owl eyes" appearance
Glandular

385. How can adamantinoma and OFD be differentiated histologically?

385. Adamantinoma: has epithelial component
OFD: looks like fibrous dysplasia but with osteoblastic rimming

386. What is the treatment for adamantinoma?

386. Wide resection

Other Commonly Tested Lesions Involving Bone

Aneurysmal Bone Cyst (ABC)

387. What age group is particularly at risk?

387. Age <20 years old

388. Is an ABC generally painful?

388. Yes

389. What are the three most common anatomic locations?

389. Femur
Tibia
Posterior spine

390. Are ABCs usually located centrally within bone?

390. No; eccentric

391. Are ABCs usually lytic or blastic?

391. Lytic with thin periosteal rim

392. Where might an ABC extend into?

392. Adjacent soft tissue

393. What is the classic MRI feature of an ABC?

393. Fluid-fluid levels

394. What are the histologic features?

394. Cavernous spaces without endothelial lining

395. What has a similar histology? Key difference?

395. Hemangioma (similar histology with epithelial lining)

396. If a very cellular stroma is present, what diagnosis must be considered?

396. Telangiectatic osteosarcoma

397. What is the usual treatment for an ABC?

397. Curettage and bone graft

398. ABCs are most likely to recur in what patients?

398. Those with open physes

Unicameral Bone Cyst

399. What two anatomic locations are most commonly affected?

399. Proximal humerus
Proximal femur

400. In what two places are unicameral bone cysts (UBCs) generally found within bone?

400. Central (compare with ABC: eccentric)
Metaphyseal (compare with giant cell tumor [GCT]: epiphyseal)

401. What are the two histologic features?

401. Clear, fluid-filled cyst lined by thin membrane of fibrous tissue
May see some multinucleated giant cells

402. What are the two components of first-line treatment?

402. Aspiration
Steroid injection

403. What is the treatment of a recurrent lesion or an impending fracture?

403. Curettage and bone graft

404. In lower extremities, consider what treatment for impending pathologic fracture?

404. ORIF

Langerhans' Cell Histiocytosis (Eosinophilic Granuloma [EG])

405. Is EG benign or malignant?

405. Benign

406. What are the two plain radiographic features?

406. Destructive (lytic) lesion with distinct margins
Generally, no associated soft tissue mass

407. How does an involved vertebral body classically appear?

407. Vertebra plana (uniformly collapsed)

408. What are the four key histologic features?

408. Eosinophils
Cigar-shaped nuclei
Pale histiocytes
Birbeck granules (racquet-shaped inclusion bodies in cytoplasm on electron microscopy)

409. Is histiocytosis generally a self-limited condition?

409. Yes

410. What are two local treatment options?

410. Observation
Curettage and bone graft

411. What are the different types of EG?

411. Single-bone disease (most common, approximately 80%)
Multiple-bone disease
Bone disease with systemic and visceral involvement

412. What are two systemic diseases?

412. Hand-Schüller-Christian disease
Letterer-Siwe disease

413. What are the three features of Hand-Schuller-Christian syndrome?

413. Exophthalmos
Diabetes insipidus
Lytic skull lesions

414. What age group is affected by Letterer-Siwe disease?

414. Children <3 years old

415. What are the four features of Letterer-Siwe?

415. Multiple bony lesions
Anemia
Bacterial infections
Hepatosplenomegaly

416. What is the prognosis?

416. Fatal

Giant Cell Tumor

417. Is giant cell tumor benign or malignant?

417. Benign but can be locally aggressive

418. What gender is more commonly affected?

418. Female (1.5:1)

419. What are the three most common anatomic locations involved?

419. Knee
Spine/sacrum
Distal radius

420. What is the typical location within bone?

420. Epiphysis

421. Are physes generally open or closed?

421. Physes are generally closed

422. Contrast with physeal status in what other disorder?

422. Chondroblastoma: physes are generally open

423. Giant cell tumors may degenerate into what lesions?

423. Aneurysmal bone cyst
Other neoplasms

424. What is the appearance of giant cell tumor on bone scan?

424. Doughnut: intense circumference, central lytic area

425. In what two ways are giant cell tumors treated?

425. Curettage and bone grafting or polymethylmethacrylate (PMMA) with adjuvant (e.g., phenol, cautery): 25% recur
Marginal resection if multiply recurrent or extensive bony destruction

426. What is the likelihood of developing metastases?

426. 3% incidence of benign pulmonary metastases

Giant Cell Reparative Granuloma

427. What two anatomic locations are most commonly involved?

427. Hands/feet
Jaw

428. What is the typical radiographic appearance?

428. Lytic, eccentric

429. Histologically, giant cell reparative granuloma may resemble what? Is there a difference?

429. Giant cell tumor
Bone is present

Myositis Ossificans

430. What population is most commonly affected by myositis ossificans (MO)?

430. Athletes

431. Where is the ossification generally seen radiographically?

431. The ossification is generally periosteally based

432. What are the histologic features of the periphery and the center?

432. Periphery: mature (eggshell)
Center: immature

433. How is MO treated?

433. Initial immobilization
Nonsteroidal antiinflammatory drugs (NSAIDs)

434. How and when should mobilization be resumed?

434. Begin active range of motion after 1 to 2 days
Avoid passive stretching

435. What is MO progressiva?

435. Autosomal dominant disorder with multiple sites of ossification

Reactive Hand/Foot Lesions

436. What is the etiology of these lesions?

436. Posttraumatic
Arise from subperiosteal hemorrhage

437. What diagnosis comes to mind if the lesion resembles callus?

437. Florid reactive periostitis

438. What diagnosis comes to mind if the lesion resembles osteochondroma with cartilage cap?

438. Bizarre parosteal osteochondromatous proliferation (BPOP)

439. What diagnosis comes to mind if the lesion is found under the nail?

439. Subungual exostosis

Tumoral Calcinosis

440. What patient population is particularly at risk?

440. African descent

441. What are the most common anatomic locations of tumoral calcinosis?

441. Extensor surfaces

442. In affected patients, what is the usual serum calcium concentration?

442. Normal

443. What is the histologic appearance?

443. Hydroxyapatite crystals

Unusual Tumors

444. How does infantile fibrosarcoma generally present?

444. Huge mass at birth

445. What is the treatment if the mass is unresectable?

445. Chemotherapy in addition to more limited surgery

446. A histology that demonstrates gray acellular cords with rare tumor cells is indicative of what?

446. Myxoid chondrosarcoma

447. What is the associated translocation for this disorder?

447. 9:22

448. What population is at risk for granuloma annulare?

448. Children

449. What are the two components of the typical clinical presentation for this disorder?

449. Multiple soft tissue masses
Scalp lesions

450. What is the treatment of granuloma annulare?

450. None usually necessary

Key Treatment Review and Clarification

451. What two treatments are recommended for UBC?

451. Aspiration
Steroid injection

452. What three treatments are recommended for giant cell tumor and chondroblastoma?

452. Curettage
Cauterize
Graft

453. What treatment is recommended for CMF and periosteal osteochondroma?

453. Marginal resection

454. What treatment is recommended for adamantinoma, parosteal osteosarcoma, and chordoma?

454. Wide resection

455. What treatment is recommended for NOF?

455. Leave alone

456. What treatment is recommended for squamous cell carcinoma secondary to chronic draining osteomyelitis?

456. Wide resection (for example, distal phalangeal amputation)

12

Rehabilitation

■ Lower Extremity

Amputations

General Principles

1. How does self-selected walking velocity vary with level of lower extremity amputation?

2. How much additional energy is required for ambulation after traumatic below-knee amputation (BKA)?

3. How much additional energy is required for ambulation after traumatic above-knee amputation (AKA)?

4. How much additional energy is required for ambulation after BKA for vascular disease?

5. How much additional energy is required for ambulation after AKA for vascular disease?

6. Is complex regional pain syndrome an indication for amputation?

7. What are myodesis and myoplasty?

8. Which is preferred in association with amputation?

9. What are two factors most predictive of health-related quality of life (HRQOL) after amputation?

10. What is the prevalence of phantom sensation/pain after amputation?

---

1. The more proximal the amputation, the slower the walking velocity

2. 25%

3. 65%

4. 40%

5. 100%

6. No

7. Myodesis: muscle attachment to bone
   Myoplasty: attachment of muscle to its antagonist

8. Myodesis

9. Pain
   Ambulation distance

10. 60 to 75%

11. Musculoskeletal pain at what site is very common after successful amputation?

11. Back pain

12. What skin complication may result from chronic limb swelling after amputation?

12. Verrucous hyperplasia

13. What is the preferred treatment for this condition?

13. Total contact casting

14. Terminal bony overgrowth classically occurs with what two amputations?

14. Diaphyseal amputations
    Pediatric humerus amputations

15. What is the preferred means of preventing terminal overgrowth?

15. Stump capping

16. If overgrowth does occur, what is the treatment of choice?

16. Revise limb

Above-Knee Amputation and Knee Disarticulation

17. How do AKA functional outcomes compare with those of through-knee amputations?

17. AKA patients generally have better functional outcomes

18. After an AKA, what hip position optimizes prosthetic fit?

18. 10 degrees hip flexion
    10 degrees hip adduction

19. What is the ideal limb length for an AKA?

19. 12 cm above knee

20. When performing a knee disarticulation, what should one do with the patellar tendon?

20. Suture patellar tendon to anterior cruciate ligament/posterior cruciate ligament (ACL/PCL)

Below-Knee Amputation

21. After a BKA, what position of the knee optimizes fit of the prosthesis?

21. 7 to 10 degrees of knee flexion

22. What is the ideal limb length for BKA?

22. 12 to 15 cm below knee

23. A cut at this level corresponds to what region of the gastrocnemius?

23. Musculotendinous junction

24. Where should the fibula be cut?

24. 1 cm shorter than the tibia

25. How large a posterior flap is required?

25. 1 cm greater than the diameter of the leg

26. After a BKA, what percentage of elderly patients regain their preoperative functional status?

26. 30 to 50%

Amputations at the Ankle and Foot

27. Where should a great toe amputation ideally be made?

27. Distal to the flexor hallucis brevis (FHB)

28. What is the prosthesis of choice after great toe amputation?

28. Steel shank and rocker bottom shoe

29. Where should a second toe amputation ideally be performed? Why?

29. Distal to the proximal phalanx metaphyseal flare

30. During ray amputations of the foot, what structure should one endeavor to preserve?

31. If more than two rays must be resected, what amputation should be considered?

32. What two procedures should be performed in conjunction with a transmetatarsal or Lisfranc amputation?

33. What are the two key things required for a successful Syme's amputation?

Prosthesis Design and Selection

Foot Considerations

34. For what patients is the single action cushioned heel (SACH) foot best suited?

35. What is the biggest disadvantage of the SACH foot?

36. What are the two main advantages of an articulated dynamic response foot?

37. What is the function of the keel?

38. What is the advantage of a split keel?

Socket and Suspension Options

39. What are the two basic requirements for use of suction-type suspension systems?

40. What is the most common socket type employed after BKA?

41. When is a supracondylar suspension system indicated after BKA?

42. What is the preferred socket design after knee disarticulation?

43. What are the two basic socket options for transfemoral amputees?

44. Ischial containment sockets are particularly useful for what patients?

45. What wall should be removable when designing a prosthesis for use after Syme's amputation?

To minimize the risk of postoperative hallux valgus

30. Plantar plate

31. Transmetatarsal

32. Achilles tendon lengthening
Transfer of tibialis anterior to the talar neck

33. Patent posterior tibial artery
Intact heel pad

34. Low demand

35. Overload of the contralateral limb

36. Improved performance on uneven surfaces
Decreased shear forces

37. Spring-like posterior component

38. Allows inversion and eversion

39. Healed wound
Stable limb

40. Patellar tendon-bearing socket

41. If residual limb length <5 cm

42. Modified quadrilateral socket

43. Quadrilateral with shelf for tuberosity (narrow anteroposterior [AP] diameter)
Ischial containment (narrow medial-lateral diameter)

44. Higher demand, active

45. Medial wall

Knee Assemblies

46. What are the two basic choices for axis of rotation?

46. Single axis (essentially a hinge joint)
Polycentric (moving center of rotation)

47. For whom is the single axis knee particularly useful and why?

47. Children
It is simple and reliable

48. What are the two reported advantages of a polycentric knee?

48. Increased stability
Improved flexion

49. What are the two basic choices for control type?

49. Stance control
Swing control

50. For what two types of patients is a stance control knee particularly useful?

50. Patients with knee instability
Patients who cannot control flexion

51. What two stance control options are available?

51. Manual lock
Stance phase weight activated

52. Which of these is the most stable and for whom may it be particularly useful?

52. Manual lock
Especially useful for household-only ambulators

53. What two swing control options are available?

53. Constant friction (one speed)
Variable friction

54. For what patient population might constant friction knees be particularly useful?

54. Elderly or low-demand patients

55. What are three examples of variable friction systems?

55. Hydraulic
Pneumatic
C-Leg (computer-controlled)

56. What are the two disadvantages of variable friction systems?

56. Generally heavier
Less durable

57. What is the preferred knee assembly after knee disarticulation?

57. Four-bar polycentric knee

Diagnosing and Treating Prosthetic Problems After Below-Knee Amputation

58. If pistoning is observed in the swing phase, it suggests a problem with what component?

58. Suspension

59. If pistoning is observed in the stance phase, it suggests a problem with what component?

59. Poor socket fit

60. What gait abnormality is seen if the prosthetic foot is too soft?

60. Excessive knee extension

61. What gait abnormality is seen if the prosthetic foot is too hard?

61. Excessive knee flexion

62. What gait abnormality is seen if the prosthetic foot is too far forward?

62. Excessive knee extension

63. What gait abnormality is seen if the prosthetic foot is too inset?

63. Circumduction gait (lateral thrust)

64. What gait abnormality is seen if the prosthetic foot is too outset?

64. Broad gait (medial thrust)

65. What gait abnormality is seen if the prosthetic foot is in too much dorsiflexion?

65. Excessive knee flexion

66. What gait abnormality is seen if the prosthetic foot is in too much equinus?

66. Excessive knee extension

Diagnosing and Treating Prosthetic Problems after Above-Knee Amputation

67. What are two potential causes of a Trendelenburg gait pattern?

67. Abducted socket
Weak hip abductors

68. What are the two potential causes of a circumduction gait pattern?

68. Prosthesis is too long
Groin irritation by the socket

69. With circumduction on the side of amputation, what gait pattern is seen on the unaffected side?

69. Vaulting (walking on toes)

70. What is the potential cause of a heel whip pattern?

70. Rotational malalignment of the knee relative to the tibia

Orthoses and Other Ambulatory Assistive Devices

71. What shoe insert provides the best shock absorption?

71. Highly cross-linked polyethylene (HCLPE) foam

72. In what hand should a cane be held?

72. In the hand opposite the affected lower extremity

73. What effect does this have on center of gravity?

73. Moves the center of gravity over the affected side

74. What is the resulting effect on joint reaction force (JRF)?

74. Decreased JRF

Effects of Brain Injury on Gait

75. What changes are seen in the gait pattern after a stroke with resultant hemiplegia?

75. Prolonged stance phase (double limb support)

76. What foot/ankle deformity commonly occurs after a stroke?

76. Equinovarus foot

77. What is the first-line treatment option?

77. Splint and physical therapy

78. What type of ankle-foot orthosis (AFO) is appropriate during the recovery period?

78. One that enables dorsiflexion
One that has a plantar flexion stop

79. In what direction does muscle function generally return after a stroke?

79. Proximal to distal

80. What is the best physical exam predictor of ambulation recovery after acquired brain injury?

80. Balance

81. If equinus persists after 6 to 12 months, then what procedure should be undertaken?

81. Achilles tendon lengthening

82. What tendon transfer can improve foot and ankle function? Why? What is it particularly indicated for?

82. Split anterior tibial tendon transfer (SPLATT)
Because anterior tibial tendon is generally spastic
Indicated for dynamic varus

83. What is the problem with performing a posterior tibial (PT) tendon transfer for foot drop?

83. PT tendon is out of phase with dorsiflexion

■ Upper Extremity Amputations and Prostheses

Wrist Disarticulation Versus Transradial Amputation

84. What are the two preferred amputations for complete brachial plexus palsy?

84. Transradial
Elbow disarticulation

85. What are the two advantages of disarticulation?

85. Increased rotation (distal radioulnar joint [DRUJ] intact)
Better suspension (distal radial flare)

86. What is the disadvantage of disarticulation?

86. Difficult prosthetic fit

87. What is the ideal length of a transradial amputation? Why?

87. Between the middle and distal thirds of forearm
Allows best myoelectric prosthesis fit

88. When is the best time to fit a prosthesis? Why?

88. Within 30 days of amputation
Improved success and prosthesis acceptance

89. In general, when is a myoelectric prosthesis preferred versus a body-driven prosthesis?

89. Myoelectric generally for sedentary activities
Body-driven prostheses for heavier labor

■ High-Yield Rehabilitation Review

Nonanatomic Procedures to Improve Function in Specific Clinical Situations

Spinal Cord Injury

90. How can the function of a patient with a C5 level injury be improved to approximate a C6 level of function?

90. Brachioradialis (BR) to extensor carpi radialis brevis (ECRB) transfer
Restores wrist extension

91. How can the function of a patient with a C5 level injury be improved to approximate a C7 level of function?

91. Deltoid to triceps transfer
Restores elbow extension

92. Quick review: how dependent is a patient with a spinal cord injury (SCI) at C4 for transfers?

92. Totally dependent

93. Compare with a C5 SCI patient.

93. Assisted transfers

94. Compare with a C6 SCI patient.

94. Independent

95. Autonomic dysreflexia is associated with SCI above what level?

95. T5

Key Lower Extremity Procedures

96. What tendon transfer may prolong ambulation in a child with muscular dystrophy?

96. PT tendon transfer

97. What tendon transfer may improve equinovarus foot in cerebral palsy?

97. SPLATT

Key Upper Extremity Procedures

98. What is the key tendon transfer for low median nerve palsy?

98. Flexor digitorum superficialis (FDS) to abductor pollicis brevis (APB)

99. What is the key tendon transfer for high median nerve palsy?

99. BR to flexor pollicis longus (FPL)

100. What are the two key tendon transfers for ulnar nerve palsy?

100. ECRB to adductor pollicis
Intrinsic transfers

101. What are the three key tendon transfers for radial nerve palsy?

101. Pronator teres to ECRB
Palmaris longus (PL) to extensor pollicis longus (EPL)
Flexor carpi ulnaris (FCU) to extensor digitorum communis (EDC)
Other permutations are also possible

102. What are the two key procedures to improve upper extremity function in an adult with upper brachial plexus injury?

102. Glenohumeral arthrodesis
Pectoralis major transfer (to restore elbow flexion)

103. What are the four key procedures to improve upper extremity function in the pediatric cerebral palsy patient?

103. Shoulder derotation osteotomy
Biceps lengthening
Wrist arthrodesis or FCU transfer to ECRB
FDS to flexor digitorum profundus (FDP) transfer; FPL lengthening

Athletic Training Terminology and Stages of Rehabilitation

Definitions

104. What is periodization? Cite an example.

104. The process of structuring training into phases

Example: designing an annual plan for workout variability

105. What is conditioning specificity? Cite an example.

105. A progression from highly general training to highly specific training
Example: training for a specific sport

106. What is prioritization? Cite an example.

106. Adaptation of a training regimen to emphasize specific areas of interest
Example: focus on improving shoulder and chest strength

107. What is conditioning?

107. Cardiovascular training, strength training, and stretching

Stages of Postinjury Rehabilitation

108. When does primary rehabilitation occur? What are its two goals? Cite examples.

108. During the acute stage of injury
Acute pain control
Avoid deconditioning
Examples: thermal modalities, immobilization, injections

109. When does secondary rehabilitation occur? What are its two goals? Cite examples.

109. After acute phase of injury or postoperatively
Prevent chronic disability
Avoid physical deconditioning, medication dependence, psychological dysfunction
Examples: joint mobilization, strengthening

110. When is tertiary rehabilitation indicated? What are its two goals?

110. Management of chronic conditions (generally >6 months in duration)
Maximize function of patients with chronic deconditioning and distress despite earlier stages of rehabilitation
Chronic pain control

13

Rapid Review of Selected Topics

■ Last-Minute Review of Commonly Tested Details

1. Name three disorders associated with G-protein defects?

   1. Fibrous dysplasia
      Calcium sensing receptor (CaSR)
      Pseudohypoparathyroidism (gene *GNAS1*)

2. What four disorders are associated with weakness of the pelvic and shoulder girdles?

   2. Temporal arteritis
      Limb girdle dystrophy
      Duchenne muscular dystrophy
      Polymyositis/dermatomyositis

3. What two disorders may affect the jaw?

   3. Caffey
      Giant cell reactive granuloma (feet and hands)

4. Hemosiderin is present on the histology of what three disorders?

   4. Nonossifying fibroma
      Pigmented villonodular synovitis (PVNS)
      Brown tumors (associated with primary hyperparathyroidism)

5. Melanin is seen with what disorder?

   5. Clear cell sarcoma

6. What three viruses may be associated with Paget's?

   6. Respiratory syncytial virus (RSV)
      Paramyxovirus
      Canine distemper

7. What virus may be associated with rheumatoid arthritis?

   7. Epstein-Barr virus (EBV)

8. High levels of type III collagen are seen in what three clinical situations?

   8. Dupuytren's
      Early ligament healing
      Developmental dysplasia of the hip (DDH)

Review of Disorders Identified on Urine Testing

9. High urinary levels of homogentisic acid are associated with what disorder?

   9. Ochronosis or alkaptonuria

10. What enzyme is deficient?

    10. Homogentisic acid oxidase

11. What is the characteristic clinical feature?

    11. Black intervertebral disks

12. High urinary levels of homocysteine are associated with what disorder?

    12. Homocystinuria

13. What enzyme is deficient?

14. What are the two characteristic clinical features?

15. What are two treatments?

16. High urinary levels of phosphoethanolamine are associated with what disorder?

17. What enzyme is deficient?

13. Cystathionine synthetase

14. Inferior lens dislocation
Osteopenia

15. Low methionine diet
Vitamin B_6

16. Hypophosphatasia

17. Alkaline phosphatase

Numbers

18. What are the key numbers for the Mangled Extremity Severity Scale (MESS) score?

19. What are the key numbers for Mirel's criteria?

18. 4
7

19. 7
10

Disorders Associated with Diaphyseal Hyperostosis

20. What population is at risk for chronic sclerosing osteomyelitis?

21. What organisms are most often responsible?

22. What is the radiographic appearance?

23. What is the treatment?

24. What population is at risk for Caffey's hyperostosis?

25. What organisms are responsible?

26. What is the radiographic appearance?

27. What is the treatment?

28. How does Caffey's differ from chronic multifocal osteomyelitis?

29. What is the inheritance pattern for Camurati-Engelmann?

30. What organisms are associated?

31. What is the radiographic appearance?

32. What is the treatment?

33. What is the radiographic appearance of periosteal osteosarcoma?

34. What are the two components of the treatment?

20. Adolescents

21. Anaerobes

22. Diaphyseal proliferation

23. Antibiotics

24. Infants after febrile illness

25. None

26. Hyperostosis of the jaw and ulna

27. Nonsteroidal antiinflammatory drugs (NSAIDs)

28. Caffeys' involves only one bone
Chronic multifocal: bilateral, symmetric involvement

29. Autosomal dominant

30. None

31. Symmetric cortical thickening of long bones

32. NSAIDs

33. Tibial or femoral diaphyseal sunburst lesions

34. Chemotherapy
Wide resection

Key Ligaments of the Hand and Foot: Quick Review and Comparison

35. What two volar radiocarpal ligaments must be repaired after volar scaphoid approach?

35. Radioscaphocapitate
Long radiolunate

36. What is the clinical significance of the short radiolunate ligament?

36. Disrupted in a Mayfield IV perilunate injury

37. What is the clinical significance of the ulnocapitate ligament?

37. Injured with lunotriquetral dissociation

38. What are the two aspects of the clinical significance of the anterior oblique ligament?

38. Primary stabilizer of the carpometacarpal (CMC)
Bennett's fracture fragment stabilizer

39. Distal tibiofibular ligaments: in what two clinical situations is the anterior inferior tibiofibular ligament (AITFL) important?

39. Syndesmotic injury
Avulsed with Tillaux fractures

40. What type of insertion do the deep deltoid ligaments have?

40. Direct (four zones)

41. What are the deep components of the deltoid ligament?

41. Anterior tibiotalar
Posterior tibiotalar

42. In which clinical situation is the anterior tibiotalar ligament particularly important?

42. Hypertrophies with recurrent ankle sprains

Miscellaneous

43. For what two surgical procedures is it especially important to perform a preoperative Allen test?

43. Radial arm flap
Revision Dupuytren's surgery

44. What is the significance of the supreme thoracic artery?

44. First branch of the axillary artery

45. What is the significance of superior thyroid artery?

45. May need to be ligated for approach to proximal anterior cervical discectomy and fusion (ACDF)